REFERENCE EDITION

ESAP™ 2023

Endocrine Society's
Endocrine Self-Assessment Program
Questions, Answers, and Discussions

Lisa R. Tannock, MD, Program Co-Chair
Professor of Medicine
University of Kentucky and
Department of Veterans Affairs

Thomas J. Weber, MD, Program Co-Chair
Professor of Medicine
Division of Endocrinology, Metabolism, and Nutrition
Duke University Medical Center

Barbara Gisella Carranza Leon, MD
Associate Professor of Medicine
Division of Diabetes, Endocrinology,
and Metabolism
Vanderbilt University Medical Center

Alice Y. Chang, MD, MSc
Assistant Professor of Medicine
Division of Endocrinology,
Diabetes, and Nutrition
Mayo Clinic

Gregory Clines, MD, PhD
Associate Professor of Internal Medicine
Metabolism, Endocrinology,
and Diabetes Division
University of Michigan

Dima Lutfi Diab, MD
Associate Professor of Clinical Medicine
University of Cincinnati

Nicole M. Ehrhardt, MD
Assistant Professor of Medicine
University of Washington
Diabetes Institute

Nazanene H. Esfandiari, MD
Professor of Medicine
Metabolism, Endocrinology,
and Diabetes Division
University of Michigan

Mathis Grossmann, MD, PhD
Professor of Medicine
University of Melbourne
Austin Health

Mark Gurnell, MBBS, MA (Med Ed), PhD
Professor of Clinical Endocrinology
& Clinical SubDean
University of Cambridge,
Wellcome Trust-MRC Institute
of Metabolic Science &
School of Clinical Medicine

Sarah E. Mayson, MD
Associate Professor of Medicine
Director of the Endocrinology
Fellowship Program
Division of Endocrinology,
Metabolism, and Diabetes
University of Colorado School of Medicine

Kevin M. Pantalone, DO
Staff Endocrinologist
Director of Diabetes Initiatives
Department of Endocrinology
Cleveland Clinic

Deepika Reddy, MD
Assistant Professor
Division of Diabetes, Endocrinology,
and Metabolism
University of Utah Healthcare

Roberto Salvatori, MD
Professor of Medicine
Medical Director, Johns
Hopkins Pituitary Center
Johns Hopkins University

Meera Shah, MB ChB
Assistant Professor of Medicine
Mayo Clinic College of Medicine
Consultant, Division of Endocrinology
Mayo Clinic – Rochester

Aniket R. Sidhaye, MD
Associate Professor of Clinical Medicine
Program Director,
Adult Endocrinology Fellowship
Johns Hopkins University
School of Medicine

Adina F. Turcu, MD, MS
Associate Professor of Internal Medicine
Metabolism, Endocrinology,
and Diabetes Division
University of Michigan

Abbie L. Young, MS, CGC, ELS(D)
Medical Editor

Endocrine Society
2055 L Street NW, Suite 600, Washington, DC 20036
1-888-ENDOCRINE • www.endocrine.org

ENDOCRINE SOCIETY
Hormone Science to Health

The Endocrine Society is the world's largest, oldest, and most active organization working to advance the clinical practice of endocrinology and hormone research. Founded in 1916, the Society now has more than 18,000 global members across a range of disciplines. The Society has earned an international reputation for excellence in the quality of its peer-reviewed journals, educational resources, meetings, and programs that improve public health through the practice and science of endocrinology.

For between-edition updates, visit us at:
endocrine.org/education-and-training/book-updates

Other publications:
endocrine.org/publications

The statements and opinions expressed in this publication are those of the individual authors and do not necessarily reflect the views of the Endocrine Society. The Endocrine Society is not responsible or liable in any way for the currency of the information, for any errors, omissions, or inaccuracies, or for any consequences arising therefrom. With respect to any drugs mentioned, the reader is advised to refer to the appropriate medical literature and the product information currently provided by the manufacturer to verify appropriate dosage, method and duration of administration, and other relevant information. In all instances, it is the responsibility of the treating physician or other health care professional, relying on independent experience and expertise, as well as knowledge of the patient, to determine the best treatment for the patient.

ISBN: 978-1-936704-20-0

Library of Congress Control Number: 2022951809

On the Cover: 3D rendering of DNA structure, abstract background.

OVERVIEW

The Endocrine Self-Assessment Program (ESAP™) is a self-study curriculum aimed at physicians wanting a self-assessment and a broad review of endocrinology. The ESAP Reference Edition consists of 120 brand-new multiple-choice questions in all areas of endocrinology, diabetes, and metabolism. There is extensive discussion of each correct answer, a comprehensive syllabus, and references. ESAP is updated annually with new questions.

The ESAP reference book is intended primarily for consultation and self-assessment of knowledge relating to endocrinology. As a reference book, educational credits are not available upon completion of the multiple-choice questions included. For information on educational products that include educational credit, please visit endocrine.org/store.

LEARNING OBJECTIVES

ESAP 2023 will allow learners to assess their knowledge of all aspects of endocrinology, diabetes, and metabolism.

Completion of this educational activity enables learners to accomplish key objectives:

- Recognize clinical manifestations of endocrine and metabolic disorders and select among current options for diagnosis, management, and therapy.
- Identify risk factors for endocrine and metabolic disorders and develop strategies for prevention.
- Evaluate endocrine and metabolic manifestations of systemic disorders.
- Use existing resources pertaining to clinical guidelines and treatment recommendations for endocrine and related metabolic disorders to guide diagnosis and treatment.

TARGET AUDIENCE

ESAP is a self-study curriculum aimed at physicians seeking initial certification or recertification in endocrinology, program directors interested in a testing and training instrument, and clinicians simply wanting a self-assessment and broad review of endocrinology.

STATEMENT OF INDEPENDENCE

The Endocrine Society has a policy of ensuring that the content and quality of this educational activity are balanced, independent, objective, and scientifically rigorous. The scientific content of this activity was developed under the supervision of the Endocrine Society's ESAP Faculty Working Group.

DISCLOSURE POLICY

The faculty, committee members, and staff who are in position to control the content of this activity are required to disclose to the Endocrine Society and to learners any relevant financial relationship(s) of the individual or spouse/partner that have occurred within the last 12 months with any commercial interest(s) whose products or services are related to the content. Financial relationships are defined by remuneration in any amount from the commercial interest(s) in the form of grants; research support; consulting fees; salary; ownership interest (eg, stocks, stock options, or ownership interest excluding diversified mutual funds); honoraria or other payments for participation in speakers' bureaus, advisory boards, or boards of directors; or other financial benefits. The intent of this disclosure is not to prevent planners with relevant financial relationships from planning or delivering content, but rather to provide learners with information that allows them to make their own judgments of whether these financial relationships may have influenced the educational activity with regard to exposition or conclusion. The Endocrine Society has reviewed all disclosures and resolved or managed all identified conflicts of interest, as applicable.

The following faculty reported relevant financial relationship(s): **Barbara Gisella Carranza Leon, MD**, is a coinvestigator for clinical trials and/or research studies for Novartis, IONIS Pharmaceutical, National Institutes of Health, FH Foundation, and Regenxbio. **Alice Y. Chang, MD, MSc**, serves on the national advisory board for Corcept Pharmaceuticals. **Nicole M. Ehrhardt, MD**, receives funding from Novo Nordisk and Merck. She serves on the advisory board for Novo Nordisk and Dexcom and is an investigator for Dexcom. **Mathis Grossmann, MD, PhD**, receives funding from Bayer Pharma and Otsuka. He is a speaker for Bayer Pharmaceuticals and is an associate editor for the *European Journal of Endocrinology*. **Mark Gurnell, MBBS, MA (Med Ed), PhD**, serves on the advisory board for AstraZeneca, HRA Pharma, and Recordati. He is on the speakers bureau for AstraZeneca and Novartis. **Kevin M. Pantalone, DO**, receives research support from Bayer, Merck, Novo Nordisk, and Twinhealth. He is a speaker for AstraZeneca, Corcept Therapeutics, Merck, and Novo Nordisk and is a consultant for AstraZeneca, Bayer, Corcept Therapeutics, Diasome, Eli Lilly, Merck, Novo Nordisk, and Sanofi. He is a principal investigator for Eli Lilly, Novo Nordisk, and Twinhealth. **Roberto Salvatori, MD**, receives grant funds from the Department of Defense. He serves on the advisory board for Novo Nordisk, Strongbridge, Ipsen, and HR Pharmaceuticals. He is a clinical trial investigator for Ascendis, Corcept, and Crinetics and is a journal editor for the Pituitary Society. **Meera Shah, MB ChB**, is a research collaborator for Pendulum Therapeutics, Inc. Compensation for her time is paid to her institution, Mayo Clinic. **Adina Turcu, MD, MS**, receives grant funds from the National Institutes of Health. She is an advisor for CinCor. She is an investigator in a sponsor-initiated clinical trial for Novartis and is a consultant for Crinetics, Poxel, Chiasma, and PhaseBio. **Thomas J. Weber, MD**, serves as a primary investigator and consultant for Ultragenyx. He is on the Sanofi adjudication committee for the Duke Clinical Research Institute on Endocrine Events, compensation for which is sent to the Duke discretionary fund.

The following faculty reported no relevant financial relationships: **Gregory A. Clines, MD, PhD; Dima Lutfi Diab, MD; Nazanene H. Esfandiari, MD; Sarah E. Mayson, MD; Deepika Reddy, MD; Aniket Sidhaye, MD; and Lisa R. Tannock, MD**.

The medical editor for this program, **Abbie L. Young, MS, CGC, ELS(D)**, reported no relevant financial relationships.

The Endocrine Society staff associated with the development of content for this activity reported no relevant financial relationships.

DISCLAIMERS

The information presented in this activity represents the opinion of the faculty and is not necessarily the official position of the Endocrine Society.

USE OF PROFESSIONAL JUDGMENT:

The educational content in this self-assessment test relates to basic principles of diagnosis and therapy and does not substitute for individual patient assessment based on the health care provider's examination of the patient and consideration of laboratory data and other factors unique to the patient. Standards in medicine change as new data become available.

DRUGS AND DOSAGES:

When prescribing medications, the physician is advised to check the product information sheet accompanying each drug to verify conditions of use and to identify any changes in drug dosage schedule or contraindications.

POLICY ON UNLABELED/OFF-LABEL USE

The Endocrine Society has determined that disclosure of unlabeled/off-label or investigational use of commercial product(s) is informative for audiences and therefore requires this information to be disclosed to the learners at the beginning of the presentation. Uses of specific therapeutic agents, devices, and other products discussed in this educational activity may not be the same as those indicated in product labeling approved by the Food and Drug Administration (FDA). The Endocrine Society requires that any discussions of such "off-label" use be based on scientific research that conforms to generally accepted standards of experimental design, data collection, and data analysis. Before recommending or prescribing any therapeutic agent or device, learners should review the complete prescribing information, including indications, contraindications, warnings, precautions, and adverse events.

ACKNOWLEDGMENT OF COMMERCIAL SUPPORT

This activity is not supported by educational grant(s) or other funds from any commercial supporter.

PUBLICATION DATE: February 2023

Laboratory Reference Ranges

Reference ranges vary among laboratories. The listed reference ranges should be used when interpreting laboratory values presented in ESAP™. Conventional units are listed first with SI units in parentheses.

Lipid Values

High-density lipoprotein (HDL) cholesterol

Optimal---------------------------->60 mg/dL (SI: >1.55 mmol/L)

Normal --------------------- 40-60 mg/dL (SI: 1.04-1.55 mmol/L)

Low--------------------------------<40 mg/dL (SI: <1.04 mmol/L)

Low-density lipoprotein (LDL) cholesterol

Optimal-- <100 mg/dL (SI: <2.59 mmol/L) (for primary prevention);

<70 mg/dL (SI: <1.81 mmol/L) (for secondary prevention)

Low---------------------- 100-129 mg/dL (SI: 2.59-3.34 mmol/L)

Borderline-high --------- 130-159 mg/dL (SI: 3.37-4.12 mmol/L)

High --------------------- 160-189 mg/dL (SI: 4.14-4.90 mmol/L)

Very high ------------------------ ≥190 mg/dL (SI: ≥4.92 mmol/L)

Non-HDL cholesterol

Optimal-------------------------- <130 mg/dL (SI: <3.37 mmol/L)

Borderline-high --------- 130-159 mg/dL (SI: 3.37-4.12 mmol/L)

High ---------------------------- ≥240 mg/dL (SI: ≥6.22 mmol/L)

Total cholesterol

Optimal-------------------------- <200 mg/dL (SI: <5.18 mmol/L)

Borderline-high --------- 200-239 mg/dL (SI: 5.18-6.19 mmol/L)

High ---------------------------- ≥240 mg/dL (SI: ≥6.22 mmol/L)

Triglycerides

Optimal-------------------------- <150 mg/dL (SI: <1.70 mmol/L)

Borderline-high --------- 150-199 mg/dL (SI: 1.70-2.25 mmol/L)

High --------------------- 200-499 mg/dL (SI: 2.26-5.64 mmol/L)

Very high ------------------------ ≥500 mg/dL (SI: ≥5.65 mmol/L)

Lipoprotein (a) --------------------------≤30 mg/dL (SI: ≤1.07 μmol/L)

Apolipoprotein B -------------------- 50-110 mg/dL (SI: 0.5-1.1 g/L)

Hematologic Values

Erythrocyte sedimentation rate ------------------------- 0-20 mm/h

Haptoglobin -------------------- 30-200 mg/dL (SI: 300-2000 mg/L)

Hematocrit------------------------- 41%-51% (SI: 0.41-0.51) (male);

35%-45% (SI: 0.35-0.45) (female)

Hemoglobin A_{1c}----------------------- 4.0%-5.6% (20-38 mmol/mol)

Hemoglobin --------------- 13.8-17.2 g/dL (SI: 138-172 g/L) (male);

12.1-15.1 g/dL (SI: 121-151 g/L) (female)

International normalized ratio --------------------------------0.8-1.2

Mean corpuscular volume (MCV) ---------80-100 μm^3 (SI: 80-100 fL)

Platelet count----------------150-450 × 10^3/μL (SI: 150-450 × 10^9/L)

Protein (total) ----------------------------6.3-7.9 g/dL (SI: 63-79 g/L)

Reticulocyte count--- 0.5%-1.5% of red blood cells (SI: 0.005-0.015)

White blood cell count-------- 4500-11,000/μL (SI: 4.5-11.0 × 10^9/L)

Thyroid Values

Thyroglobulin --------- 3-42 ng/mL (SI: 3-42 μg/L) (after surgery and radioactive iodine treatment: <1.0 ng/mL [SI: <1.0 μg/L])

Thyroglobulin antibodies -----------------≤4.0 IU/mL (SI: ≤4.0 kIU/L)

Thyrotropin (TSH) ------------------------------------0.5-5.0 mIU/L

Thyrotropin-receptor antibodies (TRAb) ----------------- ≤1.75 IU/L

Thyroid-stimulating immunoglobulin-------- ≤120% of basal activity

Thyroperoxidase (TPO) antibodies --------<2.0 IU/mL (SI: <2.0 kIU/L)

Thyroxine (T_4) (free) ----------0.8-1.8 ng/dL (SI: 10.30-23.17 pmol/L)

Thyroxine (T_4) (total)------- 5.5-12.5 μg/dL (SI: 94.02-213.68 nmol/L)

Free thyroxine (T_4) index --------------------------------------- 4-12

Triiodothyronine (T_3) (free)------2.3-4.2 pg/mL (SI: 3.53-6.45 pmol/L)

Triiodothyronine (T_3) (total)----- 70-200 ng/dL (SI: 1.08-3.08 nmol/L)

Triiodothyronine (T_3), reverse ---- 10-24 ng/dL (SI: 0.15-0.37 nmol/L)

Triiodothyronine uptake, resin -----------------------------25%-38%

Radioactive iodine uptake -- 3%-16% (6 hours); 15%-30% (24 hours)

Endocrine Values

Serum

Aldosterone-------------------- 4-21 ng/dL (SI: 111.0-582.5 pmol/L)

Alkaline phosphatase ------------ 50-120 U/L (SI: 0.84-2.00 μkat/L)

Alkaline phosphatase (bone-specific) ---------≤20 μg/L (adult male);

≤14 μg/L (premenopausal female);

≤22 μg/L (postmenopausal female)

Androstenedione - 65-210 ng/dL (SI: 2.27-7.33 nmol/L) (adult male);

30-200 ng/dL (SI: 1.05-6.98 nmol/L) (adult female)

Antimullerian hormone ------- 0.7-19.0 ng/mL (SI: 5.0-135.7 pmol/L) (male, >12 years);

0.9-9.5 ng/mL (SI: 6.4-67.9 pmol/L) (female, 13-45 years);

<1.0 ng/mL (SI: <7.1 pmol/L) (female, >45 years)

Calcitonin ----------------<16 pg/mL (SI: <4.67 pmol/L) (basal, male);

<8 pg/mL (SI: <2.34 pmol/L) (basal, female);

≤130 pg/mL (SI: ≤37.96 pmol/L) (peak calcium infusion, male);

≤90 pg/mL (SI: ≤26.28 pmol/L) (peak calcium infusion, female)

Carcinoembryonic antigen ---------------- <2.5 ng/mL (SI: <2.5 μg/L)

Chromogranin A --------------------------- <93 ng/mL (SI: <93 μg/L)

Corticosterone ---53-1560 ng/dL (SI: 1.53-45.08 nmol/L) (>18 years)

Corticotropin (ACTH) ------------- 10-60 pg/mL (SI: 2.2-13.2 pmol/L)

Cortisol (8 AM) ----------------- 5-25 μg/dL (SI: 137.9-689.7 nmol/L)

Cortisol (4 PM) --------------------2-14 μg/dL (SI: 55.2-386.2 nmol/L)

C-peptide ----------------------- 0.5-2.0 ng/mL (SI: 0.17-0.66 nmol/L)

C-reactive protein --------------0.8-3.1 mg/L (SI: 7.62-29.52 nmol/L)

Cross-linked N-telopeptide of type 1 collagen ----------------------

5.4-24.2 nmol BCE/mmol creat (male);

6.2-19.0 nmol BCE/mmol creat (female)

Dehydroepiandrosterone sulfate (DHEA-S)

Patient Age	Female	Male
18-29 years	44-332 μg/dL (SI: 1.19-9.00 μmol/L)	89-457 μg/dL (SI: 2.41-12.38 μmol/L)
30-39 years	31-228 μg/dL (SI: 0.84-6.78 μmol/L)	65-334 μg/dL (SI: 1.76-9.05 μmol/L)
40-49 years	18-244 μg/dL (SI: 0.49-6.61 μmol/L)	48-244 μg/dL (SI: 1.30-6.61 μmol/L)
50-59 years	15-200 μg/dL (SI: 0.41-5.42 μmol/L)	35-179 μg/dL (SI: 0.95-4.85 μmol/L)
≥60 years	15-157 μg/dL (SI: 0.41-4.25 μmol/L)	25-131 μg/dL (SI: 0.68-3.55 μmol/L)

Deoxycorticosterone ------ <10 ng/dL (SI: <0.30 nmol/L) (>18 years)

1,25-Dihydroxyvitamin D_3----- 16-65 pg/mL (SI: 41.6-169.0 pmol/L)

Estradiol -------------- 10-40 pg/mL (SI: 36.7-146.8 pmol/L) (male);
10-180 pg/mL (SI: 36.7-660.8 pmol/L) (follicular, female);
100-300 pg/mL (SI: 367.1-1101.3 pmol/L) (midcycle, female);
40-200 pg/mL (SI: 146.8-734.2 pmol/L) (luteal, female);
<20 pg/mL (SI: <73.4 pmol/L) (postmenopausal, female)

Estrone --------------- 10-60 pg/mL (SI: 37.0-221.9 pmol/L) (male);
17-200 pg/mL (SI: 62.9-739.6 pmol/L) (premenopausal female);
7-40 pg/mL (SI: 25.9-147.9 pmol/L) (postmenopausal female)

α-Fetoprotein--------------------------------- <6 ng/mL (SI: <6 μg/L)

Follicle-stimulating hormone (FSH) ---------------------------------
1.0-13.0 mIU/mL (SI: 1.0-13.0 IU/L) (male);
<3.0 mIU/mL (SI: <3.0 IU/L) (prepuberty, female);
2.0-12.0 mIU/mL (SI: 2.0-12.0 IU/L) (follicular, female);
4.0-36.0 mIU/mL (SI: 4.0-36.0 IU/L) (midcycle, female);
1.0-9.0 mIU/mL (SI: 1.0-9.0 IU/L) (luteal, female);
>30.0 mIU/mL (SI: >30.0 IU/L) (postmenopausal, female)

Free fatty acids ---------------- 10.6-18.0 mg/dL (SI: 0.4-0.7 nmol/L)

Gastrin---------------------------------- <100 pg/mL (SI: <100 ng/L)

Growth hormone (GH)--0.01-0.97 ng/mL (SI: 0.01-0.97 μg/L) (male);
0.01-3.61 ng/mL (SI: 0.01-3.61 μg/L) (female)

Homocysteine -------------------------- ≤1.76 mg/L (SI: ≤13 μmol/L)

β-Human chorionic gonadotropin (β-hCG) --------------------------
<3.0 mIU/mL (SI: <3.0 IU/L) (nonpregnant female);
>25 mIU/mL (SI: >25 IU/L) indicates a positive pregnancy test

β-Hydroxybutyrate ------------------ <3.0 mg/dL (SI: <288.2 μmol/L)

17-Hydroxypregnenolone ------ 29-189 ng/dL (SI: 0.87-5.69 nmol/L)

17α-Hydroxyprogesterone<220 ng/dL (SI: <6.67 nmol/L) (adult male);
<80 ng/dL (SI: <2.42 nmol/L) (follicular, female);
<285 ng/dL (SI: <8.64 nmol/L) (luteal, female);
<51 ng/dL (SI: <1.55 nmol/L) (postmenopausal, female)

25-Hydroxyvitamin D ---- <20 ng/mL (SI: <49.9 nmol/L) (deficiency);
21-29 ng/mL (SI: 52.4-72.4 nmol/L) (insufficiency);
30-80 ng/mL (SI: 74.9-199.7 nmol/L) (optimal levels);
>80 ng/mL (SI: >199.7 nmol/L) (toxicity possible)

Inhibin B -------------------------- 15-300 pg/mL (SI: 15-300 ng/L)

Insulinlike growth factor 1 (IGF-1)

Patient Age	Female	Male
18 years	162-541 ng/mL (SI: 21.2-70.9 nmol/L)	170-640 ng/mL (SI: 22.3-83.8 nmol/L)
19 years	138-442 ng/mL (SI: 18.1-57.9 nmol/L)	147-527 ng/mL (SI: 19.3-69.0 nmol/L)
20 years	122-384 ng/mL (SI: 16.0-50.3 nmol/L)	132-457 ng/mL (SI: 17.3-59.9 nmol/L)
21-25 years	116-341 ng/mL (SI: 15.2-44.7 nmol/L)	116-341 ng/mL (SI: 15.2-44.7 nmol/L)
26-30 years	117-321 ng/mL (SI: 15.3-42.1 nmol/L)	117-321 ng/mL (SI: 15.3-42.1 nmol/L)
31-35 years	113-297 ng/mL (SI: 14.8-38.9 nmol/L)	113-297 ng/mL (SI: 14.8-38.9 nmol/L)
36-40 years	106-277 ng/mL (SI: 13.9-36.3 nmol/L)	106-277 ng/mL (SI: 13.9-36.3 nmol/L)
41-45 years	98-261 ng/mL (SI: 12.8-34.2 nmol/L)	98-261 ng/mL (SI: 12.8-34.2 nmol/L)
46-50 years	91-246 ng/mL (SI: 11.9-32.2 nmol/L)	91-246 ng/mL (SI: 11.9-32.2 nmol/L)
51-55 years	84-233 ng/mL (SI: 11.0-30.5 nmol/L)	84-233 ng/mL (SI: 11.0-30.5 nmol/L)
56-60 years	78-220 ng/mL (SI: 10.2-28.8 nmol/L)	78-220 ng/mL (SI: 10.2-28.8 nmol/L)
61-65 years	72-207 ng/mL (SI: 9.4-27.1 nmol/L)	72-207 ng/mL (SI: 9.4-27.1 nmol/L)
66-70 years	67-195 ng/mL (SI: 8.8-25.5 nmol/L)	67-195 ng/mL (SI: 8.8-25.5 nmol/L)
71-75 years	62-184 ng/mL (SI: 8.1-24.1 nmol/L)	62-184 ng/mL (SI: 8.1-24.1 nmol/L)
76-80 years	57-172 ng/mL (SI: 7.5-22.5 nmol/L)	57-172 ng/mL (SI: 7.5-22.5 nmol/L)
>80 years	53-162 ng/mL (SI: 6.9-21.2 nmol/L)	53-162 ng/mL (SI: 6.9-21.2 nmol/L)

Insulinlike growth factor binding protein 3 -------------- 2.5-4.8 mg/L

Insulin------------------------- 1.4-14.0 μIU/mL (SI: 9.7-97.2 pmol/L)

Islet-cell antibody assay------- 0 Juvenile Diabetes Foundation units

Luteinizing hormone (LH)--- 1.0-9.0 mIU/mL (SI: 1.0-9.0 IU/L) (male);
<1.0 mIU/mL (SI: <1.0 IU/L) (prepuberty, female);
1.0-18.0 mIU/mL (SI: 1.0-18.0 IU/L) (follicular, female);
20.0-80.0 mIU/mL (SI: 20.0-80.0 IU/L) (midcycle, female);
0.5-18.0 mIU/mL (SI: 0.5-18.0 IU/L) (luteal, female);
>30.0 mIU/mL (SI: >30.0 IU/L) (postmenopausal, female)

Metanephrines (plasma fractionated)
Metanephrine ---------------------- <99 pg/mL (SI: <0.50 nmol/L)
Normetanephrine ---------------- <165 pg/mL (SI: <0.90 nmol/L)

75-g oral glucose tolerance test blood glucose values---------------
60-100 mg/dL (SI: 3.3-5.6 mmol/L) (fasting);
<200 mg/dL (SI: <11.1 mmol/L) (1 hour);
<140 mg/dL (SI: <7.8 mmol/L) (2 hour); between 140-200 mg/dL (SI: 7.8-11.1 mmol/L) is considered impaired glucose tolerance or prediabetes; greater than 200 mg/dL (SI: >11.1 mmol/L) is a sign of diabetes mellitus

50-g oral glucose tolerance test for gestational diabetes ---------- <140 mg/dL (SI: <7.8 mmol/L) (1 hour)

100-g oral glucose tolerance test for gestational diabetes ---------- <95 mg/dL (SI: <5.3 mmol/L) (fasting); <180 mg/dL (SI: <10.0 mmol/L) (1 hour); <155 mg/dL (SI: <8.6 mmol/L) (2 hour); <140 mg/dL (SI: <7.8 mmol/L) (3 hour)

Osteocalcin ---------- 9.0-42.0 ng/mL (SI: 9.0-42.0 µg/L)

Parathyroid hormone, intact (PTH) ---------- 10-65 pg/mL (SI: 10-65 ng/L)

Parathyroid hormone–related protein (PTHrP) ---------- <2.0 pmol/L

Progesterone ---------- ≤1.2 ng/mL (SI: ≤3.8 nmol/L) (male); ≤1.0 ng/mL (SI: ≤3.2 nmol/L) (follicular, female); 2.0-20.0 ng/mL (SI: 6.4-63.6 nmol/L) (luteal, female); ≤1.1 ng/mL (SI: ≤3.5 nmol/L) (postmenopausal, female); >10.0 ng/mL (SI: >31.8 nmol/L) (evidence of ovulatory adequacy)

Proinsulin ---------- 26.5-176.4 pg/mL (SI: 3.0-20.0 pmol/L)

Prolactin ---------- 4-23 ng/mL (SI: 0.17-1.00 nmol/L) (male); 4-30 ng/mL (SI: 0.17-1.30 nmol/L) (nonlactating female); 10-200 ng/mL (SI: 0.43-8.70 nmol/L) (lactating female)

Prostate-specific antigen (PSA) ---------- <2.0 ng/mL (SI: <2.0 µg/L) (≤40 years); <2.8 ng/mL (SI: <2.8 µg/L) (≤50 years); <3.8 ng/mL (SI: <3.8 µg/L) (≤60 years); <5.3 ng/mL (SI: <5.3 µg/L) (≤70 years); <7.0 ng/mL (SI: <7.0 µg/L) (≤79 years); <7.2 ng/mL (SI: <7.2 µg/L) (≥80 years)

Renin activity, plasma, sodium replete, ambulatory ---------- 0.6-4.3 ng/mL per h

Renin, direct concentration ---------- 4-44 pg/mL (SI: 0.1-1.0 pmol/L)

Sex hormone–binding globulin (SHBG) ---------- 1.1-6.7 µg/mL (SI: 10-60 nmol/L) (male); 2.2-14.6 µg/mL (SI: 20-130 nmol/L) (female)

α-Subunit of pituitary glycoprotein hormones ---------- <1.2 ng/mL (SI: <1.2 µg/L)

Testosterone (bioavailable) ---------- 0.8-4.0 ng/dL (SI: 0.03-0.14 nmol/L) (20-50 years, female on oral estrogen); 0.8-10.0 ng/dL (SI: 0.03-0.35 nmol/L) (20-50 years, female not on oral estrogen); 83.0-257.0 ng/dL (SI: 2.88-8.92 nmol/L) (male 20-29 years); 72.0-235.0 ng/dL (SI: 2.50-8.15 nmol/L) (male 30-39 years); 61.0-213.0 ng/dL (SI: 2.12-7.39 nmol/L) (male 40-49 years); 50.0-190.0 ng/dL (SI: 1.74-6.59 nmol/L) (male 50-59 years); 40.0-168.0 ng/dL (SI: 1.39-5.83 nmol/L) (male 60-69 years)

Testosterone (free) ---------- 9.0-30.0 ng/dL (SI: 0.31-1.04 nmol/L) (male); 0.3-1.9 ng/dL (SI: 0.01-0.07 nmol/L) (female)

Testosterone (total) ---------- 300-900 ng/dL (SI: 10.4-31.2 nmol/L) (male); 8-60 ng/dL (SI: 0.3-2.1 nmol/L) (female)

Vitamin B_{12} ---------- 180-914 pg/mL (SI: 133-674 pmol/L)

Chemistry Values

Alanine aminotransferase ---------- 10-40 U/L (SI: 0.17-0.67 µkat/L)

Albumin ---------- 3.5-5.0 g/dL (SI: 35-50 g/L)

Amylase ---------- 26-102 U/L (SI: 0.43-1.70 µkat/L)

Anion gap ---------- 3-11 mEq/L (SI: 3-11 mmol/L)

Aspartate aminotransferase ---------- 20-48 U/L (SI: 0.33-0.80 µkat/L)

Bicarbonate ---------- 21-28 mEq/L (SI: 21-28 mmol/L)

Bilirubin (total) ---------- 0.3-1.2 mg/dL (SI: 5.1-20.5 µmol/L)

Blood gases

Po_2, arterial blood ---------- 80-100 mm Hg (SI: 10.6-13.3 kPa)

Pco_2, arterial blood ---------- 35-45 mm Hg (SI: 4.7-6.0 kPa)

Blood pH ---------- 7.35-7.45

Calcium ---------- 8.2-10.2 mg/dL (SI: 2.1-2.6 mmol/L)

Calcium (ionized) ---------- 4.60-5.08 mg/dL (SI: 1.2-1.3 mmol/L)

Carbon dioxide ---------- 22-28 mEq/L (SI: 22-28 mmol/L)

CD_4 cell count ---------- 500-1400/µL (SI: 0.5-1.4 × 10^9/L)

Chloride ---------- 96-106 mEq/L (SI: 96-106 mmol/L)

Creatine kinase ---------- 50-200 U/L (SI: 0.84-3.34 µkat/L)

Creatinine ---------- 0.7-1.3 mg/dL (SI: 61.9-114.9 µmol/L) (male); 0.6-1.1 mg/dL (SI: 53.0-97.2 µmol/L) (female)

Ferritin ---------- 15-200 ng/mL (SI: 33.7-449.4 pmol/L)

Folate ---------- ≥4.0 ng/mL (SI: ≥4.0 µg/L)

Glucose ---------- 70-99 mg/dL (SI: 3.9-5.5 mmol/L)

γ-Glutamyltransferase ---------- 2-30 U/L (SI: 0.03-0.50 µkat/L)

Iron ---------- 50-150 µg/dL (SI: 9.0-26.8 µmol/L) (male); 35-145 µg/dL (SI: 6.3-26.0 µmol/L) (female)

Lactate dehydrogenase ---------- 100-200 U/L (SI: 1.7-3.3 µkat/L)

Lactic acid ---------- 5.4-20.7 mg/dL (SI: 0.6-2.3 mmol/L)

Lipase ---------- 10-73 U/L (SI: 0.17-1.22 µkat/L)

Magnesium ---------- 1.5-2.3 mg/dL (SI: 0.6-0.9 mmol/L)

Osmolality ---------- 275-295 mOsm/kg (SI: 275-295 mmol/kg)

Phosphate ---------- 2.3-4.7 mg/dL (SI: 0.7-1.5 mmol/L)

Potassium ---------- 3.5-5.0 mEq/L (SI: 3.5-5.0 mmol/L)

Prothrombin time ---------- 8.3-10.8 s

Serum urea nitrogen ---------- 8-23 mg/dL (SI: 2.9-8.2 mmol/L)

Sodium ---------- 136-142 mEq/L (SI: 136-142 mmol/L)

Transferrin saturation ---------- 14%-50%

Troponin I ---------- <0.6 ng/mL (SI: <0.6 µg/L)

Tryptase ---------- <11.5 ng/mL (SI: <11.5 µg/L)

Uric acid ---------- 3.5-7.0 mg/dL (SI: 208.2-416.4 µmol/L)

Urine

Albumin ---------- 30-300 µg/mg creat (SI: 3.4-33.9 µg/mol creat)

Albumin-to-creatinine ratio ---------- <30 mg/g creat

Aldosterone ---------- 3-20 µg/24 h (SI: 8.3-55.4 nmol/d) (should be <12 µg/24 h [SI: <33.2 nmol/d] with oral sodium loading—confirmed with 24-hour urinary sodium >200 mEq)

Calcium ---------- 100-300 mg/24 h (SI: 2.5-7.5 mmol/d)

Catecholamine fractionation

Normotensive normal ranges:

Dopamine ---------- <400 µg/24 h (SI: <2610 nmol/d)

Epinephrine ---------- <21 µg/24 h (SI: <115 nmol/d)

Norepinephrine ---------- <80 µg/24 h (SI: <473 nmol/d)

Citrate --------------------320-1240 mg/24 h (SI: 16.7-64.5 mmol/d)
Cortisol ---------------------------- 4-50 μg/24 h (SI: 11-138 nmol/d)
Cortisol following dexamethasone-suppression test (low-dose:
2 day, 2 mg daily) ----------------- <10 μg/24 h (SI: <27.6 nmol/d)
Creatinine----------------------- 1.0-2.0 g/24 h (SI: 8.8-17.7 mmol/d)
Glomerular filtration rate (estimated) ------->60 mL/min per 1.73 m^2
5-Hydroxyindole acetic acid----- 2-9 mg/24 h (SI: 10.5-47.1 μmol/d)
Iodine (random)-- >100 μg/L
17-Ketosteroids ---- 6.0-21.0 mg/24 h (SI: 20.8-72.9 μmol/d) (male);
4.0-17.0 mg/24 h (SI: 13.9-59.0 μmol/d) (female)
Metanephrine fractionation
Normotensive normal ranges:
Metanephrine --------<261 μg/24 h (SI: <1323 nmol/d) (male);
<180 μg/24 h (SI: <913 nmol/d) (female)
Normetanephrine --------------------- age and sex dependent
Total metanephrine ------------------- age and sex dependent
Osmolality -------------150-1150 mOsm/kg (SI: 150-1150 mmol/kg)
Oxalate ----------------------------- <40 mg/24 h (SI: <456 mmol/d)
Phosphate --------------------- 0.9-1.3 g/24 h (SI: 29.1-42.0 mmol/d)
Potassium ---------------------- 17-77 mEq/24 h (SI: 17-77 mmol/d)
Sodium -----------------------40-217 mEq/24 h (SI: 40-217 mmol/d)
Uric acid ----------------------------<800 mg/24 h (SI: <4.7 mmol/d)

Saliva

Cortisol (salivary), midnight ------------<0.13 μg/dL (SI: <3.6 nmol/L)

Semen

Semen analysis---------------- >20 million sperm/mL; >50% motility

Abbreviations

ACTH --corticotropin
ACE inhibitor--------------- angiotensin-converting enzyme inhibitor
ALT ---------------------------------------alanine aminotransferase
AST ------------------------------------ aspartate aminotransferase
BMI -- body mass index
CNS--------------------------------------- central nervous system
CT--computed tomography
DHEA -------------------------------------- dehydroepiandrosterone
DHEA-S---------------------------- dehydroepiandrosterone sulfate
DNA -- deoxyribonucleic acid
DPP-4 inhibitor ---------------------dipeptidyl-peptidase 4 inhibitor
DXA------------------------------dual-energy x-ray absorptiometry
FDA ----------------------------------Food and Drug Administration
FGF-23 --------------------------------- fibroblast growth factor 23
FNA ---fine-needle aspiration
FSH ------------------------------------ follicle-stimulating hormone
GH --- growth hormone
GHRH------------------------- growth hormone–releasing hormone
GLP-1 receptor agonist----- glucagonlike peptide 1 receptor agonist
GnRH -----------------------------gonadotropin-releasing hormone
hCG --------------------------------- human chorionic gonadotropin
HDL---high-density lipoprotein
HIV----------------------------------- human immunodeficiency virus
HMG-CoA reductase inhibitor---------- 3-hydroxy-3-methylglutaryl
coenzyme A reductase inhibitor
IGF-1------------------------------------- insulinlike growth factor 1
LDL --low-density lipoprotein
LH --- luteinizing hormone
MCV --------------------------------------mean corpuscular volume
MIBG------------------------------------ *meta*-iodobenzylguanidine
MRI ---------------------------------- magnetic resonance imaging
NPH insulin -------------------- neutral protamine Hagedorn insulin
PCSK9 inhibitor---- proprotein convertase subtilisin/kexin 9 inhibitor
PET ---------------------------------positron emission tomography
PSA --------------------------------------- prostate-specific antigen
PTH --parathyroid hormone
PTHrP-------------------------parathyroid hormone–related protein
SGLT-2 inhibitor -----------sodium-glucose cotransporter 2 inhibitor
SHBG -------------------------------- sex hormone–binding globulin
T_3 --- triiodothyronine
T_4 --- thyroxine
TPO antibodies ------------------------- thyroperoxidase antibodies
TRH --------------------------------- thyrotropin-releasing hormone
TRAb --------------------------------------TSH-receptor antibodies
TSH -- thyrotropin
VLDL----------------------------------- very low-density lipoprotein

QUESTIONS

ENDOCRINE SELF-ASSESSMENT PROGRAM 2023

Part I

1 A 61-year-old woman is diagnosed with osteoporosis, with an L1-L4 lumbar spine T-score of −3.1. In addition to taking calcium and vitamin D supplements, she has received denosumab, 60 mg subcutaneously every 6 months, for 5 years. Her most recent DXA scan documents a statistically significant improvement in her lumbar spine bone mineral density and stable bone mineral density in the total right hip.

As part of her work in international development, she will be spending the next 12 months in a remote village in another country. She will be unable to receive her denosumab injections during the next year but plans to restart her injection regimen once she returns. She asks for advice on how to treat osteoporosis during her travels. The patient confirms that she will be able to secure 12 months of an oral osteoporosis therapy, if prescribed.

In addition to calcium and vitamin D supplements, which of the following is the best recommendation to treat this patient's osteoporosis until she returns?

A. Abaloparatide
B. Alendronate
C. Raloxifene
D. Zoledronic acid administered before she travels, 6 months after her last denosumab injection
E. No therapy until she resumes denosumab injections when she returns

2 A 71-year-old woman is found to have a left adrenal mass while undergoing staging CT for a suspected bronchogenic carcinoma. She has had a persistent cough for the last 2 months with occasional hemoptysis. She has a history of type 2 diabetes mellitus and polymyalgia rheumatica. Her medications are atorvastatin, 40 mg daily; metformin, 1000 mg twice daily; omeprazole, 40 mg daily; prednisolone, 7.5 mg daily; and ramipril, 10 mg daily. She has a 25 pack-year history of cigarette smoking.

On physical examination, her height is 66 in (167.6 cm) and weight is 185 lb (84.1 kg) (BMI = 29.9 kg/m^2). Her blood pressure is 145/90 mm Hg, and pulse rate is 72 beats/min and regular. She has several bruises on her shins and forearms. Chest examination confirms findings consistent with collapse of the left upper lung lobe.

On adrenal CT (triple-phase), a 3.5-cm mass is observed in the left adrenal gland. Baseline density is 35 Hounsfield units. One minute following contrast, density is 105 Hounsfield units, and 15 minutes following contrast, density is 50 Hounsfield units. The right adrenal gland appears normal.

Which of the following is the most appropriate next step in this patient's management?

A. CT-guided biopsy of the left adrenal mass
B. CT-guided biopsy of the left upper lobe lung mass
C. Measurement of plasma ACTH
D. Measurement of plasma metanephrines
E. Measurement of serum cortisol following a 1-mg dexamethasone-suppression test

3 A 54-year-old man is referred from the liver unit for optimization of type 2 diabetes mellitus. He received a liver transplant 18 months ago for alcohol-related cirrhosis. Following liver transplant, he gained approximately 22 lb (10 kg). Current medications include mycophenolate mofetil, tacrolimus, basal insulin glargine, metformin, and a vitamin D supplement. His current hemoglobin A_{1c} level is 7.9% (63 mmol/mol).

Despite a well-functioning transplant, he describes low energy, weakness, and low libido. He reports a history of mumps orchitis as a teenager. He recalls normal puberty and has fathered 2 children.

On physical examination, his blood pressure is 128/76 mm Hg and pulse rate is 74 beats/min. His height is 70 in (177.8 cm), and weight is 225 lb (102.3 kg) (BMI = 32.3 kg/m^2). He has gynecomastia, reduced body hair, reduced muscle bulk, and soft testes (10 mL right, 5 mL left). Visual fields are normal.

Chart review reveals the following laboratory values 2 months before liver transplant:

Total testosterone = 72 ng/dL (300-900 ng/dL) (SI: 2.5 nmol/L [10.4-31.2 nmol/L])
LH = 1.0 mIU/mL (1.0-9.0 mIU/mL) (SI: 1.0 IU/L [1.0-9.0 IU/L])
FSH = 1.2 mIU/mL (1.0-13.0 mIU/mL) (SI: 1.2 IU/L [1.0-13.0 IU/L])

At the time, the laboratory profile was attributed to his ill health and was not assessed further.

Current laboratory profile:

Total testosterone (fasting, 8 AM) = 106 ng/dL (SI: 3.7 nmol/L)
LH = 35.0 mIU/mL (SI: 35.0 IU/L)
FSH = 42.0 mIU/mL (SI: 42.0 IU/L)

Repeated testing 8 weeks later shows similar results.

Which of the following is the best explanation for the discrepant androgenic profile before and after liver transplant?

A. Gonadal axis suppression by posttransplant weight gain
B. Gonadal axis suppression due to development of posttransplant diabetes mellitus
C. Primary hypogonadism masked by ill health before liver transplant
D. Sertoli-cell–only syndrome
E. Testicular toxicity due to tacrolimus therapy

4 A 19-year-old woman is referred for management of her lipid disorder. The patient reports that 2 months ago, she met with her primary care provider for the first time. At that visit, elevated cholesterol was documented. The patient believes she has had high cholesterol since she was a child. She has not taken any prescription medication to address this finding. She has no other medical problems and currently takes no medications. She states that multiple family members have elevated cholesterol and heart problems. Her mother underwent coronary artery bypass grafting at age 50 years, and her maternal grandfather had a myocardial infarction at age 48 years. She follows a low-fat diet.

On physical examination, her blood pressure is 122/77 mm Hg and pulse rate is 88 beats/min. Her height is 65 in (165 cm), and weight is 132 lb (60 kg) (BMI = 22 kg/m^2). She has corneal arcus bilaterally. Her breathing effort is normal, and lungs are clear to auscultation bilaterally. On cardiac examination, heart sounds are normal with a regular rate and rhythm. Her abdomen is soft and nontender. She has bilateral Achilles tendon xanthomas.

Laboratory test results:

Lipid profile	2 Months ago	Current
Total cholesterol	311 mg/dL (SI: 8.05 mmol/L)	320 mg/dL (SI: 8.29 mmol/L)
Triglycerides	142 mg/dL (SI: 1.60 mmol/L)	100 mg/dL (SI: 1.13 mmol/L)
HDL cholesterol	53 mg/dL (SI: 1.37 mmol/L)	51 mg/dL (SI: 1.32 mmol/L)
LDL cholesterol	230 mg/dL (SI: 5.96 mmol/L)	245 mg/dL (SI: 6.35 mmol/L)

Which of the following is this patient's most likely diagnosis?

A. Familial chylomicronemia syndrome
B. Familial combined hyperlipidemia
C. Familial dysbetalipoproteinemia
D. Familial hypobetalipoproteinemia
E. Heterozygous familial hypercholesterolemia

5 A 32-year-old woman returns for continued management of type 1 diabetes mellitus. Diabetes-related complications include stable nonproliferative retinopathy and microalbuminuria. She has no history of diabetic neuropathy. Type 1 diabetes was diagnosed at age 17 years, and she admits that she has not always prioritized her health. Until recently, she viewed her diabetes management as a burden, and she often skipped doses of bolus insulin. Her hemoglobin A_{1c} level has historically been near 11.0% (97 mmol/mol). She started taking her diabetes seriously after her older sister, who also had longstanding type 1 diabetes, died 1 year ago of complications related to end-stage kidney disease. She has been very diligent with her insulin regimen for the past 6 months and has been closely following the advice of a diabetes educator and a nutritionist. She is thrilled that her most recent hemoglobin A_{1c} value is 6.6% (49 mmol/mol). However, she is concerned and frustrated after being informed that her retinopathy has worsened since her last dilated eye examination 1 year ago.

Current medications include insulin aspart, insulin degludec, and lisinopril.

On physical examination, her blood pressure is 128/72 mm Hg and pulse rate is 70 beats/min. Her height is 64 in (162.6 cm), and weight is 184 lb (83.5 kg) (BMI = 31.6 kg/m^2). There is decreased sensation to 10-g monofilament testing on the distal plantar aspect of her feet bilaterally. The rest of her physical examination findings are normal.

Laboratory test results:

LDL cholesterol = 88 mg/dL (<100 mg/dL [optimal]) (SI: 2.28 mmol/L [<2.59 mmol/L])
Triglycerides = 162 mg/dL (<150 mg/dL [optimal]) (SI: 1.83 mmol/L [<1.70 mmol/L])
Electrolytes, normal
Creatinine = 0.9 mg/dL (0.6-1.1 mg/dL) (SI: 79.6 μmol/L [53.0-97.2 μmol/L])
Hemoglobin A_{1c} = 6.6% (4.0%-5.6%) (49 mmol/mol [20-38 mmol/mol])
Albumin-to-creatinine ratio = 33 mg/g creat (<30 mg/g creat)

Which of the following is the best next step in this patient's treatment?

A. Add fenofibrate
B. Add losartan
C. Initiate insulin pump therapy
D. Maximize lisinopril dosage
E. Provide reassurance and continue current therapies

6 A 47-year-old woman had a ski accident with resulting head trauma 6 months ago. Since then, she has been feeling unwell, with frequent headaches and insomnia. She has gained 30 lb (13.6 kg). She has been having periods, but they are less regular than in the past and are also heavier.

Laboratory test results (sample drawn at 8 AM):

Cortisol = 17.5 μg/dL (5-25 μg/dL) (SI: 482.8 nmol/L [137.9-689.7 nmol/L])
Free T_4 = 1.2 ng/dL (0.8-1.8 ng/mL) (SI: 15.4 pmol/L [10.30-23.17 pmol/L])
TSH = 2.3 mIU/L (0.5-5.0 mIU/L)
IGF-1 = 147 ng/mL (91-246 ng/mL) (SI: 19.3 nmol/L [11.9-32.2 nmol/L])

Her medical history is notable for insomnia and a 5-year history of hypertension. She has spent time reading on the internet and asks whether her symptoms could be due to GH deficiency.

On physical examination, her height is 66 in (168 cm) and weight is 186 lb (84.4 kg) (BMI = 29.9 kg/m^2). Her blood pressure is 125/85 mm Hg, and pulse rate is 76 beats/min. Her current medications are amitriptyline, 5 mg at bedtime, and losartan, 50 mg daily.

Which of the following is the best approach to determine whether her symptoms could be due to GH deficiency?

A. Arginine-stimulation test after stopping losartan
B. Glucagon-stimulation test
C. Macimorelin-stimulation test after stopping amitriptyline
D. Measurement of IGFBP-3
E. No stimulation test is needed (IGF-1 is normal and she is still having periods)

7 A 25-year-old woman presents for follow-up 3 months after undergoing Roux-en-Y gastric bypass. Diabetes mellitus was diagnosed at age 16 years, and metformin was initiated at that time. Insulin was started approximately 5 years ago. BMI at the time of her diabetes diagnosis was 35 kg/m^2. After numerous unsuccessful attempts at weight loss, she recently decided to undergo bariatric surgery because of a lifelong history of difficulty maintaining a healthy body weight.

The patient's diabetes regimen before bariatric surgery included metformin, 1000 mg twice daily; semaglutide, 1.0 mg once weekly; and glargine insulin, 20 units daily. Before surgery, she reported blood glucose levels that ranged from 80 to 120 mg/dL (4.4-6.7 mmol/L) fasting and 210 to 250 mg/dL (11.7-13.9 mmol/L) preprandial. Her hemoglobin A_{1c} value just before surgery was 8.5% (69 mmol/mol). The patient had not had a hemoglobin A_{1c} value less than 8.0% (<64 mmol/mol) for several years.

In the immediate postoperative period, her blood glucose values remained in the range of 180 to 220 mg/dL (4.4-12.2 mmol/L) despite minimal oral intake. She was discharged from the hospital on insulin glargine, 10 units daily, and advised to monitor glucose levels at home. Metformin and semaglutide were discontinued.

Today, 3 months after gastric bypass surgery, the patient reports a 37.5-lb (17-kg) weight loss. She is only checking fasting glucose intermittently and the values range from 100 to 150 mg/dL (5.6 to 8.3 mmol/L). She continues to administer insulin glargine, 10 units daily. She has no concerns about hypoglycemia.

On physical examination, her height is 63.4 in (161 cm) and weight is 234 lb (106 kg) (BMI = 41 kg/m^2). She has no stigmata of Cushing syndrome. There is no peripheral edema.

Laboratory test results:

Fasting glucose = 99 mg/dL (70-99 mg/dL) (SI: 5.5 mmol/L [3.9-5.5 mmol/L])
Hemoglobin A_{1c} = 6.9% (4.0%-5.6%) (52 mmol/mol [20-38 mmol/mol])

Which of the following adjustments to her diabetes management is the best next step?

A. Discontinue basal insulin and monitor blood glucose values only
B. Discontinue basal insulin and restart metformin
C. No adjustment needed; continue current basal insulin regimen
D. Reduce basal insulin dosage and restart semaglutide
E. Reduce basal insulin dosage and restart metformin

8 A 67-year-old woman was diagnosed with estrogen receptor–positive breast cancer last year and underwent a modified radical mastectomy, external-beam radiation, and chemotherapy. She was subsequently prescribed the aromatase inhibitor letrozole to reduce her risk of breast cancer recurrence, with a plan for 5 years of treatment. DXA performed to assess bone mineral density documents osteopenia, with the lowest T-score of −2.2 in the L1-L4 lumbar spine. She has not experienced a fracture, there is no family history of hip fracture, and she has no other risks for fracture.

In addition to recommending calcium and vitamin D supplements, which of the following is the best next step in managing this patient's osteopenia?

A. Prescribe denosumab
B. Prescribe raloxifene
C. Prescribe risedronate
D. Prescribe teriparatide for 2 years followed by bisphosphonate therapy
E. Recommend no therapy, as she does not have osteoporosis

9 A 21-year-old man with type 1 diabetes mellitus diagnosed at age 8 years presents for follow-up. He currently takes 10 units of insulin glargine daily and uses an insulin-to-carbohydrate ratio of 1 unit per 18 g carbohydrate for his prandial insulin and a correction factor of 1 unit per 30 mg/dL (1.7 mmol/L). Goal glucose concentration is 100 mg/dL (5.6 mmol/L) during the day. Over the last 7 days, he has averaged 25 units of insulin daily. He notes recurrent low blood glucose values at various times during the day. Overnight, his fingerstick glucose measurements are typically stable, with a drop of less than 30 mg/dL (1.7 mmol/L) while in the fasting state. He plays basketball most days of the week.

On physical examination, his blood pressure is 127/63 mm Hg and pulse rate is 59 beats/min. His height is 70 in (178 cm), and weight is 135 lb (61.2 kg) (BMI = 19.4 kg/m²).

Laboratory test results (sample drawn while fasting):

Hemoglobin A_{1c} = 6.4% (4.0%-5.6%) (46 mmol/mol [20-38 mmol/mol])
Creatinine = 0.8 mg/dL (0.7-1.3 mg/dL) (SI: 70.7 µmol/L [61.9-114.9 µmol/L])
Serum urea nitrogen = 20 mg/dL (8-23 mg/dL) (SI: 7.1 mmol/L [2.9-8.2 mmol/L])
Plasma glucose = 101 mg/dL (70-99 mg/dL) (SI: 5.6 mmol/L [3.9-5.5 mmol/L])
Sodium = 141 mEq/L (136-142 mEq/L) (SI: 141 mmol/L [136-142 mmol/L])

Which of the following is the best next step in this patient's management?

A. Change the correction factor to 1:70
B. Change the insulin-to-carbohydrate ratio to 1:30
C. Instruct the patient to eat a 30-g carbohydrate snack every 2 hours between meals to prevent low blood glucose
D. Instruct the patient to stop playing basketball
E. Reduce basal insulin by 20%

10 A 32-year-old woman with nonclassic congenital adrenal hyperplasia is referred for advice on optimization of management before in vitro fertilization embryo transfer. Nonclassic congenital adrenal hyperplasia was diagnosed when she was 15 years old and presented with irregular periods and hirsutism. Oral contraceptives were prescribed at that time to help manage hirsutism. She stopped oral contraceptives when she wanted to conceive. After 6 months of trying unsuccessfully, hydrocortisone was prescribed. Eventually, she was referred to reproductive endocrinology, and hydrocortisone was switched to prednisolone.

Laboratory test results after 1 month of prednisolone:

17-Hydroxyprogesterone = 166 ng/dL (<80 ng/dL [follicular]) (SI: 5.03 nmol/L [<2.42 nmol/L])
Progesterone = 0.6 ng/mL (≤1.0 ng/mL [follicular]) (SI: 1.9 nmol/L [≤3.2 nmol/L])
ACTH = 8 pg/mL (10-60 pg/mL) (SI: 1.8 pmol/L [2.2-13.2 pmol/L])

Follicle stimulation for egg retrieval has resulted in 1 male embryo. Her cycle day 3 follicular-phase progesterone concentration was 2 ng/mL (6.4 nmol/L) while on prednisolone. The patient has been referred to endocrinology because of an increase in follicular-phase progesterone (rising to 8 ng/mL [25.4 nmol/L]) despite bedtime prednisolone at increasing doses over the last 6 months (current dosage, 5 mg daily). A recent 17-hydroxyprogesterone measurement is 313 ng/dL (9.48 nmol/L).

She has no features of glucocorticoid excess.

Which of the following is the best next step in this patient's management?

A. Increase the prednisolone dosage to further suppress 17-hydroxyprogesterone
B. Measure progesterone by liquid chromatography–tandem mass spectrometry
C. Measure progesterone in the luteal phase
D. Proceed with embryo transfer
E. Switch glucocorticoid to dexamethasone

11 A 28-year-old woman with type 1 diabetes mellitus and hypertension seeks preconception counseling. Diabetes was diagnosed at age 15 years, and she has no known complications. Her glycemic control is excellent with a recent hemoglobin A_{1c} measurement of 6.8% (51 mmol/mol). Her management consists of continuous glucose monitoring and insulin pump therapy with predictive low glucose threshold suspend technology. She has never been pregnant. Her medications include insulin aspart delivered via an insulin pump and lisinopril.

On physical examination, her blood pressure is 122/78 mm Hg and pulse rate is 78 beats/min. Examination findings are unremarkable.

She receives counseling about glycemic targets and insulin requirements during pregnancy, the need for an updated eye examination, and folic acid supplementation.

Regarding management of this patient's hypertension, which of the following is the best next step in her care?

A. Discontinue lisinopril now; add no additional medication
B. Discontinue lisinopril now; initiate atenolol
C. Discontinue lisinopril now; initiate nifedipine
D. Discontinue lisinopril when conception is confirmed; initiate atenolol
E. Discontinue lisinopril when conception is confirmed; initiate extended-release nifedipine

12

A 51-year-old woman is referred for evaluation of an incidentally identified adrenal mass. A right adrenal mass, measuring 3.5 × 2.2 × 3.1 cm, and bilateral adrenal calcifications were noted on abdominal CT with contrast (*see image, arrows*) that was performed for abdominal pain, nausea, and vomiting. She reports losing 41 lb (18.6 kg) since her mother died 6 months ago. She was born in India and moved to the United States at age 26 years. She travels to India to see her family every few years. Her medical history includes chronic back pain, for which she takes oxycodone, 5 mg as needed (no more than once daily), sleep apnea, and obesity. Her only other medication is a daily multivitamin.

At her clinic appointment, her blood pressure is 92/68 mm Hg and pulse rate is 98 beats/min.

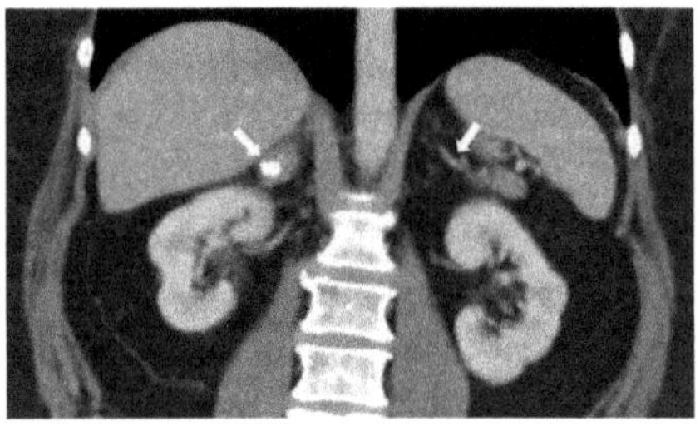

Laboratory test results:

Complete blood cell count, normal
Serum potassium = 5.5 mEq/L (3.5-5.0 mEq/L) (SI: 5.5 mmol/L [3.5-5.0 mmol/L])
Serum sodium = 134 mEq/L (136-142 mEq/L) (SI: 134 mmol/L [136-142 mmol/L])
Serum creatinine = 1.2 mg/dL (0.6-1.1 mg/dL) (SI: 106 μmol/L [53.0-97.2 μmol/L])

Which of the following is this patient's most likely diagnosis?

A. Adrenal cortical carcinoma
B. Pheochromocytoma
C. Primary adrenal insufficiency due to adrenal hemorrhage
D. Primary adrenal insufficiency due to tuberculosis
E. Secondary adrenal insufficiency due to narcotic use

13

A 36-year-old-woman presents to her primary care physician with sensation of a neck lump. Thyroid ultrasonography is ordered, and she is referred to endocrinology. She has no dysphagia or dysphonia, no history of radiation therapy to her head and neck, and no family history of thyroid cancer. Her medical history is notable for hypothyroidism and kidney stones. Her only medication is levothyroxine, 100 mcg daily.

On physical examination, her blood pressure is 116/70 mm Hg and pulse rate is 80 beats/min. Her height is 60 in (152.4 cm), and weight is 124 lb (56.3 kg) (BMI = 24.2 kg/m^2). Palpation of her neck reveals a normal-sized thyroid gland with no nodularity. There is no cervical lymphadenopathy. The rest of her examination findings are normal.

Laboratory test results:

Serum TSH = 1.6 mIU/L (0.5-5.0 mIU/L)
Pregnancy test, negative

Thyroid ultrasonography documents a 0.6 × 1.0 × 2.50-cm hypoechoic lesion (*see images*).

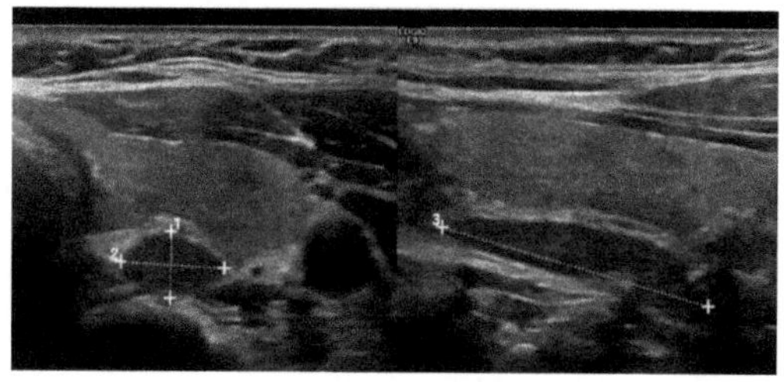

Which of the following is the best next step in this patient's management?

A. Measure serum thyroglobulin
B. Measure serum TPO antibodies
C. Obtain comprehensive metabolic panel
D. Perform neck CT
E. Perform ^{123}I-thyroid scan

14 A 66-year-old woman presents for evaluation and management of osteoporosis. Osteoporosis was diagnosed at age 65 years when she sustained a right hip fracture after a fall. At the time, DXA revealed T-scores of −3.3 in the left femoral neck and −3.0 in the left proximal one-third radius. She took alendronate briefly but stopped it because of upper gastrointestinal adverse effects. She has been on abaloparatide for the past 2 months and reports that she has been adherent to her medication and takes it at bedtime. She has had 2 falls in the past month due to dizziness. She has adequate calcium and vitamin D intake. She takes no medications for hypertension.

On physical examination, her blood pressure is 110/60 mm Hg and she is orthostatic. She is unable to stand without assistance.

Laboratory test results:

Serum calcium = 10.1 mg/dL (8.2-10.2 mg/dL) (SI: 2.5 mmol/L [2.1-2.6 mmol/L])
Serum phosphate = 3.7 mg/dL (2.3-4.7 mg/dL) (SI: 1.2 mmol/L [0.7-1.5 mmol/L])
Serum creatinine = 1.8 mg/dL (0.6-1.1 mg/dL) (SI: 159.1 μmol/L [53.0-97.2 μmol/L])
Glomerular filtration rate (estimated) = 30 mL/min per 1.73 m^2 (>60 mL/min per 1.73 m^2)
Serum 25-hydroxyvitamin D = 32 ng/mL (30-80 ng/mL [optimal]) (SI: 79.9 nmol/L [74.9-199.7 nmol/L])
Serum albumin = 4.1 g/dL (3.5-5.0 g/dL) (SI: 41 g/L [35-50 g/L])

Which of the following is the best recommendation now?

A. Continue abaloparatide
B. Discontinue abaloparatide
C. Switch to denosumab
D. Switch to raloxifene
E. Switch to zoledronic acid

15 A 48-year-old man with a history of a 2-cm nonfunctioning pituitary macroadenoma was initially evaluated 5 years ago. At that time, he had normal pituitary function, a borderline-elevated prolactin concentration (28.8 ng/mL [1.3 nmol/L]), and normal visual field testing. MRI in 1 year was recommended, but he was lost to follow-up. He now presents to the emergency department with a severe headache that has lasted 24 hours and blurry vision for the last week. He takes no medications.

On physical examination, his blood pressure is 129/75 mm Hg, pulse rate is 68 beats/min, and temperature is 98.2°F (36.8°C). He has bitemporal hemianopsia.

Precontrast MRI images are shown (*left, coronal; right, sagittal*).

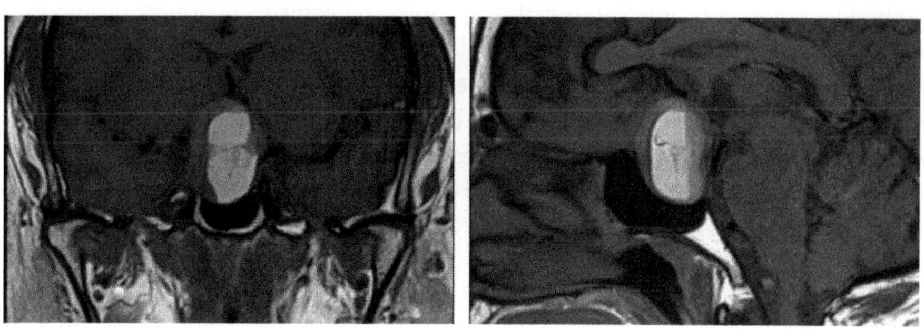

Which of the following is the best next step in this patient's management?

A. Formal visual field testing with optical coherence tomography
B. Intravenous glucocorticoid administration
C. Measurement of prolactin after dilution
D. Measurement of serum cortisol
E. Transsphenoidal surgical decompression

16 A 42-year-old woman returns for continued management of type 1 diabetes mellitus, which was diagnosed at age 11 years. She was recently hospitalized for diabetic ketoacidosis. Her glycemic control has slowly deteriorated over the last 6 months, and she notes that it has acutely worsened over the past 3 weeks. She does not know what is causing the markedly higher blood glucose values. She has lost 6 lb (2.7 kg) over the past 3 months. She is frustrated that her hemoglobin A_{1c} level (measured during her hospital stay) was 11.5% (102 mmol/mol). She has not had a hemoglobin A_{1c} measurement above 7.0% (>53 mmol/mol) for nearly 4 years, and she is adamant that she has continued to adhere to her current treatment regimen.

The only change in her life is that she moved in with her boyfriend to help him maintain his sobriety, as he struggles with addiction issues. She has been working from home during the COVID-19 pandemic, and this has allowed her to focus more on her diabetes management and eating healthy. She stores her unused insulin vials in the fridge and, once opened, keeps them at room temperature until the vial is empty or the expiration date passes, whichever comes first. While money has been tight, and the cost of her diabetes medications and supplies seem to continually be increasing, she always prioritizes her medications, no matter the cost.

Current medications include insulin aspart and insulin degludec.

On physical examination, her blood pressure is 118/72 mm Hg and pulse rate is 68 beats/min. Her height is 68 in (172.7 cm), and weight is 145 lb (65.8 kg) (BMI = 22 kg/m^2). No lipohypertrophy is noted at the usual sites of insulin administration.

Laboratory test results:

Electrolytes, normal
Albumin-to-creatinine ratio = 35 mg/g creat (<30 mg/g creat)
Creatinine = 1.1 mg/dL (0.6-1.1 mg/dL) (SI: 97.3 μmol/L [53.0-97.2 μmol/L])
Hemoglobin A_{1c} = 11.5% (4.0%-5.6%) (102 mmol/mol [20-38 mmol/mol])

Which of the following interventions is the best next step in this patient's management?

A. Add a GLP-1 receptor agonist
B. Measure serum 1,5-anhydroglucitol
C. Measure serum fructosamine
D. Obtain and initiate a new supply of her existing insulin therapies
E. Refer for counseling

17 A 70-year-old woman with adrenocortical carcinoma is admitted to the hospital. She has a history of right adrenalectomy and partial left adrenalectomy with left nephrectomy and is maintained on oral mitotane. Two days ago, she presented to the emergency department with an adrenal crisis. Her symptoms included nausea, vomiting, and syncope in the context of a urinary tract infection and missing 2 doses of her home prednisone regimen. She was initially treated with intravenous fluids, appropriate antibiotic therapy, and hydrocortisone. Her treatment has subsequently been tapered to prednisone, 10 mg twice daily, and fludrocortisone, 0.1 mg twice daily.

Today the patient reports that she is feeling better overall but continues to have mild nausea, as well as longstanding constipation and fatigue of several months' duration.

On physical examination, her height is 67 in (170.2 cm), and weight is 155 lb (70.5 kg) (BMI = 24.3 kg/m^2). Her blood pressure is 120/80 mm Hg supine and 116/76 mm Hg standing, and pulse rate is 68 beats/min supine and 74 beats/min standing. Examination findings are unremarkable.

Laboratory test results:

TSH = 0.5 mIU/L (0.5-5.0 mIU/L)
Complete blood cell count, normal
Serum sodium = 135 mEq/L (136-142 mEq/L) (SI: 130 mmol/L [136-142 mmol/L])

Results of a complete metabolic panel, including serum potassium and creatinine measurements, are otherwise normal.

Which of the following is the best next step in this patient's management?

A. Discontinue prednisone, restart intravenous hydrocortisone
B. Increase the prednisone dosage
C. Measure serum free T_4
D. Measure serum tissue transglutaminase antibodies
E. Perform CT of the abdomen and pelvis with contrast

18 A 19-year-old man of East Asian ancestry seeks evaluation for a 2-year history of left arm weakness and tremor. The symptoms were mild at first, but they have progressed over the past 2 years. He regularly goes to the gym and finds he cannot build up left arm muscle mass. He has a history of type 1 diabetes mellitus since age 7 years. His diabetes is well controlled, with hemoglobin A_{1c} values in the range of 6.0% to 6.6% (42 to 49 mmol/mol) over the past 3 years. He uses insulin aspart via an insulin pump. He has no other relevant medical history and takes no other medications. His family history is notable for myasthenia gravis in his paternal grandfather.

On physical examination, his height is 70 in (178 cm) and weight is 147 lb (66.8 kg) (BMI = 21.1 kg/m^2). His blood pressure is 112/70 mm Hg, and pulse rate is 72 beats/min. He has weakness of the left upper extremity, most prominent in the triceps. He has left upper-extremity tremor and atrophy of the interosseus muscles of the hand. No sensory abnormalities are noted, and reflexes are normal. The rest of the physical examination findings are normal.

Electromyography and a nerve conduction study show evidence of chronic denervation of C7-C8 innervated muscles and a decrease in compound muscle action potential.

Which of the following is this patient's most likely diagnosis?

A. Carpal tunnel syndrome
B. Monomelic amyotrophy
C. Myasthenia gravis
D. Stiff-person syndrome
E. Treatment-induced neuropathy of diabetes

19 A 23-year-old man is referred for further evaluation of hypertension that was first detected during a routine medical assessment for a pilot's license. His medical history is otherwise unremarkable, and he is not taking any medications. Both his father and paternal grandfather were diagnosed with hypertension at a young age; his grandfather died suddenly at age 42 years, and his father had a myocardial infarction at age 38 years. The patient does not smoke cigarettes, drink alcohol, or consume licorice.

On physical examination, his height is 72 in (182.9 cm) and weight is 180 lb (81.6 kg) (BMI = 24.4 kg/m^2). His blood pressure is 185/92 mm Hg, and pulse rate 68 beats/min and regular. Physical examination findings are unremarkable.

Laboratory test results:

Serum sodium = 143 mEq/L (136-142 mEq/L) (SI: 143 mmol/L [136-142 mmol/L])
Serum potassium = 3.0 mEq/L (3.5-5.0 mEq/L) (SI: 3.0 mmol/L [3.5-5.0 mmol/L])
Serum bicarbonate = 31 mEq/L (21-28 mEq/L) (SI: 31 mmol/L [21-28 mmol/L])
Serum creatinine = 1.0 mg/dL (0.7-1.3 mg/dL) (SI: 88.4 μmol/L [61.9-114.9 μmol/L])
Plasma renin activity = 0.05 ng/mL per h (0.6-4.3 ng/mL per h)
Plasma aldosterone concentration = <2.5 ng/dL (4-21 ng/dL) (SI <69.4 pmol/L [111-582.5 pmol/L])
Urinary free cortisol = 40 μg/24 h (4-50 μg/24 h) (SI: 110.4 nmol/d [11-138 nmol/d])

Which of the following is the most likely cause of this patient's presentation?

A. Congenital adrenal hyperplasia due to 11β-hydroxylase deficiency
B. Glucocorticoid resistance syndrome
C. Liddle syndrome
D. Pseudohypoaldosteronism type 2 (Gordon syndrome)
E. Syndrome of apparent mineralocorticoid excess

20 Endocrinology is consulted regarding a 62-year-old man with recent-onset hyponatremia. Seventy-two hours ago, he was admitted to the hospital via the emergency department with sudden-onset severe frontal and occipital headache. CT on admission demonstrated a subarachnoid hemorrhage, but no intracranial aneurysm was identified on subsequent cerebral angiography. Following initial treatment, his condition stabilized, but within the past 24 hours he has developed hyponatremia. His medical history includes hypertension and benign prostatic hyperplasia, treated with amlodipine and finasteride, respectively.

On physical examination, his Glasgow Coma Scale score is 15/15. His blood pressure is 110/70 mm Hg, and resting pulse rate is 88 beats/min and regular. He is clinically euvolemic. Findings on neurologic examination are unremarkable.

Laboratory test results:

Serum sodium = 124 mEq/L (136-142 mEq/L) (SI: 124 mmol/L [136-142 mmol/L])
Serum potassium = 4.2 mEq/L (3.5-5.0 mEq/L) (SI: 4.2 mmol/L [3.5-5.0 mmol/L])
Serum creatinine = 0.72 mg/dL (0.7-1.3 mg/dL) (SI: 63.6 μmol/L [61.9-114.9 μmol/L])
Serum urea nitrogen = 8.3 mg/dL (8-23 mg/dL) (SI 3.0 mmol/L [2.9-8.2 mmol/L])
Plasma glucose = 68 mg/dL (70-99 mg/dL) (SI: 3.8 mmol/L [3.9-5.5 mmol/L])
Serum osmolality = 266 mOsm/kg (275-295 mOsm/kg) (SI: 266 mmol/kg [275-295 mmol/kg])
Urine osmolality = 410 mOsm/kg (150-1150 mOsm/kg) (SI: 410 mmol/kg [150-1150 mmol/kg])
Spot urine sodium = 104 mEq/L (SI: 104 mmol/L)
TSH = 0.4 mIU/L (0.5-5.0 mIU/L)
Free T_4 = 0.75 ng/dL (0.8-1.8 ng/dL) (SI: 9.65 pmol/L [10.30-23.17 pmol/L])

Which of the following is the most appropriate next step in this patient's management?

A. Restrict oral fluids to ≤750 mL per 24 hours
B. Start 3% sodium chloride intravenous infusion
C. Start hydrocortisone
D. Start levothyroxine
E. Start tolvaptan

21 A patient with a 10-year history of type 2 diabetes mellitus calls to say he has had higher than expected morning blood glucose values (150-169 mg/dL [8.3-9.4 mmol/L]) for the past 4 days. His treatment regimen was recently changed from insulin glargine, 16 units daily, to NPH insulin, 10 units twice daily, as he lost his health insurance and could not afford insulin glargine. He also takes glimepiride and metformin. He notes that the NPH insulin appears cloudy and has some sediment at the bottom; he asks what to do.

Which of the following is the best next step in this patient's management?

A. Increase the evening insulin dose to 18 units
B. Return the insulin bottle to the pharmacy and get a new one
C. Roll the insulin bottle between his hands until it is uniformly cloudy, then inject usual dose
D. Shake the insulin bottle until it is clear, then inject usual dose
E. Store the insulin bottle in the refrigerator between uses

22 A 45-year-old woman with hypothyroidism, type 2 diabetes mellitus, fibromyalgia, and bipolar disorder returns for follow-up. The patient reports having a difficult time the past several months. She chose to stop valproate and subsequently had several episodes of mania. She also stopped taking her other prescribed medications. She has resumed valproate and would like to re-start her other long-term medications, which include metformin and levothyroxine. Review of systems is notable for fatigue, weight gain, joint pain, constipation, hoarseness, and cold intolerance.

On physical examination, her blood pressure is 134/85 mm Hg and pulse rate is 60 beats/min. Her height is 66 in (167 cm), and weight is 229 lb (104 kg) (BMI = 37 kg/m^2). She is in no distress. On neck examination, she has a goiter. Her breathing effort is normal, and breath sounds are normal. On cardiac examination, heart sounds are normal with a regular rate and rhythm. Her abdomen is soft and nontender. She has no pitting edema on her lower extremities.

Laboratory test results:

Creatinine = 0.77 mg/dL (0.6-1.1 mg/dL) (SI: 68.1 μmol/L [53.0-97.2 μmol/L])
Hemoglobin A_{1c} = 7.0% (4.0%-5.6%) (53 mmol/mol [20-38 mmol/mol])
TSH = 211.0 mIU/L (0.5-5.0 mIU/L)
Total cholesterol = 402 mg/dL (<200 mg/dL [optimal]) (SI: 10.41 mmol/L [<5.18 mmol/L])
Triglycerides = 1506 mg/dL (<150 mmol/L [optimal]) (SI: 17.02 mmol/L [<1.70 mmol/L])
HDL cholesterol = 33 mg/dL (>60 mg/dL [optimal]) (SI: 0.85 mmol/L [>1.55 mmol/L])
Direct LDL cholesterol = 180 mg/dL (<100 mg/dL [optimal]) (SI: 4.66 mmol/L [<2.59 mmol/L])
Urine albumin-to-creatinine ratio = 15 mg/g creat (<30 mg/g creat)

Which of the following medications should be started first to address this patient's hypertriglyceridemia?

A. Atorvastatin
B. Fenofibrate
C. Icosapent ethyl
D. Levothyroxine
E. PCSK9 inhibitor

23 A 45-year-old man presents with a 1-year history of fatigue and lethargy and a recent of loss of libido and decreased need to shave. There is no associated vision disturbance or headaches and no complaints suggestive of a systemic etiology for his symptoms. He has been taking various opioids, including initially high-dosage fentanyl patches and oxycodone, for the past 6 months to ease back pain. His current medications include pregabalin, 150 mg daily; duloxetine, 60 mg daily; and extended-release tramadol, 150 mg daily. He states he has never used anabolic steroids. He has not received any glucocorticoid injections for his back pain.

On physical examination, his blood pressure is 129/81 mm Hg (lying down) and 115/75 mm Hg (standing). Pulse rate is 78 beats/min (lying down) and 88 beats/min (standing). His height is 68 in (172.7 cm), and weight is 230 lb (104.5 kg) (BMI = 35.0 kg/m^2). He has bilateral palpable gynecomastia, sparse body hair, and normal testicular volume. Visual fields are intact.

Current laboratory test results (8 AM, fasting):

Serum testosterone = 50 ng/dL (300-900 ng/dL) (SI: 1.7 nmol/L [10.4-31.2 nmol/L])
LH = 2.8 mIU/mL (1.0-9.0 mIU/mL) (SI: 2.8 IU/L [1.0-9.0 IU/L])
FSH = 3.5 mIU/mL (1.0-13.0 mIU/mL) (SI: 3.5 IU/L [1.0-13.0 IU/L])
TSH = 2.2 mIU/L (0.5-5.0 mIU/L)
Free T_4 = 1.6 ng/dL (0.8-1.8 ng/dL) (SI: 20.6 pmol/L [10.30-23.17 pmol/L])
Cortisol = 1.0 μg/dL (5-25 μg/dL) (SI: 27.6 nmol/L [137.9-689.7 nmol/L])
ACTH = 4.1 pg/mL (10-60 pg/mL) (SI: 0.9 pmol/L [2.2-13.2 pmol/L])
Hemoglobin = 12.5 g/dL (13.8-17.2 g/dL) (SI: 125 g/L [138-172 g/L])

Iron studies, ACE measurement, prolactin measurement, and findings on pituitary-directed MRI are normal.

In addition to starting hydrocortisone and testosterone replacement, which of the following is the most important next step in this patient's management?

A. Perform another pituitary MRI in 6 months
B. Perform urinary anabolic steroid testing
C. Recommend genetic testing for idiopathic hypogonadotropic hypogonadism
D. Refer to a dietician for weight-loss measures
E. Wean analgesic medications, especially opioids

24 A 59-year-old woman was diagnosed with a seizure disorder in her 20s and has been on phenytoin since her diagnosis. Her seizures are very well controlled and attempts to transition to other antiseizure medications have failed and led to more seizures. Osteoporosis was diagnosed 10 years ago, and her last DXA documented a spine T-score of –2.7. Four years ago, she experienced acute lower back pain after picking up a box and was subsequently found to have an L2 vertebral compression fracture.

Results of a complete metabolic panel are normal.

Which of the following is the most likely mechanism of increased fractures in this patient?

A. Direct effects of phenytoin on the osteoblast to reduce bone formation
B. Hypercalciuria
C. Primary hyperparathyroidism
D. Increase in falls
E. Increase in vitamin D catabolism due to phenytoin

25 A 68-year-old man with type 2 diabetes mellitus and end-stage kidney disease receiving nocturnal peritoneal dialysis presents for consultation. His diabetes has been well controlled for the past 5 years on metformin and insulin glargine; however, he recently stopped metformin because of declining kidney function. Since initiating peritoneal dialysis 3 months ago, his glycemic control has deteriorated with only once-daily insulin glargine. His most recent hemoglobin A_{1c} value is 9.2% (77 mmol/mol). He is frustrated because his hemoglobin A_{1c} level has historically been less than 7.0% (<53 mmol/mol). Despite adhering to insulin glargine taken once daily in the morning and his nutrition plan, his blood glucose is running high, particularly in the morning.

Over the past 3 months, his primary care provider increased his insulin glargine dose from 32 units to 50 units, but this change has not improved his glycemic control. With this dosage increase, he has been having frequent low blood glucose values in the midafternoon and early evening, which was never a problem before starting dialysis. The hypoglycemia is most frequent when he delays or skips meals or while he is exercising. When his blood glucose concentration is greater than 250 mg/dL (>13.9 mmol/L), he often skips a meal or avoids snacking to decrease his blood glucose.

He brings his blood glucose log to the appointment, which lists the following values:

Day	Prebreakfast	Prelunch	Predinner	At bedtime (when cycle of peritoneal dialysis is initiated)
1	262 mg/dL (SI: 14.5 mmol/L)	240 mg/dL (SI: 13.3 mmol/L)	82 mg/dL (SI: 4.6 mmol/L)	140 mg/dL (SI: 7.8 mmol/L)
2	305 mg/dL (SI: 16.9 mmol/L)	222 mg/dL (SI: 12.3 mmol/L)	174 mg/dL (SI: 9.7 mmol/L)	164 mg/dL (SI: 9.1 mmol/L)
3	245 mg/dL (SI: 13.6 mmol/L)	210 mg/dL (SI: 11.7 mmol/L)	64 mg/dL (SI: 3.6 mmol/L)	144 mg/dL (SI: 8.0 mmol/L)
4	284 mg/dL (SI: 15.8 mmol/L)	187 mg/dL (SI: 10.4 mmol/L)	52 mg/dL (SI: 2.9 mmol/L)	158 mg/dL (SI: 8.8 mmol/L)
5	330 mg/dL (SI: 18.3 mmol/L)	248 mg/dL (SI: 13.8 mmol/L)	110 mg/dL (SI: 6.1 mmol/L)	168 mg/dL (SI: 9.3 mmol/L)

On physical examination, his blood pressure is 138/64 mm Hg and pulse rate is 78 beats/min. His height is 68 in (172.7 cm), and weight is 185 lb (83.9 kg) (BMI = 28.1 kg/m^2). His peritoneal dialysis catheter does not have surrounding erythema or induration. There is no lipohypertrophy at sites of insulin administration.

Laboratory test results:

Hemoglobin A_{1c} = 9.2% (4.0%-5.6%) (77 mmol/mol [20-38 mmol/mol])
Hemoglobin = 10.8 g/dL (13.8-17.2 g/dL) (SI: 108 g/L [138-172 g/L])
Electrolytes, normal
Glutamic acid decarboxylase 65 antibodies, undetectable

Which of the following is the best next step in this patient's management?

A. Change the insulin glargine dosing to twice daily
B. Reduce the dosage of insulin glargine and add glimepiride
C. Reduce the dosage of insulin glargine and add meal-time insulin lispro
D. Stop insulin glargine and administer NPH insulin at the start of peritoneal dialysis
E. Switch insulin glargine administration to the evening

26 A 62-year-old woman is hospitalized after undergoing total pancreatectomy 6 days ago for the treatment of locally advanced pancreatic adenocarcinoma. Extensive resection was performed, and a feeding jejunostomy tube was placed at the time of surgery. The patient is currently on intravenous central parenteral nutrition and receiving tube feeding via the jejunostomy tube. She does not take in anything by mouth. All medications, including pancreatic enzyme supplementation, are administered through the feeding jejunostomy tube.

The patient's central parenteral nutrition program currently infuses for 24 hours a day and contains 150 g of dextrose. Her tube-feeding program consists of an infusion of a semi-elemental tube-feeding formulation at a rate of 20 mL per hour over 12 hours, from 8 AM to 8 PM. The tube-feeding formula contains 150 g of carbohydrate per L. Her current insulin regimen consists of 15 units of regular insulin (included in the central parenteral nutrition formulation), 5 units of insulin glargine, and insulin aspart as needed.

The patient's her height is 63 in (160 cm), and weight is 128 lb (58 kg) (BMI = 22.7 kg/m^2). She has normal kidney function.

The patient's glucose meter readings and insulin use for the previous 2 days are shown in the *table.*

	Postoperative day 4						Postoperative day 5					
Time	1:15 AM	5:00 AM	8:20 AM	12:35 PM	4:00 PM	8:50 PM	12:30 AM	4:10 AM	8:05 AM	1:00 PM	5:00 PM	9:30 PM
Glucose, mg/dL (mmol/L)	290 (16.1)	166 (9.2)	158 (8.8)	315 (17.5)	76 (4.2)	165 (9.2)	200 (11.1)	165 (9.2)	120 (6.7)	250 (13.9)	230 (12.8)	220 (12.2)
Insulin	4 units insulin aspart	1 unit insulin aspart	5 units insulin glargine	6 units insulin aspart	—	—	1 unit insulin aspart	—	5 units insulin glargine	4 units insulin aspart	2 units insulin aspart	2 units insulin aspart
Notes			Tube feeding start		Treated with juice	Tube feeding end			Tube feeding start			Tube feeding end

The plan is to continue her current nutrition regimen (ie, combination of central parenteral nutrition and tube feeding at the current rate). She is receiving no other source of dextrose.

Which of the following changes should be made to this patient's glycemic management?

A. Discontinue insulin glargine; start NPH insulin, 4 units twice daily; and maintain parenteral nutrition insulin at 15 units daily
B. Increase insulin glargine to 6 units and maintain parenteral nutrition insulin at 15 units
C. Increase insulin in parenteral nutrition to 20 units and maintain insulin glargine at 5 units daily
D. No changes necessary; continue 15 units regular insulin in parenteral nutrition, 5 units insulin glargine, and insulin aspart as needed for hyperglycemia
E. Start NPH insulin, 6 units daily, with tube feeding, in addition to 15 units regular insulin in parenteral nutrition and 5 units insulin glargine

27

A 29-year-old woman is referred for an elevated testosterone measurement. She had been on oral contraceptive pills for a prolonged period until she discontinued them a year ago when she decided to try for pregnancy. She had a positive pregnancy test 2 months later and subsequently had a spontaneous miscarriage the next month. Since stopping oral contraceptive pills, her periods have been irregular. Workup for irregular periods documented an elevated total testosterone concentration of 76 ng/dL (2.6 nmol/L). Over the course of the year, testosterone continued to rise to the most recent value of 179 ng/dL 6.2 nmol/L) by liquid chromatography–tandem mass spectrometry. She has no clinical symptoms of hyperandrogenism, but she has not been able to conceive again. She has gained approximately 10 lb (4.5 kg) over the last year. In discussing her history, she states that her periods were regular in adolescence.

On physical examination, her blood pressure is 121/84 mm Hg and pulse rate is 80 beats/min. Her height is 65.5 in (166.5 cm), and weight is 144.3 lb (65.6 kg) (BMI = 23.6 kg/m^2). There is no evidence of significant terminal hair growth and no clitoromegaly.

Laboratory test results:

Prolactin = 9.7 ng/mL (4-30 ng/mL) (SI: 0.42 nmol/L [0.17-1.30 nmol/L])
TSH = 1.0 mIU/L (0.5-5.0 mIU/L)
DHEA-S = 281 µg/dL (44-332 µg/dL) (SI: 7.62 µmol/L [1.19-9.00 µmol/L])
17-Hydroxyprogesterone = 71.9 ng/dL (<80 ng/dL [follicular]) (SI: 2.18 nmol/L [<2.42 nmol/L])
FSH = 4.6 mIU/mL (2.0-12.0 mIU/mL [follicular]) (SI: 4.6 IU/L [2.0-12.0 IU/L])
LH = 6.1 mIU/mL (1.0-9.0 mIU/mL [follicular]) (SI: 6.1 IU/L [1.0-9.0 IU/L])

On pelvic ultrasonography, the uterus is normal in appearance. Both ovaries contain more than 20 follicles; the right ovary is 11.5 cc and the left ovary is 16.3 cc. These findings are consistent with polycystic ovary syndrome. Findings on abdominal CT are normal with no adrenal masses.

Which of the following is the best next step in this patient's management?

A. 48-Hour dexamethasone-suppression test
B. Letrozole for ovulation induction
C. Metformin
D. Ovarian/adrenal venous sampling
E. Ovarian drilling

28

A 34-year-old man of Japanese ancestry presents to clinic with concerns about hypoglycemia. Over the past month, he has developed postprandial sweats, shakiness, and sometimes confusion. The symptoms resolve about 15 to 30 minutes after drinking juice. He has been able to check fingerstick blood glucose when he is symptomatic, and the measurements are typically 60 to 65 mg/dL (3.3 to 3.6 mmol/L). His primary care physician had him wear a continuous glucose monitor for a week, and the observed pattern was hyperglycemia immediately after meals followed by more delayed hypoglycemia. The same pattern of glucose changes was seen following a mixed-meal challenge. Other medical history includes Graves disease diagnosed 4 months ago (treated with methimazole), asthma, and seasonal allergies. In addition to methimazole, current medications include a budesonide inhaler and albuterol inhaler. He does not smoke cigarettes and has minimal alcohol intake (1 beer a month).

On physical examination, vital signs and examination findings are normal.

Laboratory test result (sample drawn at 8 AM following 12-hour fast):

Glucose = 72 mg/dL (70-99 mg/dL) (SI: 4.0 mmol/L [3.9-5.5 mmol/L])

Which of the following is the best test to determine the etiology of this patient's hypoglycemia?

A. 8-AM cortisol measurement
B. 72-Hour fast
C. Gastric-emptying study
D. Hypoglycemia panel (sulfonylurea and meglitinide screen)
E. Insulin autoantibody measurement

29

A 45-year-old man undergoes total thyroidectomy for a multinodular goiter that is complicated by postsurgical hypoparathyroidism. He is initially prescribed calcitriol and calcium citrate with dosages titrated to maintain a serum calcium concentration between 8.0 and 8.5 mg/dL (2.0 and 2.1 mmol/L). His current dosages are calcitriol, 0.5 mcg twice daily, and calcium citrate, 500 mg 4 times daily. He also takes chlorthalidone, 12.5 mg daily, to reduce urinary calcium excretion and has no symptoms of hypocalcemia. He does not take a medication for gastroesophageal reflux disease.

Laboratory test results:

Calcium = 8.4 mg/dL (8.2-10.2 mg/dL) (SI: 2.0 mmol/L [2.1-2.6 mmol/L])
Albumin = 4.1 g/dL (3.5-5.0 g/dL) (SI: 41 g/L [35-50 g/L])
Creatinine = 0.9 mg/dL (0.7-1.3 mg/dL) (SI: 79.6 µmol/L [61.9-114.9 µmol/L])
Phosphate = 6.7 mg/dL (2.3-4.7 mg/dL) (SI: 1.8 mmol/L [0.7-1.5 mmol/L])
Magnesium = 1.7 mg/dL (1.5-2.3 mg/dL) (SI: 0.7 mmol/L [0.6-0.9 mmol/L])
Intact PTH = <6 pg/mL (10-65 pg/mL) (SI: <6 ng/L [10-65 ng/L])
Urinary calcium = 278 mg/24 h (100-300 mg/24 h) (SI: 7.0 mmol/d [2.5-7.5 mmol/d])

In addition to recommending a lower-phosphate diet, which of the following is the best next step?

A. Change calcium citrate to calcium carbonate
B. Decrease the calcitriol dosage to 0.5 mcg once daily
C. Increase the chlorthalidone dosage to 25 mg daily
D. Prescribe magnesium oxide
E. Prescribe sevelamer

30

A 61-year-old man who underwent Roux-en-Y gastric bypass 10 months ago has been referred for evaluation of new symptoms. Approximately 6 months after surgery, his wife started to notice episodes of agitation, verbal aggression, and slurring of speech. She notes that he smells as if he were drinking alcohol during these episodes. The patient, however, very firmly states that he has not consumed any alcohol since surgery. The episodes typically happen twice weekly, but he can also go for longer than a week without an episode. Blood glucose values during an episode (via glucose meter) are always greater than 75 mg/dL (>4.2 mmol/L). He does not think the episodes correlate to a particular food or activity.

Approximately 1 month ago, he had a severe episode that led to his wife calling the police because she feared for her safety. A breathalyzer was administered, and it was positive for ethanol. Again, the patient stated he had not consumed any alcohol. He was taken to the emergency department for evaluation because of mental status changes. Serum ethanol measured at that time was elevated at 146 mg/dL (reference range, <10 mg/dL). A comprehensive toxicology screen was otherwise negative.

At today's appointment, he is noted to have lost approximately 30% of his body weight and currently weighs 176 lb (80 kg) (BMI = 22.7 kg/m^2). He reports taking vitamin and mineral supplementation as prescribed and reiterates that he has not been drinking alcohol.

Which of the following is the most likely diagnosis?

A. Autobrewery syndrome secondary to Roux-en-Y gastric bypass
B. Autonomic neuropathy secondary to rapid weight loss after Roux-en-Y gastric bypass
C. Dumping syndrome secondary to Roux-en-Y gastric bypass
D. New-onset psychosis secondary to nutritional deficiency after Roux-en-Y gastric bypass
E. Nondisclosure of alcohol consumption

31 A 70-year-old man is referred for counseling in the context of commencing adjuvant androgen-deprivation therapy for localized prostate cancer. His urologist has recommended this therapy, but he is concerned about adverse effects on cardiometabolic health.

Which of the following is the most likely effect of starting androgen-deprivation therapy in this patient?

A. Decrease in fat mass
B. Decrease in insulin resistance
C. Decrease in LDL cholesterol
D. Increase in HDL cholesterol
E. Increase in muscle mass

32 A 24-year-old pregnant woman with gestational diabetes mellitus presents for a follow-up appointment at 32 weeks' gestation during her third pregnancy. She has had gestational diabetes with each pregnancy. After her prior deliveries, her blood glucose returned to normal. She does not adhere closely to her insulin treatment regimen. She frequently skips insulin doses out of fear of hypoglycemia because she had a very severe hypoglycemic episode during her last pregnancy. Her current insulin regimen consists of regular insulin with meals and once-daily insulin detemir. Her diet is highly variable, and she does not always restrict her carbohydrate content at meals as instructed. She has received nutritional counseling twice during her current pregnancy.

On physical examination, her blood pressure is 122/60 mm Hg and pulse rate is 110 beats/min. Her height is 64 in (162.6 cm), and weight is 210 lb (95.3 kg) (BMI = 36 kg/m^2). Her prepregnancy weight was 185 lb (84.1 kg) (BMI = 31.8 kg/m^2).

Fetal ultrasonography is notable for a normal fetal heart rate and anatomic structures, but measurements are concerning for fetal macrosomia.

Recent laboratory test results document a hemoglobin A_{1c} measurement of 7.8% (62 mmol/mol). Her point-of-care glucose concentration at today's appointment is 194 mg/dL (10.8 mmol/L).

Which of the following is the best next step in this patient's management?

A. Refer back to nutritional counseling
B. Start a DPP-4 inhibitor
C. Start carbohydrate counting
D. Start glyburide
E. Start metformin

33 A 67-year-old man seeks evaluation for a longstanding history of hypertension and intermittent hypokalemia. His blood pressure has become increasingly difficult to control over the past year, and he is currently taking 4 antihypertensive medications: amlodipine, 10 mg daily; lisinopril, 40 mg daily; hydrochlorothiazide, 25 mg daily; and metoprolol XL, 50 mg daily.

Hormonal workup confirms primary aldosteronism. He is interested in curative surgical treatment, and he is a good surgical candidate. Abdominal CT shows a 1-cm left adrenal mass (5 Hounsfield units on unenhanced images).

Laboratory test results:

Aldosterone = 27 ng/dL (4-21 ng/dL) (SI: 749.0 pmol/L [111.0-582.5 pmol/L])
Direct renin mass concentration = <2 pg/mL (4-44 pg/mL) (SI: 0.5 pmol/L [0.1-1.0 pmol/L])
ACTH = 13 pg/mL (10-60 pg/mL) (SI: 2.8 pmol/L [2.2-13.2 pmol/L])
Cortisol = 10 μg/dL (5-25 μg/dL) (SI: 275.9 nmol/L [137.9-689.7 nmol/L])
Urinary cortisol = 33 μg/24 h (4-50 μg/24 h) (SI: 91.1 nmol/d [11-138 nmol/d])

Results of a 1-mg overnight dexamethasone-suppression test:

Cortisol = 2.1 μg/dL (<1.8 μg/dL) (SI: 57.9 nmol/L [<49.7 nmol/L])
ACTH = <5 pg/mL (SI: <1.1 pmol/L)

The patient undergoes adrenal venous sampling:

		Time	
Location	**Measurement**	**Value prior to cosyntropin**	**Value 10 minutes after cosyntropin**
Inferior vena cava	Cortisol	13.7 μg/dL (SI: 378 nmol/L)	19.3 μg/dL (SI: 532 nmol/L)
	Aldosterone	11.0 ng/dL (SI: 305 pmol/L)	23.0 ng/dL (SI: 638 pmol/L)
	Aldosterone/cortisol	0.8	1.19
Right adrenal vein (RAV)	Cortisol	449 μg/dL (SI: 12,387 nmol/L)	1741 μg/dL (SI: 40,031 nmol/L)
	Aldosterone	59.0 ng/dL (SI: 1637 pmol/L)	1890 ng/dL (SI: 52,429 pmol/L)
	Aldosterone/cortisol	0.13	1.08
Left adrenal vein (LAV)	Cortisol	389 μg/dL (SI: 10,732 nmol/L)	1465 μg/dL (SI: 40,416 nmol/L)
	Aldosterone	533 ng/dL (SI: 14,785 pmol/L)	9340 ng/dL (SI: 259,092 pmol/L)
	Aldosterone/cortisol	1.37	6.37
Lateralization index	$\frac{(\text{Aldosterone/cortisol})_{LAV}}{(\text{Aldosterone/cortisol})_{RAV}}$	**10.54**	**5.85**

Which of the following is the best next step in this patient's management?

A. Adrenal nodule biopsy
B. Initiation of a mineralocorticoid receptor antagonist
C. Left adrenalectomy
D. Midnight salivary cortisol measurement
E. Right adrenalectomy

34 A 76-year-old man with osteoporosis returns for follow-up. He took alendronate for 5 years, having completed therapy approximately 5 years ago, and has been taking teriparatide for the past year. DXA reveals improving bone mineral density in the spine and hips, with a lowest T-score of −2.7 in the left femoral neck. He reports recurrent kidney stones over the past year and is taking hydrochlorothiazide for this. His dietary calcium intake is estimated to be 1000 to 1200 mg daily, and he does not take any calcium supplements. He takes over-the-counter cholecalciferol, 1000 IU daily. He has gastroparesis due to diabetes mellitus. He had a myocardial infarction 6 months ago.

On physical examination, he has no costovertebral angle or spine tenderness to palpation or percussion.

Laboratory test results:

- Serum calcium = 10.2 mg/dL (8.2-10.2 mg/dL) (SI: 2.5 mmol/L [2.1-2.6 mmol/L])
- Serum phosphate = 3.0 mg/dL (2.3-4.7 mg/dL) (SI: 1.0 mmol/L [0.7-1.5 mmol/L])
- Serum creatinine = 1.2 mg/dL (0.7-1.3 mg/dL) (SI: 106.1 µmol/L [61.9-114.9 µmol/L])
- Glomerular filtration rate (estimated) = 60 mL/min per 1.73 m^2 (>60 mL/min per 1.73 m^2)
- Serum 25-hydroxyvitamin D = 39 ng/mL (30-80 ng/mL [optimal]) (SI: 97.3 nmol/L [74.9-199.7 nmol/L])
- Serum albumin = 4.3 g/dL (3.5-5.0 g/dL) (SI: 43 g/L [35-50 g/L])
- Urinary calcium = 380 mg/24 h (100-300 mg/24 h) (SI: 9.5 mmol/d [2.5-7.5 mmol/d])

Which of the following is the best recommendation now?

A. Continue teriparatide
B. Switch to alendronate
C. Switch to abaloparatide
D. Switch to romosozumab
E. Switch to zoledronic acid

35 An 18-year-old woman is referred for evaluation of primary amenorrhea. Thelarche and pubarche occurred at age 11 years, but she has never menstruated. She also reports progressive weight gain since her early teenage years. There is no history of acne, hirsutism, galactorrhea, or polyuria, and she has not experienced headaches or vision disturbance. She is not taking any regular medications or over-the-counter preparations.

On physical examination, her blood pressure is 142/80 mm Hg. Her height is 66 in (167.6 cm) (within midparental height range), and weight is 214 lb (97.1 kg) (BMI = 34.8 kg/m^2). She is clinically euthyroid and euadrenal. Breast and pubic hair development are both Tanner stage 3. Visual acuity is 20/20 (6/6) in both eyes, and visual fields are normal on formal testing.

Laboratory test results:

- Prolactin = 72 ng/mL (4-30 ng/mL) (SI: 3.13 nmol/L [0.17-1.30 nmol/L])
- TSH = 2.0 mIU/L (0.5-5.0 mIU/L)
- Free T_4 = 0.9 ng/dL (0.8-1.8 ng/dL) (SI: 11.58 pmol/L [10.30-23.17 pmol/L])
- Serum cortisol (9 AM) = 19.5 µg/dL (5-25 µg/dL) (SI: 538.0 nmol/L [137.9-689.7 nmol/L])
- IGF-1 = 201 ng/mL (162-541 ng/mL) (SI: 26.3 nmol/L [21.2-70.9 nmol/L])
- FSH = 0.5 mIU/mL (2.0-12.0 mIU/mL [follicular]) (SI: 0.5 IU/L [2.0-12.0 IU/L])
- LH = 0.3 mIU/mL (1.0-18.0 mIU/mL [follicular]) (SI: 0.3 IU/L [1.0-18.0 IU/L])
- Estradiol = <10 pg/mL (10-180 pg/mL [follicular]) (SI: <36.7 pmol/L [36.7-660.8 pmol/L])

MRI of the sella is shown (*see images*).

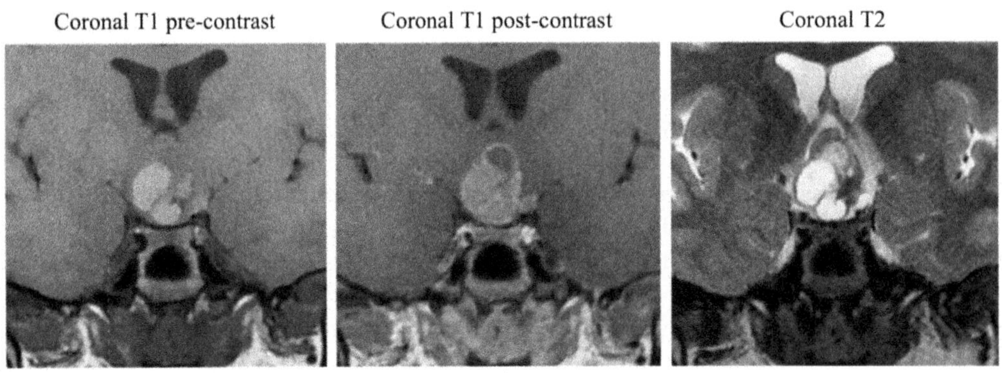

Sagittal T1 pre-contrast

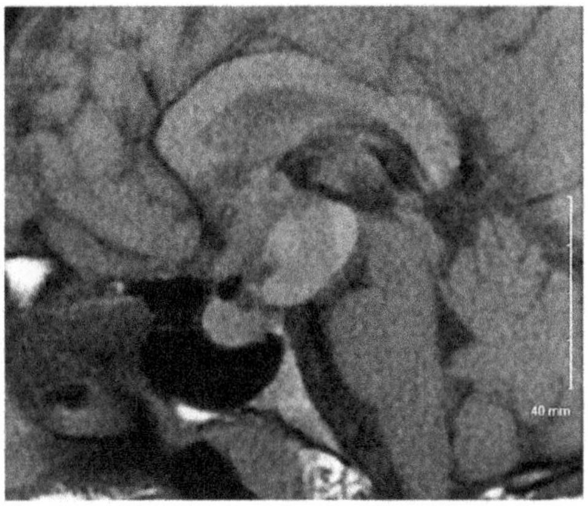

Sagittal T1 post-contrast

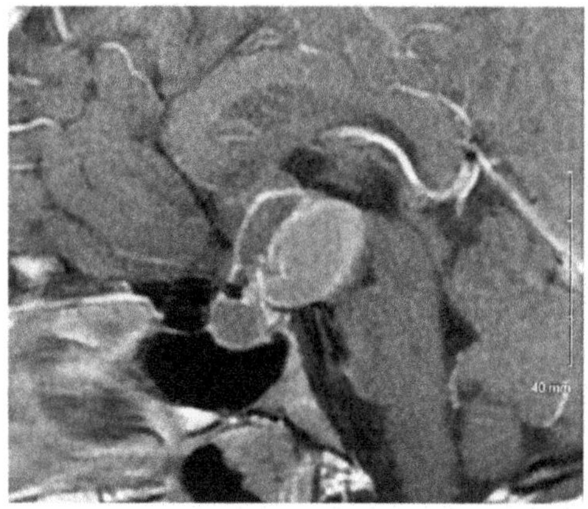

Which of the following is this patient's most likely diagnosis?

A. Craniopharyngioma
B. Cystic macroprolactinoma
C. Germ-cell tumor
D. Rathke cleft cyst
E. Suprasellar meningioma

36 A 50-year-old woman with heterozygous familial hypercholesterolemia, type 2 diabetes mellitus, gout, and coronary artery disease status post percutaneous coronary intervention is referred for management of her cholesterol disorder. Very high cholesterol was diagnosed at age 18 years. Over the years, she tried various cholesterol-lowering medications, including several statins at different dosages and administration frequencies, a cholesterol-absorption inhibitor, bile-acid sequestrants, and niacin. All of these medications caused severe cramping and myalgias, which led to their discontinuation. For several years, she has been undergoing LDL apheresis. Her prior endocrinologist retired, and she is here to establish care. She has read that new nonstatin LDL-cholesterol–lowering medications are available and she wants to try one with the hope that she could stop undergoing LDL apheresis. Her other medications include metformin, empagliflozin, carvedilol, amlodipine, aspirin, allopurinol, and clopidogrel.

On physical examination, her blood pressure is 115/59 mm Hg and pulse rate is 68 beat/min. Her height is 68 in (173 cm), and weight is 188 lb (85.5 kg) (BMI = 29 kg/m^2). She is in no distress. Her breathing effort is normal, and lungs are clear to auscultation bilaterally. On cardiac examination, heart sounds are normal with a regular rate and rhythm. Her abdomen is soft and nontender. She has no lower-extremity edema and no xanthomas. There is an arteriovenous fistula on her left upper extremity.

Laboratory test results:

Lipid profile	Before LDL apheresis	After LDL apheresis
Total cholesterol	316 mg/dL (SI: 8.18 mmol/L)	103 mg/dL (SI: 2.67 mmol/L)
Triglycerides	127 mg/dL (SI: 1.44 mmol/L)	78 mg/dL (SI: 0.88 mmol/L)
HDL cholesterol	48 mg/dL (SI: 1.24 mmol/L)	40 mg/dL (SI: 1.04 mmol/L)
LDL cholesterol	243 mg/dL (SI: 6.29 mmol/L)	47 mg/dL (SI: 1.22 mmol/L)

Given her history, which of the following is the best treatment recommendation for this patient?

A. Alirocumab
B. Bempedoic acid
C. Evinacumab
D. Lomitapide
E. Mipomersen

37 A 45-year-old-woman with a 4-cm right cystic thyroid nodule presents for a second opinion regarding management. She describes a feeling of constant pressure and pain over the right side of her neck. The nodule has been aspirated several times, but it recurs after each aspiration. She declined recommended thyroid surgery in the past. She is otherwise healthy and takes no medications. Thyroid ultrasonography documents the 4-cm cystic nodule in the right thyroid lobe and a 7-mm spongiform left thyroid nodule with no cervical adenopathy.

Laboratory test results:

Serum TSH = 1.5 mIU/L (0.5-5.0 mIU/L)
Basic metabolic panel, normal

Which of the following is the best next step in the management of this thyroid nodule?

A. Levothyroxine suppressive therapy
B. Neck CT
C. Percutaneous ethanol ablation
D. Thyroid scan
E. Total thyroidectomy

38 A 58-year-old woman with a history of non–small cell lung cancer is undergoing treatment with the anti-PD-1 antibody nivolumab. The treatment course has been complicated by rash and colitis, but she has been able to continue therapy despite these adverse effects. After 1 year of therapy, she now describes tiredness, loss of appetite, and weight loss. Her free T_4 and TSH concentrations are normal, but she has a low morning cortisol concentration of 1.9 µg/dL (52.4 nmol/L) and an ACTH concentration less than 5 pg/mL (<1.1 pmol/L). Her oncologist has prescribed hydrocortisone, 15 mg in the morning and 5 mg in the afternoon, with almost immediate improvement of her symptoms and no negative effects. She feels well and has no headaches, tremors, insomnia, neck pain, polyuria, polydipsia, shortness of breath, or chest pain. Her physical examination findings are normal.

Which of the following is the most likely finding on pituitary-directed MRI?

A. Diffuse pituitary enlargement
B. Empty sella
C. Large pituitary mass suspicious for pituitary metastasis
D. Normal pituitary gland
E. Thickening of the pituitary stalk

39 A 54-year-old woman with type 1 diabetes mellitus presents for follow-up. She has peripheral neuropathy and gastroparesis. Her diabetes has been well controlled for the past few years on a regimen of multiple daily insulin injections. She takes insulin lispro at the start of meals and once-daily insulin degludec at bedtime. Metoclopramide previously improved symptoms of gastroparesis, but lately it has not helped. She notes early satiety and some nausea with meals. She has recently developed frequent hypoglycemia 60 to 90 minutes after meals.

On physical examination, her blood pressure is 142/76 mm Hg and pulse rate is 84 beats/min. Her height is 62 in (157.5 cm), and weight is 162 lb (73.5 kg) (BMI = 29.6 kg/m^2). She has decreased sensation to 10-g monofilament on the distal plantar aspect of her feet bilaterally. No lipohypertrophy is noted at sites of insulin administration.

Laboratory test results:

Hemoglobin A_{1c} = 7.8% (4.0%-5.6%) (62 mmol/mol [20-38 mmol/mol])
Serum creatinine = 1.2 mg/dL (0.6-1.1 mg/dL) (106.1 µmol/L [53.0-97.2 µmol/L])
Estimated glomerular filtration rate = 52 mL/min per 1.73 m^2 (>60 mL/min per 1.73 m^2)

Which of the following is the best next step in this patient's management?

A. Reduce the dose of insulin degludec
B. Reduce the dose of insulin lispro at meals
C. Switch insulin degludec to insulin glargine
D. Switch insulin lispro to insulin lispro-aabc
E. Switch insulin lispro to regular insulin

40

A 19-year-old woman presents for follow-up of thyroid nodules that were initially diagnosed 2 years ago. Neck ultrasonography at that time revealed 2 solid thyroid nodules in the right thyroid lobe, including a 7 × 6 × 5-mm right upper pole nodule, a 5 × 3 × 2-mm right midpole nodule, and no abnormal lymph nodes. Follow-up with clinical visits and ultrasonography was recommended.

The patient's medical history is notable for a stage 1A Sertoli-Leydig–cell tumor of the right ovary with poor differentiation diagnosed at age 15 years after initial presentation with secondary amenorrhea and an elevated serum testosterone level. She was treated surgically, which included bilateral oophorectomy, and she has had no recurrence. Current medications include an oral contraceptive pill daily.

Her family history is notable for thyroid nodules and a granulosa-cell tumor in her mother at age 17 years. The patient's maternal grandmother died of metastatic ovarian cancer at age 68 years. A maternal aunt had a lung tumor resected during infancy. There is no family history of adrenal tumors.

On physical examination, her blood pressure is 115/71 mm Hg, and pulse rate is 90 beats/min. Her height is 65 in (165 cm), and weight is 132 lb (60 kg) (BMI = 22 kg/m^2). She has no palpable thyroid nodules or cervical lymphadenopathy. The rest of the examination findings, including those from dermatologic examination, are normal.

Neck ultrasonography performed 2 weeks ago demonstrated 3 right thyroid nodules and no abnormal cervical lymph nodes (*see image*).

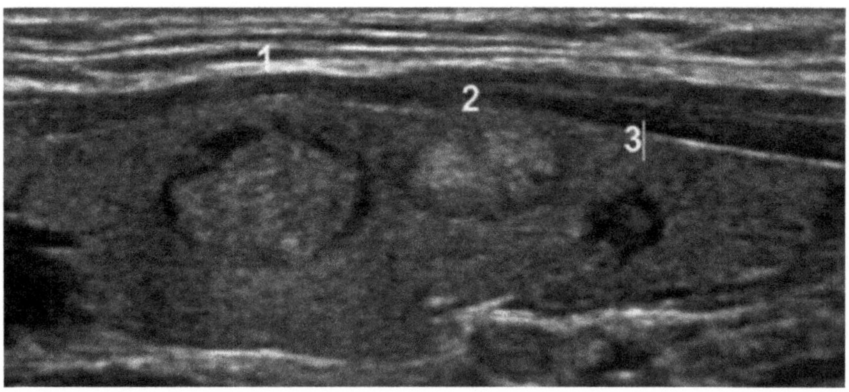

Dimensions: nodule 1: 11 × 10 × 8 mm; nodule 2: 5 × 3 × 2 mm; nodule 3: 2 × 2 × 1 mm.

The TSH concentration is 0.85 mIU/L (0.5-5.0 mIU/L).

The patient undergoes ultrasound-guided FNA biopsy of the largest right thyroid nodule (*nodule 1*), and cytopathology findings demonstrate papillary thyroid carcinoma (Bethesda VI).

Which of the following is this patient's most likely diagnosis?

A. Carney complex
B. DICER1 syndrome
C. Multiple endocrine neoplasia type 2B
D. PTEN hamartoma tumor syndrome (Cowden syndrome)
E. Werner syndrome

41 A 38-year-old woman is referred for management of hypertriglyceridemia. The patient reports that 4 months ago, she was able to obtain health insurance. At her initial visit with her primary care provider, type 2 diabetes mellitus, gastroesophageal reflux disease, and hypertension were diagnosed. The following medications were prescribed: metformin, ranitidine, amlodipine, ethinyl estradiol, and norgestimate. One week ago, her primary care provider ordered blood work, which documented elevated triglycerides. The patient does not know if this is a new problem, as she had not seen a physician since childhood. She does not drink alcohol. She has no other health problems and has no known family history of elevated triglycerides.

On physical examination, her blood pressure is 124/83 mm Hg and pulse rate is 80 beats/min. Her height is 65.5 in (166.4 cm), and weight is 256 lb (116 kg) (BMI = 42 kg/m^2). She is in no distress. On cardiac examination, heart sounds are normal with a regular rate and rhythm. Breath sounds are clear bilaterally. Her abdomen is soft, and bowel sounds are normal. There is no distention or tenderness. She has no lower-extremity edema.

Laboratory test results:

Total cholesterol = 201 mg/dL (<200 mg/dL [optimal]) (SI: 5.21 mmol/L [<5.18 mmol/L])
Triglycerides = 1628 mg/dL (<150 mmol/L [optimal]) (SI: 18.40 mmol/L [<1.70 mmol/L])
HDL cholesterol = 21 mg/dL (>60 mg/dL [optimal]) (SI: 0.54 mmol/L [>1.55 mmol/L])

Which of the following medications is a major contributor to this patient's elevated triglycerides?

A. Amlodipine
B. Ethinyl estradiol
C. Metformin
D. Norgestimate
E. Ranitidine

42 A 67-year-old man is referred for assessment and management of osteoporosis. He presented to his primary care physician with significant back pain in the context of an exacerbation of chronic obstructive pulmonary disease. Chest x-ray (*see image*) revealed no evidence of pneumonia, but a midthoracic compression fracture was noted. His primary care physician also ordered DXA (*see images*).

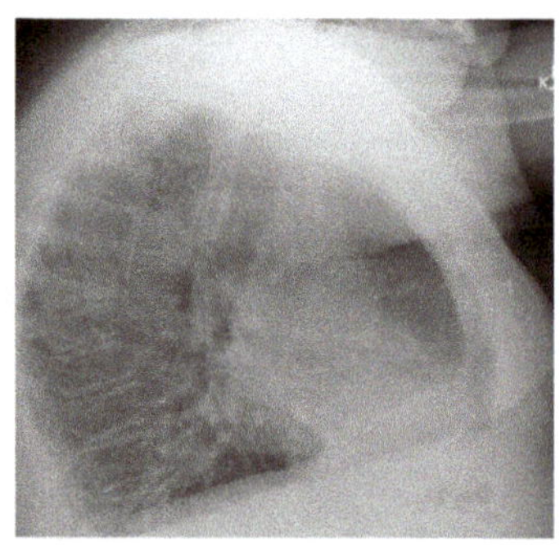

T-scores are as follows: −2.8 at the lumbar spine, −2.5 at the femoral neck, and −2.4 at the total hip.

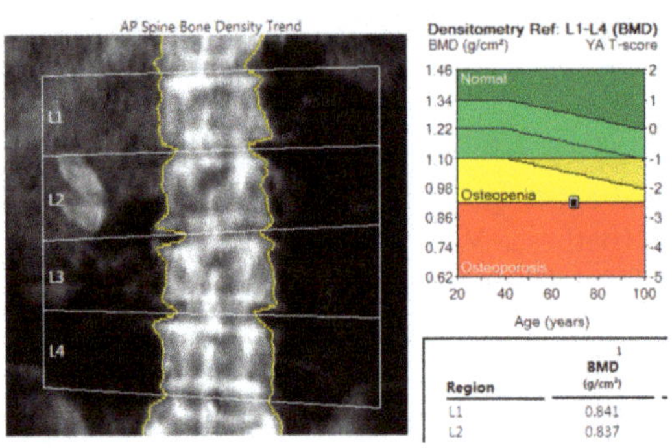

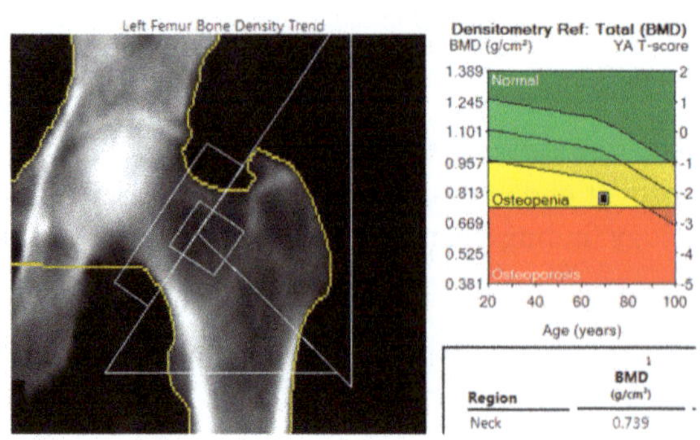

Comorbidities include chronic obstructive pulmonary disease for which he has received several courses of oral glucocorticoids over the last few years and depression that has been treated with electroconvulsive therapy on several occasions, most recently 6 months ago. Current medications include inhaled fluticasone, salmeterol, and tiotropium; sertraline, 100 mg daily; and prednisolone, 15 mg daily (on a weaning schedule). His primary care physician conducted screening for secondary causes of osteoporosis, which documented the following laboratory values:

Serum testosterone = 50 ng/dL (300-900 ng/dL) (SI: 1.7 nmol/L [10.4-31.2 nmol/L])
LH = 39.2 mIU/mL (1.0-9.0 mIU/mL) (SI: 39.2 IU/L [1.0-9.0 IU/L])
FSH = 66.6 mIU/mL (1.0-13.0 mIU/mL) (SI: 66.6 IU/L [1.0-13.0 IU/L])

On physical examination, his height is 72 in (183 cm) and weight is 236 lb (107.3 kg) (BMI is 32 kg/m^2). He has rounded facies, thin skin with several cutaneous bruises, kyphosis, mild gynecomastia, and loss of proximal muscle bulk. Testicular volume is 3 mL bilaterally, and testes feel firm to palpation.

Which of the following is the most likely cause of this patient's hypogonadism?

A. Advanced age
B. Depression
C. Glucocorticoid exposure
D. Klinefelter syndrome
E. Obesity

43 A 70-year-old man was diagnosed with Paget disease of bone 4 years ago when a whole-body technetium ^{99}Tc bone scan documented increased scintigraphic uptake in the left femur, left pelvis, and sternum. He reported a vague aching discomfort in his left femur for many years. His serum total alkaline phosphatase concentration was also noted to be elevated (184 U/L [3.07 μkat/L]). In addition to calcium and vitamin D supplements, zoledronic acid (5 mg intravenously) was administered and this promptly resolved his femur discomfort. Three months later, his total alkaline phosphatase level decreased to the normal range.

The patient now contacts the clinic because the discomfort in his left femur has returned. The total alkaline phosphatase level remains normal. He receives a second zoledronic acid infusion, but in contrast to the beneficial effects of the first infusion, his discomfort persists.

Which of the following is the best next step in this patient's management?

A. Administer a third zoledronic acid infusion, 5 mg intravenously
B. Order x-ray of the left femur
C. Prescribe calcitonin nasal spray
D. Recommend acetaminophen for 2 weeks
E. Repeat the nuclear medicine bone scan

44 An 18-year-old woman with type 1 diabetes mellitus seeks to establish care. Diabetes was diagnosed at age 13 years when she presented to the emergency department with the following laboratory values:

Blood glucose = 329 mg/dL (70-99 mg/dL) (SI: 18.3 mmol/L [3.9-5.5 mmol/L])
Bicarbonate = 24 mEq/L (21-28 mEq/L) (SI: 24 mmol/L [21-28 mmol/L])
Urine ketones, negative
Hemoglobin A_{1c} = 12.3% (4.0%-5.6%) (111 mmol/mol [20-38 mmol/mol])

Before the emergency department visit, she had 2 weeks of polyuria and polydipsia, as well as a 10-lb (4.5-kg) weight loss. Her family history at the time was notable for type 1 diabetes in her father and paternal grandfather and type 2 diabetes in her maternal grandmother. Her brother had reactive hypoglycemia. A basal-bolus insulin regimen was initiated, and her glycemic control was excellent on only modest doses of insulin (insulin glargine,

5 units, and insulin aspart, 1 to 5 units with meals). Assessment of glutamic acid decarboxylase 65 antibodies and nonspecific islet antibodies was negative. Her regimen was thus transitioned to metformin as the sole therapy for 10 months, but her glycemic control was suboptimal the entire time with hemoglobin A_{1c} levels ranging from 9.0% to 10.0% (75 to 86 mmol/mol). Insulin pump therapy was then initiated at age 15 years. Since her initial emergency department visit, she has not had any hospitalizations or episodes of diabetic ketoacidosis.

Her medical history is otherwise notable for attention-deficit/hyperactivity disorder. She was born at 34 4/7 weeks' gestation with a birth weight of 7 lb (3500 g). She was transiently hypoglycemic in the neonatal period.

Her current medications include insulin aspart delivered via insulin pump and sertraline.

On physical examination, her blood pressure is 113/75 mm Hg and pulse rate is 89 beats/min. Her height is 69.5 in (176.5 cm), and weight is 168 lb (76.1 kg) (BMI = 24.5 kg/m^2).

Laboratory test results:

C-peptide = 2.2 ng/mL (0.5-2.0 ng/mL) (SI: 0.73 nmol/L [0.17-0.66 nmol/L])
Glucose = 189 mg/dL (70-99 mg/dL) (SI: 10.5 mmol/L [3.9-5.5 mmol/L])
Hemoglobin A_{1c} = 6.9% (4.0%-5.6%) (52 mmol/mol [20-38 mmol/mol])
Urinalysis, normal

Based on the available information, which of the following is this patient's most likely diagnosis?

A. *GCK* (maturity-onset diabetes of the young type 2)
B. *HNF1A* (maturity-onset diabetes of the young type 3)
C. *HNF1B* (maturity-onset diabetes of the young type 5)
D. *HNF4A* (maturity-onset diabetes of the young type 1)
E. Type 2 diabetes mellitus

45 A 24-year-old woman has an 8-month history of bilateral galactorrhea and secondary amenorrhea. She also reports intermittent headaches, with associated blurring of vision in her right eye, that are longstanding but have worsened in the last 3 to 4 weeks. She has a history of relapsed juvenile-onset Graves disease and underwent total thyroidectomy at age 20 years. She currently takes levothyroxine, 300 mcg daily, but has persistent tiredness and lethargy. She does not take any other regular medications or over-the-counter preparations.

On physical examination, her blood pressure is 145/85 mm Hg and resting pulse rate is 60 beats/min and regular. Her height is 67 in (170.2 cm), and weight is 209 lb (95 kg) (BMI = 32.7 kg/m^2). There is no palpable thyroid remnant. She has normal secondary sexual characteristics. Breast examination confirms bilateral galactorrhea. Visual acuity is 20/25 (6/7.5) in both eyes.

Visual field assessment is shown (*see image*).

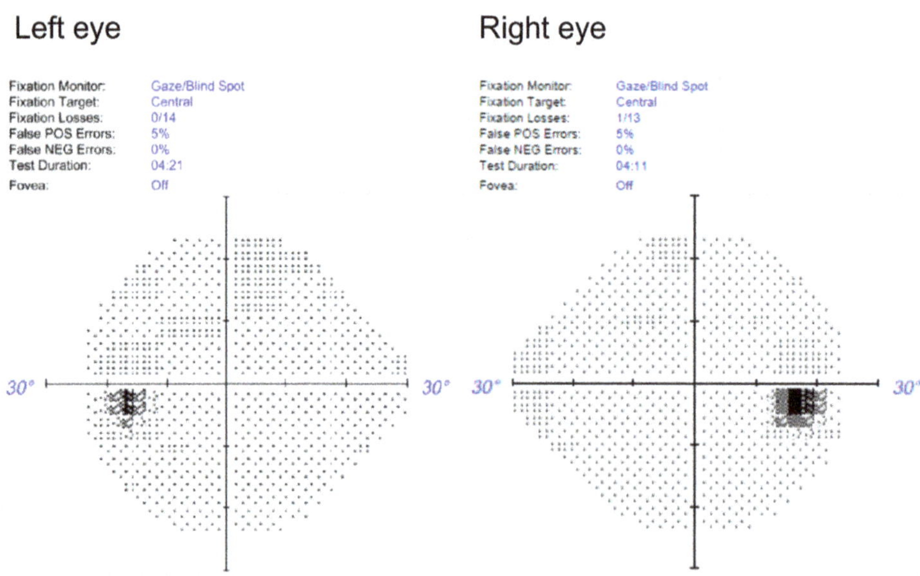

Laboratory test results:

Prolactin = 69 ng/mL (4-30 ng/mL) (SI: 3.00 nmol/L [0.17-1.30 nmol/L])
TSH = 87.1 mIU/L (0.5-5.0 mIU/L)
Free T_4 = 2.0 ng/dL (0.8-1.8 ng/dL) (SI: 25.74 pmol/L [10.30-23.17 pmol/L])
Serum cortisol (9 AM) = 16.5 μg/dL (5-25 μg/dL) (SI: 455.2 nmol/L [137.9-689.7 nmol/L])
IGF-1 = 221 ng/mL (116-341 ng/mL) (SI: 29.0 nmol/L [15.2-44.7 nmol/L])
FSH = 0.7 mIU/mL (2.0-12.0 mIU/mL [follicular]) (SI: 0.7 IU/L [2.0-12.0 IU/L])
LH = 0.6 mIU/mL (1.0-18.0 mIU/mL [follicular]) (SI: 0.6 IU/L [1.0-18.0 IU/L])
Estradiol = 30 pg/mL (10-180 pg/mL [follicular]) (SI: 110.1 pmol/L [36.7-660.8 pmol/L])

There is no evidence of interference in TSH or free T_4 assays.

MRI of the sella is shown (*see image*).

Coronal T1 postcontrast

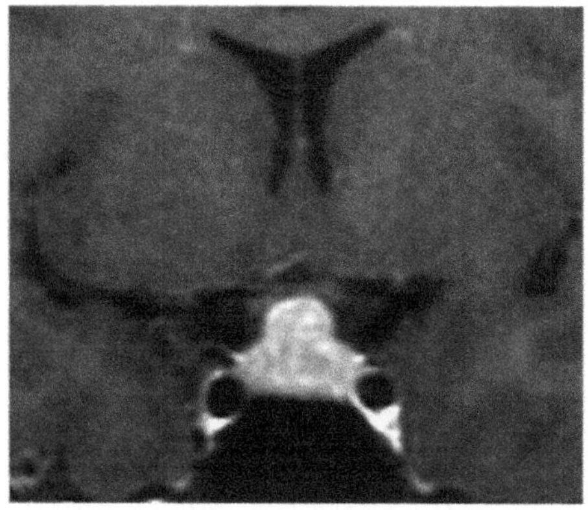

Which of the following treatments is most likely to shrink the pituitary mass and restore normal pituitary function?

A. Dopamine agonist
B. Levothyroxine
C. Radiotherapy
D. Somatostatin receptor ligand
E. Transsphenoidal surgery

46 A 55-year-old man with a 5-year history of type 2 diabetes mellitus presents for follow-up. He is currently taking 35 units of insulin glargine every evening and has been instructed to take 10 units of insulin aspart with each meal. He also takes metformin, 500 mg XR 2 tablets twice daily, and semaglutide weekly. He reports his morning blood glucose levels range from 100 to 125 mg/dL (5.6 to 6.9 mmol/L), but by dinner they range from 200 to 250 mg/dL (11.1 to 13.9 mmol/L). He has difficulty taking insulin at lunchtime while at work, as he often forgets his insulin pen at home. Lunch is usually his largest meal of the day, and he frequently eats fast food. He has occasional low glucose values in the evenings after dinner if he takes a long walk.

On physical examination, his blood pressure is 142/73 mm Hg and pulse rate is 80 beats/min. His height is 70 in (177.8 cm), and weight is 218 lb (99.1 kg) (BMI = 31.3 kg/m^2).

Laboratory test results (sample drawn while fasting):

Hemoglobin A_{1c} = 8.5% (4.0%-5.6%) (69 mmol/mol [20-38 mmol/mol])
Creatinine = 0.7 mg/dL (0.7-1.3 mg/dL) (SI: 61.9 μmol/L [61.9-114.9 μmol/L])
Serum urea nitrogen = 25 mg/dL (8-23 mg/dL) (SI: 8.9 mmol/L [2.9-8.2 mmol/L])
Plasma glucose = 101 mg/dL (70-99 mg/dL) (SI: 5.6 mmol/L [3.9-5.5 mmol/L])
Sodium = 141 mEq/L (136-142 mEq/L) (SI: 141 mmol/L [136-142 mmol/L])

Which of the following is the best next step in this patient's management?

A. Convert insulin to a simple continuous subcutaneous insulin infusion (CSII) "patch-like therapy," which delivers a fixed dose of hourly insulin and adjustable dose of meal-time insulin
B. Convert to mixed insulin NPH/insulin aspart 70/30, 55 units twice daily with breakfast and lunch
C. Increase the basal insulin dosage to 38 units
D. Increase the prandial insulin dose to 12 units with meals
E. Instruct the patient to stop exercising in the evening

47 A 53-year-old woman is referred by her primary care physician for evaluation of an elevated hCG value of 25.9 mIU/mL (25.9 IU/L) that was measured in preparation for cryoablation of a left shoulder supraspinatus fibroelastoma (3.5 × 7.6 × 3.6 cm). Her last menstrual period was 7 years ago.

Repeated laboratory test results:

- TSH = 2.6 mIU/L (0.5-5.0 mIU/L)
- FSH = 52.0 mIU/mL (>30.0 mIU/mL [postmenopausal]) (SI: 41.0 IU/L [>30.0 IU/L])
- Estradiol, undetectable
- hCG (different commercial assay) = 11.0 mIU/mL (<3.0 mIU/mL) (SI: 11.0 IU/L [<3.0 IU/L])
- α-Fetoprotein = <8.4 ng/mL (SI: <8.4 µg/L)

On pelvic ultrasonography, the uterus measures 3.1 × 3.4 × 5.1 cm. There is a 3.0-cm, posteriorly located fibroid in the myometrium. The endometrium is normal within the uterine fundus. Cystic changes are observed, including nabothian cysts within the cervix and lower uterine endometrium. Endometrial thickness is 4 mm. The right ovary is not visualized, most likely secondary to ovary position and intervening bowel gas. The left ovary appears normal with a volume of 3 cc. There is no intraperitoneal fluid.

Which of the following is the most likely etiology of this patient's elevated hCG?

A. Antibody interference with assay
B. Ectopic pregnancy
C. Germ-cell tumor
D. Menopause
E. Shoulder fibroelastoma

48

An 88-year-old woman with hypertension and chronic kidney disease is hospitalized for severe hypercalcemia. She reports memory loss, decreased appetite, constipation, joint pain, and muscle weakness. She is not anuric. She has no history of fragility fractures or kidney stones. Her dietary calcium intake is approximately 600 mg daily, and she does not take calcium or vitamin D supplements. She has no known family history of calcium or parathyroid disease.

On physical examination, she is awake and alert. Her respiratory effort is normal, and there is no spine tenderness to palpation.

Laboratory test results:

- Serum calcium = 14.1 mg/dL (8.2-10.2 mg/dL) (SI: 3.5 mmol/L [2.1-2.6 mmol/L])
- Serum phosphate = 4.1 mg/dL (2.3-4.7 mg/dL) (SI: 1.3 mmol/L [0.7-1.5 mmol/L])
- Serum creatinine = 3.3 mg/dL (0.6-1.1 mg/dL) (SI: 291.7 µmol/L [53.0-97.2 µmol/L])
- Glomerular filtration rate (estimated) = 14 mL/min per 1.73 m^2 (>60 mL/min per 1.73 m^2)
- Serum intact PTH = 403 pg/mL (10-65 pg/mL) (SI: 403 ng/L [10-65 ng/L])
- Serum 25-hydroxyvitamin D = 31 ng/mL (30-80 ng/mL [optimal]) (SI: 77.4 nmol/L [74.9-199.7 nmol/L])
- Serum albumin = 3.9 g/dL (3.5-5.0 g/dL) (SI: 39 g/L [35-50 g/L])

In addition to adequate hydration, which of the following is the most appropriate next step in the management of this patient's hypercalcemia?

A. Initiate oral cinacalcet
B. Initiate oral furosemide
C. Initiate subcutaneous denosumab
D. Refer for dialysis
E. Treat with intravenous zoledronic acid

49

A 47-year-old woman with no notable medical history has been having irregular periods. Her gynecologist orders prolactin measurement, which is borderline elevated (30.9 ng/mL [1.3 nmol/L]). Pituitary-directed MRI with gadolinium shows a normal pituitary gland. Her serum IGF-1 concentration is elevated (312 ng/mL [13.6 nmol/L]), and she is referred to endocrinology. At the time of her appointment, her menses have returned to being regular. She notes some change in the size of her fingers, as she can no longer wear her rings, although she reports that when she loses weight they seem to fit again. Her shoes feel a little tight. She has no history of excessive sweating, although she occasionally has hot flushes. She has noticed some acne. Her husband reports that she snores loudly. Her only medication is vitamin D supplementation.

On physical examination, her blood pressure is 141/94 mm Hg, pulse rate is 95 beats/min, and temperature is 98.6°F (37°C). Her height is 66 in (167.6 cm), and weight is 201.3 lb (91.3 kg) (BMI = 32.5 kg/m²). Her pupils are round. There is no increased space between her teeth; her tongue looks large. Her palms appear sweaty.

Laboratory test results:

IGF-1 = 339 ng/mL (91-246 ng/mL) (SI: 44.4 nmol/L [11.9-32.2 nmol/L])
Prolactin = 23 ng/mL (4-30 ng/mL) (SI: 1.0 nmol/L [0.17-1.30 nmol/L])
Plasma GHRH, normal

Results of a 75-g oral glucose-suppression test are shown.

	Time				
Measurement	**Baseline**	**30 minutes**	**60 minutes**	**90 minutes**	**120 minutes**
Glucose	90 mg/dL (SI: 5.0 mmol/L)	132 mg/dL (SI: 7.3 mmol/L)	117 mg/dL (SI: 6.5 mmol/L)	107 mg/dL (SI: 5.9 mmol/L)	97 mg/dL (SI: 5.4 mmol/L)
GH	2.0 ng/mL (SI: 2.0 µg/L)	1.0 ng/mL (SI: 1.0 µg/L)	1.1 ng/mL (SI: 1.1 µg/L)	1.0 ng/mL (SI: 1.0 µg/L)	1.2 ng/mL (SI: 1.2 µg/L)

Which of the following is the most appropriate next step?

A. Initiate therapy with a somatostatin receptor agonist
B. Initiate therapy with cabergoline
C. Initiate therapy with pegvisomant
D. Reassure the patient that acromegaly is ruled out
E. Refer to neurosurgery for transsphenoidal surgery

50 A 29-year-old man with type 1 diabetes mellitus requests help with managing his glucose levels in the setting of exercise. He has had diabetes for 17 years and his only complication is mild nonproliferative diabetic retinopathy without macular edema. Over the last 2 to 3 years, his hemoglobin A_{1c} level has ranged from 7.2% to 7.9% (55 to 63 mmol/mol). He has always been moderately active, jogging once or twice per week for 20 to 30 minutes and lifting weights once per week. He now plans to train for a half-marathon and would like to run 3 to 4 times per week. He aims for a glucose concentration of 125 to 175 mg/dL (6.9 to 9.7 mmol/L) before starting any exercise, but he found he was having hypoglycemia occurring during runs. Therefore, he now suspends his insulin pump and eats a packet of candy before each running session. However, as the intensity and duration of runs have increased, he finds that 1 to 2 hours after a run, his glucose concentration ranges from 220 to 250 mg/dL (12.2 to 13.9 mmol/L).

Instead of suspending his pump, he is advised to initiate an 80% reduction in the basal rate 90 minutes before each run and to resume the typical basal rate after the run is over.

If postexercise hyperglycemia persists, which of the following strategies is most likely to be effective?

A. Administer a correction bolus after the exercise to correct for high glucose levels
B. Consume 20 g of high–glycemic index carbohydrates during exercise (every 30 minutes during a run)
C. Perform a low-intensity cool-down routine for 10 to 15 minutes after each run
D. Perform light weightlifting for 10 to 15 minutes before each run
E. Resume consumption of candy before each run

51 A 43-year-old woman is admitted to the hospital with cellulitis of the right leg that has progressed despite oral antimicrobial therapy. She has had severe eosinophilic asthma since childhood, with frequent exacerbations despite maximal medical therapy. Four months ago, she started biological therapy (antiinterleukin-5 receptor monoclonal antibody). This has led to marked improvement in her asthma and allowed down-titration of other medications, which are currently beclometasone/formoterol 100/6 combined inhaler, 1 puff twice daily, and salbutamol inhaler as needed.

On physical examination, her height is 67 in (170.2 cm) and weight is 191 lb (86.8 kg) (BMI = 29.9 kg/m^2). Her temperature is 100.9°F (38.3°C), blood pressure is 100/55 mm Hg, and pulse rate is 110 beats/min and regular. On auscultation of the chest, there is good air entry throughout with only occasional scattered expiratory wheezes. There is marked cellulitis of the right leg extending above the knee.

Laboratory test results:

Hemoglobin = 13.6 g/dL (12.1-15.1 g/dL) (SI: 136 g/L [121-151 g/L])
White blood cell count = 23,100/µL (4500-11,000/µL) (SI: 23.1 × 10^9/L [4.5-11.0 × 10^9/L])
Platelet count = 262 × 10^3/µL (150-450 × 10^3/µL) (SI: 262 × 10^9/L [150-450 × 10^9/L])
C-reactive protein = 28.5 mg/L (0.8-3.1 mg/L) (SI: 271.4 nmol/L [7.62-29.52 nmol/L])
Serum sodium = 127 mEq/L (136-142 mEq/L) (SI: 127 mmol/L [136-142 mmol/L])
Serum potassium = 4.0 mEq/L (3.5-5.0 mEq/L) (SI: 4.0 mmol/L [3.5-5.0 mmol/L])
Serum urea nitrogen = 8.3 mg/dL (8-23 mg/dL) (SI: 3.0 mmol/L [2.9-8.2 mmol/L])
Serum creatinine = 0.7 mg/dL (0.6-1.1 mg/dL) (SI: 61.9 µmol/L [53.0-97.2 µmol/L])
Serum osmolality = 267 mOsm/kg (275-295 mOsm/kg) (SI: 267 mmol/kg [275-295 mmol/kg])
Urine osmolality = 610 mOsm/kg (150-1150 mOsm/kg) (SI: 610 mmol/kg [150-1150 mmol/kg])
Spot urine sodium = 48 mEq/L (SI: 48 mmol/L)

Which of the following is the most likely cause of this patient's hyponatremia?

A. Hyperglycemia
B. Hypocortisolism
C. Increased serum immunoglobulins
D. Primary polydipsia
E. Syndrome of inappropriate antidiuretic hormone secretion

52 A 54-year-old woman with a history of follicular thyroid carcinoma presents for follow-up. She describes severe lower back pain, and lumbosacral spine x-rays show lytic lesions at L3 and L4 and degenerative changes at the level of L5 and S1. Findings on ^{131}I scan, which demonstrate intensely focal radioactive iodine uptake in T6, T7, T8, L3, and L4 vertebral bodies, are consistent with skeletal metastasis. No other abnormalities are seen on radioiodine scan.

Her medical history is notable for postsurgical hypothyroidism and gastroesophageal reflux disease. She takes levothyroxine, 150 mcg daily, and omeprazole, 20 mg daily.

On physical examination, her blood pressure is 116/74 mm Hg and pulse rate is 70 beats/min. There is a well-healed scar at the base of her neck with no palpable mass or cervical adenopathy. Her thoracic spine is not tender to touch, but she has pain with palpation of her lumbar spine.

Laboratory test results:

TSH = 0.80 mIU/L (0.5-5.0 mIU/L)
Free T_4 = 1.4 ng/dL (0.8-1.8 ng/dL) (SI: 18.0 pmol/L [10.30-23.17 pmol/L])
Basic metabolic panel, normal
Thyroglobulin= 365 ng/mL (3-42 ng/mL) (SI: 365 µg/L [3-42 µg/L]) (after surgery and radioactive iodine treatment: <1.0 ng/mL [SI: <1.0 µg/L])
Thyroglobulin antibodies, negative

In addition to increasing her levothyroxine dosage and prescribing radioiodine treatment, which of the following is the best next step in this patient's management?

A. Intravenous bisphosphonate therapy
B. External radiotherapy
C. PET/CT
D. Tyrosine kinase inhibitor
E. Whole-body bone scan

53 A 21-year-old woman with a medical history of attention-deficit/hyperactivity disorder presents to the emergency department with nausea, vomiting, and weight loss and is found to be in diabetic ketoacidosis. There is no history of steroid use, and she states that her only medication is amphetamine/dextroamphetamine. She has no family history of type 1 diabetes mellitus, but her maternal grandmother has type 2 diabetes. She does not smoke cigarettes and reports drinking 1 to 2 beers a day on weekends.

On physical examination, her height is 65 in (165 cm) and weight is 140 lb (63.6 kg) (BMI = 23.3 kg/m^2). Her blood pressure is 113/75 mm Hg, and pulse rate is 106 beats/min. Examination findings are unremarkable except for dry mucous membranes and tachycardia.

Laboratory test results at hospital admission:

Glucose = 647 mg/dL (70-99 mg/dL) (SI: 35.9 mmol/L [3.9-5.5 mmol/L])
Hemoglobin A_{1c} = 16.0% (4.0%-5.6%) (SI: 151 mmol/mol [20-38 mmol/mol])

Insulin is initiated, and she is seen in clinic 2 weeks after hospital discharge.

Laboratory test results on follow-up:

Glutamic acid decarboxylase 65 antibodies = <5.0 U/mL (0-5 U/mL)
Insulinoma-associated protein (IA-2) antibodies = <7.5 U/mL (<7.5 U/mL)
Zinc transporter (ZnT8) antibodies = <10 U/mL (0-15 U/mL)
Glucose = 151 mg/dL (70-99 mg/dL) (SI: 8.4 mmol/L [3.9-5.5 mmol/L])
C-peptide = 0.4 ng/mL (0.5-2.0 ng/mL) (SI: 0.13 nmol/L [0.17-0.66 nmol/L])
Creatinine = 1.1 mg/dL (0.6-1.1 mg/dL) (SI: 97.2 μmol/L [53.0-97.2 μmol/L])

Which of the following is the most likely cause of this patient's hyperglycemia?

A. Alcohol-induced hyperglycemia
B. Latent autoimmune diabetes of adulthood
C. Maturity-onset diabetes of the young type 3 (pathogenic variant in *HNF1A* gene)
D. Type 1 diabetes mellitus
E. Type 2 diabetes mellitus

54 A 38-year-old man presents for a weight-loss consultation. He has been trying to reduce his caloric intake for the last 3 years but has not achieved meaningful weight loss. In the time between high school graduation and college graduation, he lost approximately 140 lb (63.6 kg). He was able to maintain his weight for a few years without much difficulty. However, his weight has slowly increased over time, and he attributes this to stress, changes in activity, and starting a family. He has been at his current weight for about 1 year. He records his food intake in a journal and consumes approximately 2500 calories per day. He limits carbohydrate consumption. For the last 2 years, he has walked 2.5 miles at a brisk pace 3 times per week. He averages 8000 to 10,000 steps per day. He does not describe himself as sedentary. His wife reports that he frequently snores and sometimes awakens at night. He takes no regular medications.

On physical examination, his height is 74 in (188 cm) and weight is 310 lb (141 kg) (BMI = 39.8 kg/m^2). There is no thyroid enlargement. He has no peripheral stigmata of hypercortisolism and no facial plethora.

Laboratory test results:

Fasting glucose = 99 mg/dL (70-99 mg/dL) (SI: 5.6 mmol/L [3.9-5.5 mmol/L])
Hemoglobin A_{1c} = 5.3% (4.0%-5.6%) (34 mmol/mol [20-38 mmol/mol])
TSH = 5.1 mIU/L (0.5-5.0 mIU/L)

Results of resting energy expenditure obtained via indirect calorimetry under steady state conditions:

Component	Result
Resting energy expenditure, measured value	2110 kcal/24 h
Resting energy expenditure, predicted value	2750 kcal/24 h
Resting energy expenditure, predicted	77%

Which of the following is the best next step to help this patient achieve his weight-loss goals?

A. Advise a high-protein diet, aiming for 1.2 g/kg body weight
B. Evaluate for sleep apnea and start treatment if indicated
C. Obtain 24-hour urine collection to measure free cortisol
D. Prescribe a physical activity regimen focused on resistance exercises
E. Start levothyroxine supplementation at a dosage of 0.8 mcg/kg body weight (112 mcg daily)

55 A 19-year-old transgender man with a history of type 2 diabetes mellitus is referred for gender-affirming hormone therapy. Gender dysphoria began at puberty. Gender dysphoria was diagnosed by a behavioral health provider using standards of care from the World Professional Association for Transgender Health, and he meets criteria for gender-affirming hormone therapy. Lack of family support for his gender transition has limited his ability to access care and proceed with gender-affirming therapy, including withdrawal of family support if they find out he is taking testosterone. He would like to become more independent, but he has social anxiety about being misgendered, which limits his interest in and ability to get a job.

The focus of his past health care visits has been type 2 diabetes rather than gender transition. His new primary care provider prescribed metformin, but the patient did not fill the prescription due to fear of misgendered experiences at the clinic and pharmacy, with a resultant hemoglobin A_{1c} increase from 8.7% to 10.2% (72 to 88 mmol/mol).

In discussing his treatment goals, he is looking forward to hormonal and surgical masculinization, including chest masculinizing surgery, understanding that his surgical outcomes would improve by treating his type 2 diabetes. His new primary care provider is very affirming, and this support is part of the reason he agreed to the referral to endocrinology.

On physical examination, his height is 64 in (162.5 cm) and weight is 240 lb (109 kg) (BMI = 41.2 kg/m^2). His blood pressure is 135/92 mm Hg. There is terminal hair growth on the upper lip, chin, abdomen, and thighs with a Ferriman-Gallwey score of 12. No acanthosis or other pertinent findings are noted on examination.

Which of the following is the best next step in this patient's management?

A. Evaluate for and treat polycystic ovary syndrome
B. Identify local resources for support groups and gender therapists
C. Initiate a GLP-1 receptor agonist
D. Initiate testosterone therapy to treat dysphoria
E. Refer to behavioral health/social work services

56 A 33-year-old man presents for evaluation of bilateral adrenal masses, which were found incidentally on abdominal CT performed after a car crash. Both adrenal glands were enlarged and nodular (*see image, arrows*). The patient reports that he is generally healthy. He is sometimes fatigued, particularly after intense physical activity in hot and humid weather. He has been married for 5 years, but he and his wife have been unsuccessful in conceiving a child.

On physical examination, his height is 67 in (170 cm) and weight is 190 lb (86.4 kg) (BMI = 29.8 kg/m^2). His blood pressure is 102/75 mm Hg, and pulse rate is 90 beats/min. He is well virilized. His skin is warm, dry, and tan, without plethora, striae, or bruises. Acne is noted on his chest and back. His testes are firm and heterogenous, with a volume of approximately 25 mL bilaterally.

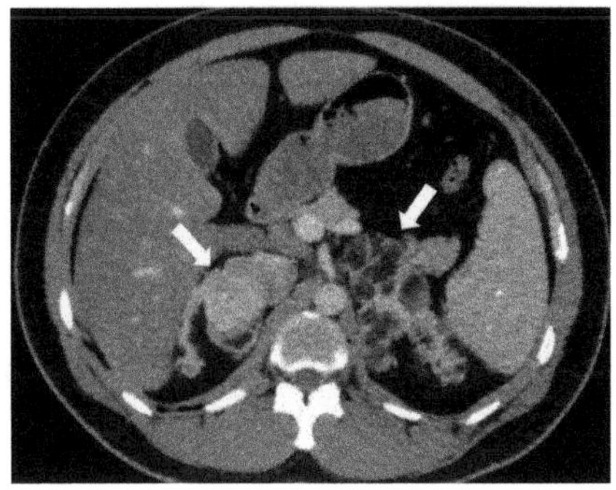

Laboratory test results (sample collected at 8 AM):

- Serum cortisol = 5 µg/dL (5-25 µg/dL) (SI: 137.9 nmol/L [137.9-689.7 nmol/L])
- ACTH = 709 pg/mL (10-60 pg/mL) (SI: 156 pmol/L [2.2-13.2 pmol/L])
- Serum aldosterone = 5.8 ng/dL (4-21 ng/dL) (SI: 161 pmol/L [111.0-582.5 pmol/L])
- Plasma renin activity = 31.9 ng/mL per h (0.6-4.3 ng/mL per h)
- DHEA-S = 83 µg/dL (65-334 µg/dL) (SI: 2.2 µmol/L [1.76-9.05 µmol/L])
- TSH = 4.06 mIU/L (0.5-5.0 mIU/L)
- Free T_4 = 1.1 ng/dL (0.8-1.8 ng/dL) (SI: 14.4 pmol/L [10.30-23.17 pmol/L])
- Testosterone = 703 ng/dL (300-900 ng/dL) (SI: 24.4 nmol/L [10.4-31.2 nmol/L])
- LH = <0.1 mIU/mL (1.0-9.0 mIU/mL) (SI: <0.1 IU/L [1.0-9.0 IU/L])
- FSH = <0.3 mIU/mL (1.0-13.0 mIU/mL) (SI: <0.3 IU/L [1.0-13.0 IU/L])

Which of the following is the best test to confirm this patient's suspected diagnosis?

A. Adrenal biopsy
B. Cosyntropin-stimulation test
C. FDG-PET scan
D. Pituitary-directed MRI
E. Serum 17-hydroxyprogesterone measurement

57

A 40-year-old woman (G1P1) presents for follow-up of Graves disease. Hyperthyroidism was diagnosed 16 months ago. At that time, she was prescribed methimazole, 20 mg daily, and her dosage was gradually tapered over the next 4 months. She has been taking methimazole, 5 mg daily, for the past 12 months with no perceived adverse effects. She reports no symptoms today and is satisfied with her current treatment approach.

On physical examination, her blood pressure is 102/74 mm Hg, and pulse rate is 61 beats/min. Her height is 65 in (165 cm), and weight is 129 lb (58.5 kg) (BMI = 21.5 kg/m^2). Findings on eye examination are notable for no lid lag, chemosis, or proptosis. Her thyroid gland is 20 g without nodules. The rest of her examination findings are normal.

Laboratory test results:

Measurement	At diagnosis	Today	Reference range
TSH	0.02 mIU/L	1.05 mIU/L	0.5-5.0 mIU/L
Free T_4	2.66 ng/dL (SI: 34.2 pmol/L)	1.17 ng/dL (SI: 15.1 pmol/L)	0.8-1.8 ng/dL (SI: 10.30-23.17 pmol/L)
Total T_3	300 ng/dL (SI: 4.62 nmol/L)	125 ng/dL (SI: 1.93 nmol/L)	70-200 ng/dL (SI: 1.08-3.08 nmol/L)
TRAb	2.6 IU/L	2.4 IU/L	≤1.75 IU/L

Which of the following is the best next step in this patient's management?

A. Continue methimazole at the current dosage
B. Discontinue methimazole and monitor thyroid function
C. Increase the methimazole dosage and start levothyroxine
D. Refer for radioactive iodine therapy
E. Refer for thyroidectomy

58 A 28-year-old man is referred for evaluation of his lipid disorder. Three months ago, he established care with a primary care provider, and the only abnormal values on laboratory testing were related to his cholesterol panel and hemoglobin A_{1c} level. Other than prediabetes, he has no health problems. Metformin was recently prescribed. He has noticed small bumps on his elbows and white-orange spots on his hands. He reports an extensive family history of heart disease. His father had a myocardial infarction at age 50 years, his paternal aunt underwent coronary artery bypass grafting at age 55 years, his paternal uncle underwent percutaneous coronary intervention at age 49 years, and his paternal grandmother died of a myocardial infarction at age 53 years.

On physical examination, his blood pressure is 135/84 mm Hg and pulse rate is 69 beats/min. His height is 72 in (183 cm), and weight is 236 lb (107 kg) (BMI = 32 kg/m^2). He has bilateral palmar crease xanthomas (*see image*) and tuberoeruptive xanthomas on his elbows. His breathing effort and breath sounds are normal. On cardiac examination, his heart sounds are normal with a regular rate and rhythm. He has no lower-extremity edema.

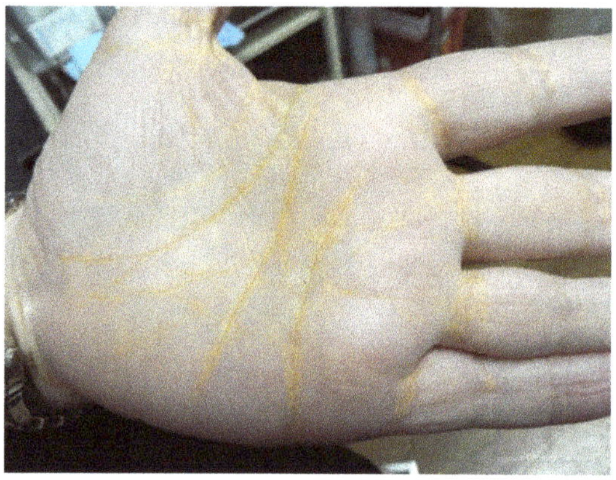

Laboratory test results:

Total cholesterol = 454 mg/dL (<200 mg/dL [optimal]) (SI: 11.76 mmol/L [<5.18 mmol/L])
Triglycerides = 519 mg/dL (<150 mmol/L [optimal]) (SI: 5.86 mmol/L [<1.70 mmol/L])
HDL cholesterol = 46 mg/dL (>60 mg/dL [optimal]) (SI: 1.19 mmol/L [>1.55 mmol/L])
Hemoglobin A_{1c} = 6.0% (4.0%-5.6%) (42 mmol/mol [20-38 mmol/mol])

Which of the following apolipoproteins is associated with this patient's lipid disorder?

A. Apolipoprotein A-1
B. Apolipoprotein (a)
C. Apolipoprotein B_{100}
D. Apolipoprotein C-II
E. Apolipoprotein E

59 A 50-year-old woman with postablative hypothyroidism and an 8-year history of type 2 diabetes mellitus is referred because of difficulty maintaining her serum TSH in the normal range despite several levothyroxine dosage adjustments. In addition, her lipid panel shows new elevations in total cholesterol, triglycerides, and LDL cholesterol. She takes liraglutide, metformin, atorvastatin, and losartan. She reports that she takes her levothyroxine on an empty stomach and waits 1 to 2 hours before eating or drinking. She does not take any over-the-counter supplements. Her mother also has hypothyroidism. She has no known drug allergies.

On physical examination, her blood pressure is 135/80 mm Hg and pulse rate is 70 beats/min. The thyroid gland is not palpable and there is no cervical adenopathy. Her abdomen is soft and nontender. There is edema in her lower extremities but no lesions on her feet.

Laboratory test results:

Fasting glucose = 120 mg/dL (70-99 mg/dL) (SI: 6.7 mmol/L [3.9-5.5 mmol/L])
Creatinine = 1.0 mg/dL (0.6-1.1 mg/dL) SI: 88.4 μmol/L [53.0-97.2 μmol/L])
Albumin = 2.4 g/dL (3.5-5.0 g/dL) (SI: 24 g/L [35-50 g/L])
Total cholesterol = 280 mg/dL (<200 mg/dL [optimal]) (SI: 7.25 mmol/L [<5.18 mmol/L])
LDL cholesterol = 170 mg/dL (<100 mg/dL [optimal]) (SI: 4.40 nmol/L [<2.59 mmol/L])
25-Hydroxyvitamin D = 25 ng/mL (30-80 ng/mL [optimal]) (SI: 64.9 nmol/L [74.9-199.7 nmol/L])
TSH = 10.0 mIU/L (0.5-5.0 mIU/L)
Free T_4 = 1.0 ng/dL (0.8-1.8 ng/dL) (SI: 12.87 pmol/L [10.30-23.17 pmol/L])
Hemoglobin A_{1c} = 8.0% (4.0%-5.6%) (SI: 64 mmol/mol [20-38 mmol/mol])
Urinary albumin = 400 μg/mg creat (30-300 μg/mg creat) (SI: 45.2 μg/mol creat [3.4-33.9 μg/mol creat])

Which of the following is the most likely cause of this patient's increasing thyroid hormone dosage requirement?

A. Biotin interference
B. Celiac disease
C. Metformin treatment
D. Nephrotic syndrome
E. Nonadherence to levothyroxine therapy

60 A 72-year-old woman with a 12-year history of type 2 diabetes mellitus returns for follow-up. For the first decade after diabetes was diagnosed, her glycemic control was good with hemoglobin A_{1c} values in the range of 6.5% to 7.5% (48-58 mmol/mol). When she was initially diagnosed, she worked closely with a diabetes educator to learn about the role of diet and exercise in the management of diabetes. Over the past 2 years, she has had rising blood glucose concentrations with hemoglobin A_{1c} levels between 8.5% and 10.0% (69 and 86 mmol/mol). She also has a history of hypertension and hyperlipidemia. She has experienced no weight loss and reports no change in bowel function. Current medications include metformin, dulaglutide, insulin glargine, lisinopril, and atorvastatin.

She is unable to identify barriers to diabetes care. She is flustered, as she arrived 15 minutes late because she thought her appointment was scheduled at a later time. She has no difficulty with sleep and reports usual interest in activities. She is frustrated with her inability to control her blood glucose levels.

On physical examination, she is alert, does not seem distressed, and is well groomed. Her blood pressure is 152/90 mm Hg, and pulse rate is 84 beats/min. Heart sounds are regular in rate and rhythm. Lungs are clear to auscultation with good air movement in all lung fields. The rest of the examination findings are normal.

Which of the following is the most likely cause of this patient's deterioration in glycemic control?

A. Dementia
B. Depression
C. Hypothyroidism
D. Pancreatic cancer
E. Poor comprehension of management in diabetes

61 A 34-year-old man is referred for evaluation of hypogonadism. He presented to his primary care physician with low libido, fatigue, anxiety, and mild depression. A fasting morning serum testosterone concentration was documented to be 153 ng/dL (5.3 nmol/L). He takes a vitamin D supplement and a variety of over-the-counter supplements. He reports normal puberty. He has not attempted to have children and currently has no paternity plans. He smokes 30 cigarettes daily and marijuana 3 times weekly, but he does not drink alcohol. He has never taken anabolic steroids. He has no headaches or vision symptoms. He reports nodding off when watching television, and his partner notes that he snores loudly and gasps for air several times during the night.

On physical examination, his height is 73 in (185.4 cm) and weight is 320 lb (145.5 kg) (BMI = 42.2 kg/m^2). He has prominent, soft breasts and reduced muscle bulk. Genital examination is difficult to conduct because of a large apron of adipose tissue, but he appears to have normal sexual hair, normal penile length, and testicular volume of 15 mL bilaterally. He has full range of eye movements, and visual fields are normal to confrontation.

Current laboratory test results (8 AM, fasting):

Serum testosterone = 176 ng/dL (300-900 ng/dL) (SI: 6.1 nmol/L [10.4-31.2 nmol/L])
SHBG = 1.1 µg/mL (1.1-6.7 µg/mL) (SI: 10 nmol/L [10-60 nmol/L])
Calculated free testosterone= 7.5 ng/dL (9.0-30.0 ng/dL) (SI: 0.26 nmol/L [0.31-1.04 nmol/L])
LH = 2.8 mIU/mL (1.0-9.0 mIU/mL) (SI: 2.8 IU/L [1.0-9.0 IU/L])
FSH = 2.5 mIU/mL (1.0-13.0 mIU/mL) (SI: 2.5 IU/L [1.0-13.0 IU/L])
Hemoglobin = 17.5 g/dL (13.8-17.2 g/dL) (SI: 175 g/L [138-172 g/L])
Hematocrit = 52% (41%-51%) (SI: 0.52 [0.41-0.51])

Thyroid function studies, prolactin measurement, iron studies, and findings on pituitary-directed MRI are normal. He is awaiting a sleep study.

Which of the following is the best strategy to address this patient's hypogonadism?

A. Clomiphene
B. Intramuscular testosterone treatment
C. Regular phlebotomy (venesection)
D. Topical testosterone treatment
E. Very low-energy diet and referral for bariatric surgery

62 A 70-year-old man is referred for evaluation and management of elevated alkaline phosphatase documented on routine blood testing. He does not have any bony pain and has not had any fractures. He takes a daily supplement containing 800 mg of calcium and 1000 IU of cholecalciferol. He has no family history of bone disease.

On physical examination, there are no palpable bony abnormalities and there is no tenderness to palpation of his spine and hips.

Laboratory test results:

Serum calcium = 9.6 mg/dL (8.2-10.2 mg/dL) (SI: 2.4 mmol/L [2.1-2.6 mmol/L])
Serum creatinine = 1.1 mg/dL (0.7-1.3 mg/dL) (SI: 97.2 μmol/L [61.9-114.9 μmol/L])
Serum 25-hydroxyvitamin D = 24.9 ng/mL (30-80 ng/mL [optimal]) (SI: 62.2 nmol/L [74.9-199.7 nmol/L])
Serum albumin = 4.5 g/dL (3.5-5.0 g/dL) (SI: 45 g/L [35-50 g/L])
Serum intact PTH = 65 pg/mL (10-65 pg/mL) (SI: 65 ng/L [10-65 ng/L])
TSH = <0.02 mIU/L (0.5-5.0 mIU/L)
Serum total alkaline phosphatase = 180 U/L (50-120 U/L) (SI: 3.01 μkat/L [0.84-2.00 μkat/L])
Serum bone-specific alkaline phosphatase = 74.3 μg/L (≤20 μg/L)

His imaging results are shown (*see images*).

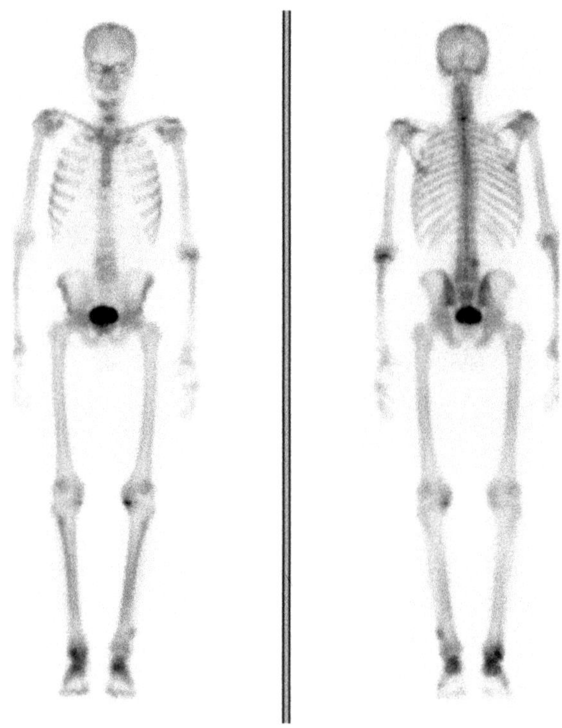

Bone scan.

Which of the following most likely explains this patient's findings?

A. Hyperthyroidism
B. Metastasis
C. Paget disease
D. Primary hyperparathyroidism
E. Vitamin D deficiency

63 A 57-year-old woman with type 2 diabetes mellitus is referred for a weight management evaluation. She has fatty liver disease (stage 2 fibrosis) and sleep apnea treated with continuous positive airway pressure. She also has hyperlipidemia and hypertension.

Despite adhering to a carbohydrate-consistent, calorie-restricted food plan for several years, her weight has not significantly changed. She is active during the day in her work, but she does not participate in a structured exercise program. Although bariatric surgery has been recommended, she would prefer to pursue other management options. In the past, she took exenatide to treat type 2 diabetes, but she discontinued the medication after 1 month because of nausea.

On physical examination, her height is 63.5 in (161 cm) and weight is 234 lb (106.4 kg) (BMI = 41 kg/m^2). Her blood pressure is 152/88 mm Hg, and pulse rate is 82 beats/min. There is no peripheral edema. She has increased abdominal girth, relatively lean extremities, and no dorsocervical fat pad. She has no evidence of hirsutism.

Her current medication regimen consists of the following:

Metformin, 1000 mg twice daily
Insulin glargine, 48 units at bedtime
Semaglutide, 1 mg subcutaneously weekly
Hydrochlorothiazide, 25 mg daily
Lisinopril, 20 mg daily
Simvastatin, 20 mg daily

Her hemoglobin A_{1c} value is 6.1% (4.0%-5.6%) (43 mmol/mol [20-38 mmol/mol]).

In addition to decreasing insulin dosing, which of the following is most likely to benefit this patient in her weight-loss efforts?

A. Increase the semaglutide dosage to 2.4 mg weekly as tolerated
B. Start extended-release phentermine/topiramate
C. Start recombinant leptin therapy
D. Stop semaglutide and start liraglutide (goal dosage: 3 mg daily)
E. Use a meal replacement program

64

A 66-year-old woman presents for evaluation of a nodule in the left thyroid lobe that was detected incidentally on chest CT. The patient has no symptoms, no personal history of head or neck radiation, and no family history of thyroid cancer.

On physical examination, her blood pressure is 130/80 mm Hg and pulse rate is 78 beats/min. Her height is 62 in (157.5 cm), and weight is 180 lb (81.8 kg) (BMI = 32.9 kg/m^2). She has a firm, 3-cm nodule in the left thyroid lobe. The rest of the findings are normal.

The TSH concentration is 0.9 mIU/L (0.5-5.0 mIU/L).

Neck ultrasonography demonstrates a 3.2 × 2.0 × 2.2-cm nodule in the left thyroid lobe (*see image*). The background thyroid parenchyma is homogeneous with normal vascularity. No abnormal cervical lymph nodes or additional thyroid nodules are observed.

The patient undergoes ultrasound-guided FNA biopsy, and cytopathology demonstrates a follicular lesion of undetermined significance (FLUS; Bethesda III). Molecular testing is completed at the time of initial biopsy. The results are positive, demonstrating an *NRAS* pathogenic variant.

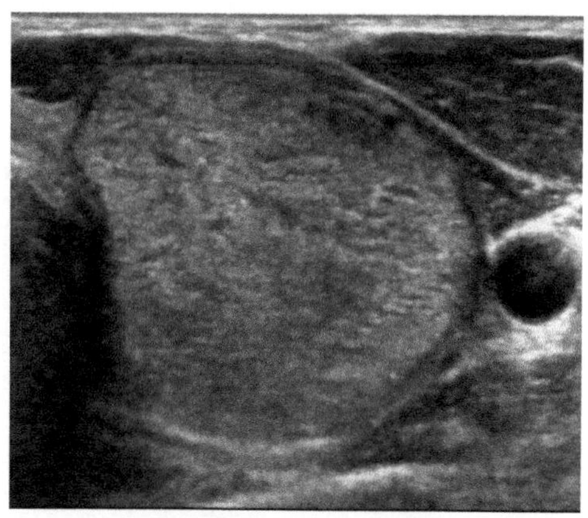

Which of the following is the most appropriate management for this patient?

A. Left hemithyroidectomy
B. Neck CT
C. Radioactive iodine uptake and scan
D. Total thyroidectomy
E. Total thyroidectomy and central neck dissection

65

A 45-year-old woman who moved to the United States from Mexico 5 years ago presents for management of type 2 diabetes mellitus. She is referred to the endocrinology clinic because of persistent suboptimal glycemic control. Type 2 diabetes was diagnosed 4 years ago. Since then, her hemoglobin A_{1c} level has been consistently greater than 9.0% (>75 mmol/mol). Diabetes complications are not known, as she has not had an eye examination and laboratory evaluation has not been completed in 3 years. Review of her medical records documents nonadherence to medical recommendations. She has seen a diabetes educator and nutritionist twice over the past year.

Her medications include metformin, basal insulin, and bolus insulin (using an insulin-to-carbohydrate ratio plus correction dosing). Other medications such as GLP-1 receptor agonists have not been prescribed because she lacks insurance coverage. Review of her blood glucose log shows she is not using correction insulin when her blood glucose is elevated.

Which of the following is the best next step in this patient's management?

A. Administer the Diabetes Numeracy Test (DNT)
B. Administer the Patient Health Questionnaire (PHQ) 9
C. Review the correction scale
D. Schedule a follow-up appointment with a certified diabetes educator
E. Switch to a smart insulin pen to help with carbohydrate counting and insulin administration

66

While on a road trip in the southern United States, a 69-year-old man presents to a local hospital emergency department with abdominal pain and nausea, which he has had on and off for 2 days. His medical history includes type 2 diabetes mellitus, dyslipidemia, hypertension, coronary artery disease, and atrial fibrillation. His medications include metformin, sitagliptin, metoprolol, lisinopril, amlodipine, simvastatin, and warfarin.

On physical examination, his blood pressure is 98/65 mm Hg and pulse rate is 102 beats/min. Oxygen saturation on room air is 98%. Several bruises are noted on his arms. He has no hyperpigmentation or plethora.

Laboratory test results:

Sodium = 134 mEq/L (136-142 mEq/L) (SI: 134 mmol/L [136-142 mmol/L])
Potassium = 5.2 mEq/L (3.5-5.0 mEq/L) (SI: 5.2 mmol/L [3.5-5.0 mmol/L])
Creatinine = 1.1 mg/dL (0.6-1.1 mg/dL) (SI: 97.2 μmol/L [53.0-97.2 μmol/L])
Serum urea nitrogen = 27 mg/dL (8-23 mg/dL) (SI: 9.6 mmol/L [2.9-8.2 mmol/L])
Glucose = 176 mg/dL (70-99 mg/dL) (SI: 9.8 mmol/L [3.9-5.5 mmol/L])
Calcium = 10.1 mg/dL (8.2-10.2 mg/dL) (SI: 2.5 mmol/L [2.1-2.6 mmol/L])
Albumin = 4.6 g/dL (3.5-5.0 g/dL) (SI: 46 g/L [35-50 g/L])
Chloride = 110 mEq/L (96-106 mEq/L) (SI: 110 mmol/L [96-106 mmol/L])
Carbon dioxide = 18 mEq/L (22-28 mEq/L) (SI: 18 mmol/L [22-28 mmol/L])

Abdominal CT (unenhanced) is shown (*see images*).

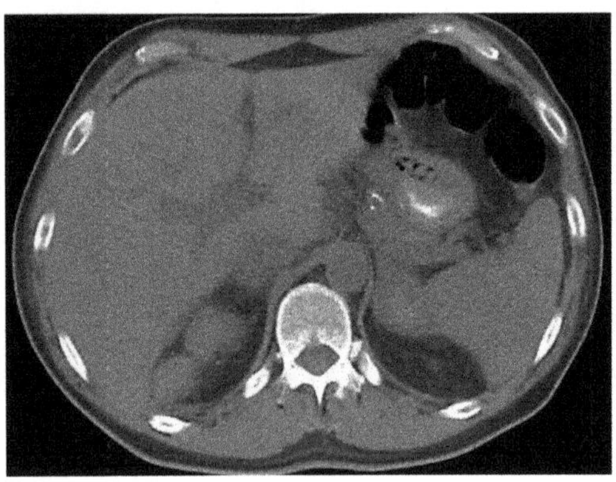

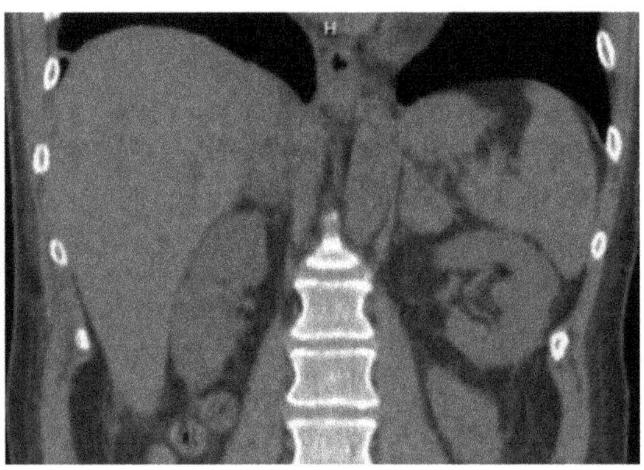

The patient is treated with intravenous fluids and hydrocortisone. The next day, he is discharged on a regimen of hydrocortisone, 20 mg in the morning and 10 mg at 2 PM, and fludrocortisone, 0.1 mg daily.

Which of the following evaluations would best inform decisions about this patient's management?

A. Adrenal biopsy
B. FDG-PET/CT
C. Follow-up abdominal CT in 3 months
D. 17-Hydroxyprogesterone measurement
E. Serum ACE measurement

67 A 23-year-old woman is referred for evaluation of polymenorrhea, menorrhagia, and pelvic pain. Following menarche at age 12 years, her menses were regular, including while taking a combined oral contraceptive preparation between ages 18 and 21 years. However, for the past 12 months she has experienced more frequent menses with menorrhagia and intermittent severe pelvic pain. There is no other notable medical history. She takes ibuprofen and tranexamic acid for symptom relief.

On physical examination, her height is 68 in (172.7 cm) and weight is 157 lb (71.4 kg) (BMI = 23.9 kg/m^2). Her blood pressure is 110/70 mm Hg. She is clinically euthyroid and euadrenal. She has normal secondary sexual characteristics. Pelvic examination is limited due to pain and bleeding.

Laboratory test results:

Prolactin = 75 ng/mL (4-30 ng/mL) (SI: 3.26 nmol/L [0.17-1.30 nmol/L])
TSH = 5.4 mIU/L (0.5-5.0 mIU/L)
Free T_4 = 0.7 ng/dL (0.8-1.8 ng/dL) (SI: 9.01 pmol/L [10.30-23.17 pmol/L])
Serum cortisol (9 AM) = 8.5 µg/dL (5-25 µg/dL) (SI: 234.5 nmol/L [137.9-689.7 nmol/L])
IGF-1 = 185 ng/mL (116-341 ng/mL) (SI: 24.2 nmol/L [15.2-44.7 nmol/L])
FSH = 23.5 mIU/mL (2.0-12.0 mIU/mL [follicular]) (SI: 23.5 IU/L [2.0-12.0 IU/L])
LH = 0.9 mIU/mL (1.0-18.0 mIU/mL [follicular]) (SI: 0.9 IU/L [1.0-18.0 IU/L])
Estradiol = 348 pg/mL (10-180 pg/mL [follicular]) (SI: 1277.5 pmol/L [36.7-660.8 pmol/L])

Ultrasonography of the pelvis shows bilateral multiloculated adnexal cysts. Endometrial thickness is 10 mm.

Which of the following is the most likely cause of her presentation?

A. Functioning gonadotroph adenoma
B. hCG-secreting germ-cell tumor
C. Hypothyroidism
D. Incipient ovarian failure
E. Pathogenic variant in the FSH receptor gene

68 A 34-year-old woman who is 26 weeks pregnant is referred for management of hypertriglyceridemia. At her last visit with her primary care provider, a fasting lipid panel documented elevated triglycerides. The patient has no personal or family history of hypertriglyceridemia. She does not have type 2 diabetes mellitus, thyroid disease, or kidney disease. She has had no episodes of pancreatitis. Her current medications include a prenatal vitamin, vitamin D, and iron. She does not smoke cigarettes or drink alcohol. She has no dietary restrictions.

On physical examination, her blood pressure is 120/80 mm Hg and pulse rate is 90 beats/min. She looks comfortable and is in no distress. Her lungs are clear to auscultation bilaterally, and heart sounds are normal with a regular rate and rhythm. She has white stretch marks on her abdomen. On palpation, her abdomen is nontender and bowel sounds are present. Her uterus is palpable halfway between the umbilicus and the xyphoid process of the sternum. She has 1+ pitting edema on both lower extremities.

Laboratory test results:
Total cholesterol = 178 mg/dL (<200 mg/dL [optimal]) (SI: 4.61 mmol/L [<5.18 mmol/L])
Triglycerides = 626 mg/dL (<150 mmol/L [optimal]) (SI: 7.07 mmol/L [<1.70 mmol/L])
HDL cholesterol = 31 mg/dL (>60 mg/dL [optimal]) (SI: 0.80 mmol/L [>1.55 mmol/L])
Fasting plasma glucose = 95 mg/dL (70-99 mg/dL) (SI: 5.3 mmol/L [3.9-5.5 mmol/L])

Which of the following is the best next step in this patient's management?

A. Admit her to the hospital and start parenteral nutrition
B. Refer for therapeutic plasma exchange
C. Start a carbohydrate- and fat-restricted diet
D. Start atorvastatin
E. Start gemfibrozil

69 A 51-year-old woman undergoes thyroid ultrasonography, which confirms a 3.6-cm (largest dimension), isoechoic, right thyroid nodule without increased vascularity or microcalcifications. FNA biopsy of this nodule diagnoses a follicular neoplasm (Bethesda IV). Molecular testing confirms the presence of a *RAS* pathogenic variant. After right hemithyroidectomy, the pathology report describes noninvasive follicular thyroid neoplasm with papillary-like nuclear features with no capsular or vascular invasion. There are no psammoma bodies. She is referred for further treatment options. She has no history of radiation exposure or family history of thyroid cancer. She has no other relevant medical history and takes no medications.

On physical examination, she has normal vital signs. There is a well-healed scar at the base of her neck. Her left thyroid lobe is not palpable. There is no cervical adenopathy. The rest of her examination findings are normal.

Laboratory test results:
TSH = 1.8 mIU/L (0.5-5.0 mIU/L)
Basic metabolic panel, normal

Which of the following is the best next step in this patient's management?

A. Initiate levothyroxine
B. Order neck CT
C. Order neck ultrasonography in 6 to 12 months
D. Perform completion thyroidectomy
E. Perform recombinant human TSH-stimulated radioactive iodine (^{131}I) whole-body scan

70 A 34-year-old woman returns for continued management of type 1 diabetes mellitus. Diabetes was diagnosed at age 6 years, and she has been on insulin pump therapy for the past 14 years. She is using a non–closed-loop system, as she thought her glycemic control was better in manual mode than when her device was in automode, and she became tired of the frequent alarms and being regularly exited from automode. Her diabetes-related complications include stable nonproliferative retinopathy and microalbuminuria.

Her current treatment regimen consists of 1 unit of insulin aspart for every 16 g of carbohydrate at meals, along with correction insulin doses of 1 unit for every 35 mg/dL (1.9 mmol/L) blood glucose is above 130 mg/dL (>7.2 mmol/L).

Her basal insulin rates are as follows:
Midnight to 6 AM = 0.45 units/h
6 AM to 4 PM = 0.55 units/h
4 PM to midnight = 0.70 units/h

She notes her blood glucose peaks about 60 to 90 minutes after her largest meals, usually lunch and dinner, when she consumes around 60 g of carbohydrate. Her hemoglobin A_{1c} level has consistently been in the range of 6.8% to 7.0% (52-53 mmol/mol), and her time in range is 70% to 75% with minimal hypoglycemia (<2%). However, she is frustrated by the postprandial glucose spikes that are preventing more time in range. This is not an issue after breakfast when she typically consumes minimal carbohydrate (<15 to 20 g). Her blood glucose levels generally run in the range of 80 to 110 mg/dL (4.4-6.1 mmol/L) until lunch.

Other than insulin therapy, her only medication is lisinopril.

On physical examination, her height is 65 in (165.1 cm) and weight is 155 lb (70.5 kg) (BMI = 25.8 kg/m^2). Her blood pressure is 118/70 mm Hg, and pulse rate is 78 beats/min. No lipohypertrophy is noted at the usual sites of insulin infusion.

Laboratory test results:

Albumin-to-creatinine ratio = 52 mg/g creat (<30 mg/g creat)
Creatinine = 0.8 mg/dL (0.6-1.1 mg/dL) (SI: 70.7 µmol/L [53.0-97.2 µmol/L])
Hemoglobin A_{1c} = 7.1% (4.0%-5.6%) (54 mmol/mol [20-38 mmol/mol])

Which of the following interventions is the best next step in this patient's management?

A. Add correction dose of insulin aspart 60 minutes after meals
B. Adjust her insulin-to-carbohydrate ratio to 1 unit for every 18 g of carbohydrate
C. Administer insulin aspart 15 minutes after her larger meals containing carbohydrate
D. Increase her basal insulin rate to 0.65 units/h from 11 AM to 4 PM
E. Switch from insulin aspart to fast-acting insulin aspart

71

A 38-year-old woman with a history of depression, anxiety disorder, and gastroesophageal reflux disease presents for evaluation of a right neck lump that she first noticed 2 months ago. The lump has subsequently increased in size. She describes difficulty swallowing and hoarseness of her voice since she noticed the lump. Review of systems is notable for sore throat, increased heart rate, anxiety, night sweats, malaise, and generalized body aches. She has no personal history of head or neck radiation and no family history of thyroid malignancy. Her sister has hypothyroidism, and her father died of lymphoma.

On physical examination, her blood pressure is 128/79 mm Hg and pulse rate is 101 beats/min. Her height is 65 in (165 cm), and weight is 152 lb (69.1 kg) (BMI = 25.3 kg/m^2). There is a nontender right thyroid mass measuring approximately 5 cm that extends past midline. There is no palpable cervical lymphadenopathy. The rest of the examination findings are normal.

Her TSH concentration is 2.05 mIU/L (0.5-5.0 mIU/L).

Neck ultrasonography demonstrates a hypoechoic solid nodule measuring 3.4 × 4.7 × 5.8 cm in the right lower pole of the thyroid gland (*see image*). This mass partially encases the ipsilateral carotid artery and compresses the right internal jugular vein. No abnormal or enlarged lymph nodes are observed.

The patient undergoes ultrasound-guided FNA biopsy, and findings are consistent with chronic lymphocytic thyroiditis. Flow cytometry reveals a low viability specimen without flow cytometric evidence of monoclonality, plasma cell dyscrasia, or nonHodgkin lymphoma.

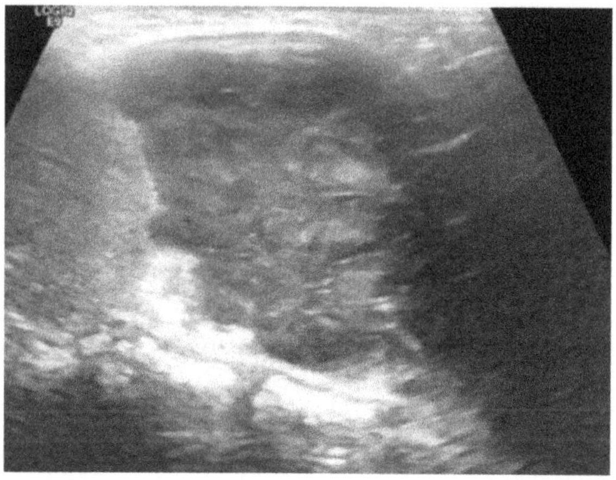

Which of the following is the most appropriate next step in this patient's management?

A. Measure serum calcitonin
B. Measure TPO antibodies
C. Perform core biopsy
D. Perform total thyroidectomy
E. Perform another ultrasound-guided FNA biopsy for cytopathology and rapid *BRAF* V600E genetic testing

72 A 46-year-old man of Asian Indian descent seeks consultation regarding type 2 diabetes mellitus. He has no known microvascular complications. Diabetes was diagnosed at age 35 years when elevated glucose was documented on bloodwork done for workup of headaches. His current treatment regimen includes sitagliptin and glimepiride.

Today, the patient's main question is whether he needs to take atorvastatin, which was previously prescribed to him. He tried taking it for about 1 month and it caused substantial heartburn that went away when he discontinued the medication. He is also worried that it may worsen his glycemic control, which he has recently improved with lifestyle modifications. He has no worrisome symptoms and, specifically, he has no exertional angina, dyspnea, or atypical symptoms and no symptoms suggestive of peripheral neuropathy or gastroparesis.

His medical history is unremarkable. His family history is notable for type 2 diabetes in both parents who were also diagnosed between ages 35 and 45 years. There is no family history of early-onset heart disease. He has a somewhat stressful job and has always had poor exercise habits. However, within the last 6 months, he initiated a regimen of walking 30 to 40 minutes 3 to 4 times per week and riding a stationary bike 3 to 4 times per week. He has a remote history of cigarette smoking (5 pack-years). He consumes 3 to 4 alcoholic beverages per week and has no history of illicit substance use. He takes no other medications.

On physical examination, his blood pressure is 133/82 mm Hg and pulse rate is 71 beats/min. His height is 71 in (180.3 cm), and weight is 173 lb (78.6 kg) (BMI = 24 kg/m^2). There are no other remarkable findings.

Laboratory test results:

Hemoglobin A_{1c} = 7.2% (4.0%-5.6%) (55 mmol/mol [20-38 mmol/mol])
Total cholesterol = 178 mg/dL (<200 mg/dL [optimal]) (SI: 4.61 mmol/L [<5.18 mmol/L])
Triglycerides = 126 mg/dL (<150 mg/dL [optimal]) (SI: 1.42 mmol/L [<1.70 mmol/L])
HDL cholesterol = 49 mg/dL (>60 mg/dL [optimal]) (SI: 1.27 mmol/L [>1.55 mmol/L])
LDL cholesterol (calculated) = 106 mg/dL (<100 mg/dL [optimal]) (SI: 2.75 mmol/L [<2.59 mmol/L])

Results of urinary albumin excretion and a basic metabolic panel are within normal limits.

He is advised to continue engaging in lifestyle improvements and to add metformin to his daily regimen. He expresses reluctance to restart moderate-intensity statin therapy because he read in his electronic medical record that his 10-year risk, according to the American College of Cardiology Atherosclerotic Cardiovascular Disease (ASCVD) Risk Estimator, is 3.9%.

Which of the following is the best next step toward understanding this patient's coronary heart disease risk in a way that would assist in shared decision-making about statin treatment?

A. Advise him that the ASCVD Risk Estimator underestimates the risk in persons of south Asian descent
B. Measure high-sensitivity C-reactive protein
C. Measure lipoprotein (a)
D. Order exercise stress echocardiography
E. Perform coronary artery calcium scoring with noncontrast CT

73 An 18-year-old woman with a history of anxiety disorder presents for evaluation and management of abnormal thyroid function. Testing was completed by her psychiatrist in the context of weight loss and increased anxiety. The patient first developed an anxiety disorder 3 years ago. This has been managed with cognitive behavioral therapy and sertraline. She also reports alternating diarrhea and constipation, a decrease in appetite from baseline, and 10-lb (4.5-kg) weight loss over the last couple of years. She has an intrauterine device for contraception. Her family history is remarkable for hypothyroidism due to Hashimoto thyroiditis in her maternal aunt.

On physical examination, her blood pressure is 125/71 mm Hg and pulse rate is 75 beats/min. Her height is 69 in (175.3 cm), and weight is 126 lb (57.3 kg) (BMI = 18.6 kg/m^2). Findings on thyroid examination are normal without enlargement or nodules. Deep tendon reflexes are 2+. The rest of the examination findings are normal.

Laboratory test results:

TSH = 0.87 mIU/L (0.5-5.0 mIU/L)
Total T_4 = 4.0 µg/dL (5.5-12.5 µg/dL) (SI: 51.5 nmol/L [94.02-213.68 nmol/L])
Total T_3 = 76 ng/dL (70-200 ng/dL) (SI: 1.17 nmol/L [1.08-3.08 nmol/L])
Free T_4 = 1.6 ng/dL (0.8-1.8 ng/dL) (SI: 20.6 pmol/L [10.30-23.17 pmol/L])
Cortisol = 12 µg/dL (5-25 µg/dL) (SI: 331.1 nmol/L [137.9-689.7 nmol/L])

Which of the following tests would support this patient's most likely diagnosis?

A. Heterophile antibody measurement
B. Pituitary MRI with and without contrast
C. *THRB* gene sequencing
D. Thyroxine-binding globulin measurement
E. TPO antibody measurement

74 An 18-year-old woman developed headaches and secondary amenorrhea 1 year ago. Menarche was at age 13 years, and her periods were always regular until 1 year ago. Her headaches occur daily, are mostly frontal, moderate in intensity, and respond to acetaminophen. Her primary care physician measured prolactin, which was found to be elevated (89 ng/mL [4-30 ng/mL] [SI: 3.87 nmol/L (0.17-1.30 nmol/L)]). β-hCG is negative. Pituitary MRI shows a sellar lesion (*see images*).

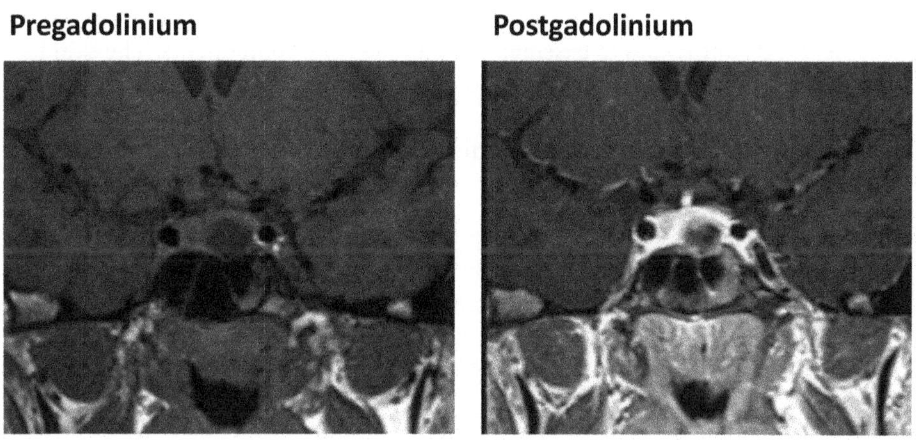

Macroprolactin testing documents that 85% of the prolactin is monomeric. Cabergoline, 0.25 mg orally twice weekly, is initiated. Six weeks later, her periods resume. Six months later, repeated MRI is unchanged, and her prolactin concentration is normal (23 ng/mL [1.00 nmol/L]).

Which of the following is this patient's most likely diagnosis?

A. Arachnoid cyst
B. Craniopharyngioma
C. Cystic prolactinoma
D. Nonfunctioning pituitary adenoma with cystic degeneration
E. Rathke cleft cyst

75 A 68-year-old man with a 6-year history of type 2 diabetes mellitus presents for follow-up. He has been on a stable regimen of oral hypoglycemic agents for the past 2 years. His last hemoglobin A_{1c} measurement 6 months ago was 7.3% (56 mmol/mol). His only diabetes-related complication is nephropathy. Since his last visit in endocrinology, he was seen by a dermatologist because of a 2-month history of a pruritic rash on his abdomen, back, and extremities (*see image*). He underwent biopsy of one of the lesions.

Current medications are saxagliptin, 2.5 mg once daily; metformin, 1000 mg twice daily; dapagliflozin, 10 mg daily; lisinopril, 40 mg daily; and amlodipine, 10 mg daily.

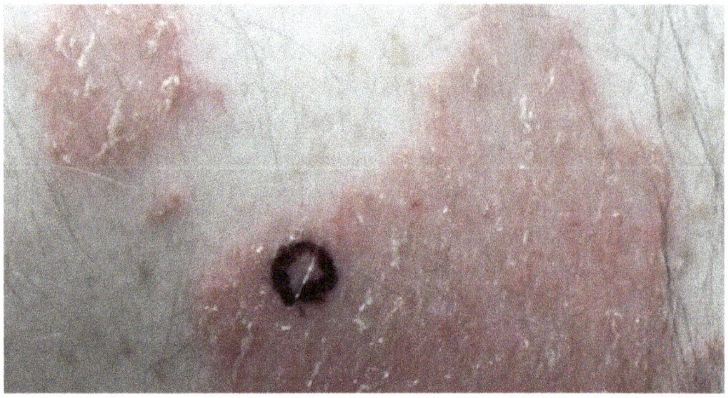

On physical examination, his height is 72 in (183 cm) and weight is 208 lb (94.5 kg) (BMI = 28.2 kg/m^2). His blood pressure is 148/82 mm Hg, and pulse rate is 67 beats/min. Skin examination shows erythematous patches of different sizes on his abdomen, back, and extremities. The largest lesion is on his back.

Laboratory test results:

Creatinine = 1.35 mg/dL (0.7-1.3 mg/dL) (SI: 119.3 µmol/L [61.9-114.9 µmol/L])
Estimated glomerular filtration rate = 52 mL/min per 1.73 m^2 (>60 mL/min per 1.73 m^2)
Urinary albumin-to-creatinine ratio = 60 mg/g creat (<30 mg/g creat)

Immune testing documents IgG antibodies to basement membrane zone components. The skin biopsy report describes spongiotic dermatitis with eosinophilic spongiosis. Bullous pemphigoid is diagnosed.

Which of the following medications should be discontinued first?

A. Amlodipine
B. Dapagliflozin
C. Lisinopril
D. Metformin
E. Saxagliptin

76 A 21-year-old man is referred for evaluation of gynecomastia. He reports entering puberty somewhat later (around age 14 years) than his friends of the same age. He is otherwise healthy and takes no regular medications or over-the-counter supplements. Breast enlargement began at the start of puberty, progressed for 1 year, and then stabilized. There is no family history of gynecomastia or infertility.

On physical examination, he has normal body proportions. His blood pressure is 122/68 mm Hg, and pulse rate is 72 beats/min. His height is 68 in (173 cm), and weight is 159 lb (72 kg) (BMI = 24.1 kg/m^2). Upper-to-lower body segment ratio is 1.1 (eunuchoidal <1.0), and arm span is 67 in (170 cm) (eunuchoidal arm span >2 in [5 cm] greater than height). Eye movements are full to confrontation, and there is no clinical visual field defect. Breast development is estimated to be Tanner stage 3 bilaterally. He has sparse body and axillary hair. On genital examination, he has sparse pubic hair and slightly reduced penile size (stretched penile length 4.3 in [11 cm]); <1 SD). Testicular volume is 15 mL bilaterally, and no masses are detected.

Current laboratory test results (8 AM, fasting):

Serum testosterone = 1245 ng/dL (300-900 ng/dL) (SI: 43.2 nmol/L [10.4-31.2 nmol/L])
Repeated measurement 1 week later with a different assay platform = 1345 ng/dL (SI: 46.7 nmol/L)
SHBG = 6.7 µg/mL (1.1-6.7 µg/mL) (SI: 60 nmol/L [10-60 nmol/L])
Serum estradiol = 47 pg/mL (10-40 pg/mL) (SI: 173 pmol/L [36.7-146.8 pmol/L])
LH = 15.8 mIU/mL (1.0-9.0 mIU/mL) (SI: 15.8 IU/L [1.0-9.0 IU/L])
FSH = 14.4 mIU/mL (1.0-13.0 mIU/mL) (SI: 14.4 IU/L [1.0-13.0 IU/L])

Which of the following is the best next step in this patient's management?

A. Genetic testing for pathogenic variants in the androgen receptor gene
B. Genetic testing for pathogenic variants in the estradiol α gene
C. Measurement of DHEA-S
D. Measurement of free testosterone
E. Pituitary-directed MRI

77 A 39-year-old man with a history of bipolar disorder is referred for evaluation of polydipsia and polyuria. He reports waking several times per night to urinate, and he often has to stop daily activities to void his bladder. His symptoms started about 6 months ago. He takes aripripazole, 10 mg daily, which was prescribed 12 months ago after he had been on lithium for several years.

Laboratory test results:

Urine volume = 5.2 L/24 h
Serum glucose, normal
Serum calcium, normal
Prolactin = 1 ng/mL (4-23 ng/mL) (SI: 0.04 nmol/L [0.17-1.00 nmol/L])
Testosterone (8 AM) = 285 ng/dL (300-900 ng/dL) (SI: 9.9 nmol/L [10.4-31.2 nmol/L])

On physical examination, he is in no distress. His blood pressure is 130/80 mm Hg, and pulse rate is 88 beats/min. His height is 67 in (170 cm), and weight is 198 lb (90 kg) (BMI = 31 kg/m^2). He has no notable features on examination.

Results after an overnight 12-hour water-deprivation test:

Morning serum sodium = 146 mEq/L (SI: 146 mmol/L)
Serum osmolality = 296 mOsm/Kg (275-295 mOsm/kg) (SI: 296 mmol/kg [275-295 mmol/kg])
Urine osmolality = 380 mOsm/kg (150-1150 mOsm/kg) (SI: 380 mmol/kg [150-1150 mmol/kg])

Which of the following is the best test to determine the cause of this patient's polyuria and polydipsia?

A. Kidney ultrasonography
B. Measurement of plasma antidiuretic hormone
C. Measurement of serum copeptin
D. Measurement of urinary sodium
E. Pituitary MRI

78 A 41-year-old woman is referred for evaluation of hypophosphatemia. She reports fatigue, muscle weakness, and bone and joint pain over the past several months. She has no nausea, vomiting, or diarrhea. She has a history of anemia due to heavy uterine bleeding and has been receiving intravenous iron infusions. She has very good dietary calcium intake (~900 mg daily) but does not take any calcium or vitamin D supplements. She is adopted.

On physical examination, she has decreased muscle strength in the upper and lower extremities.

Laboratory test results:

Serum calcium = 8.6 mg/dL (8.2-10.2 mg/dL) (SI: 2.2 mmol/L [2.1-2.6 mmol/L])
Serum phosphate = 1.5 mg/dL (2.3-4.7 mg/dL) (SI: 0.48 mmol/L [0.7-1.5 mmol/L])
Serum creatinine = 0.9 mg/dL (0.6-1.1 mg/dL) (SI: 79.6 µmol/L [53.0-97.2 µmol/L])
Serum intact PTH = 88 pg/mL (10-65 pg/mL) (SI: 88 ng/L [10-65 ng/L])
Serum 25-hydroxyvitamin D = 22 ng/mL (30-80 ng/mL [optimal]) (SI: 54.9 nmol/L [74.9-199.7 nmol/L])
Serum 1,25-dihydroxyvitamin D = 10 pg/mL (16-65 pg/mL) (SI: 26.0 pmol/L [41.6-169.0 pmol/L])
Serum albumin = 3.8 g/dL (3.5-5.0 g/dL) (SI: 38 g/L [35-50 g/L])

Which of the following is this patient's most likely diagnosis?

A. Hereditary resistance to vitamin D
B. Intravenous iron-induced hypophosphatemia
C. Nutritional osteomalacia
D. Tumor-induced osteomalacia
E. X-linked hypophosphatemia

79 A 66-year-old man with an 18-year history of type 2 diabetes mellitus complicated by stage 3A kidney disease presents for follow-up. He currently takes insulin glargine, 30 units every evening, and prandial insulin, 10 units with each meal. He also takes metformin, 500 mg XR 1 tablet twice daily. He reports being distressed after seeing his recent hemoglobin A_{1c} value in the patient portal (7.4% [57 mmol/mol]), as his measurements are typically lower than 7.0% (<53 mmol/mol). Over the years, physicians have told him that his hemoglobin A_{1c} goal is 6.5% (48 mmol/mol). His kidney disease has been stable over the last 2 years.

On physical examination, his blood pressure is 142/73 mm Hg and pulse rate is 80 beats/min. His height is 71 in (180.3 cm), and weight is 175 lb (79.5 kg) (BMI = 24.4 kg/m²).

Laboratory test results (sample drawn while fasting):

Hemoglobin A_{1c} = 7.4% (4.0%-5.6%) (57 mmol/mol [20-38 mmol/mol])
Creatinine = 1.9 mg/dL (0.7-1.3 mg/dL) (SI: 168.0 µmol/L [61.9-114.9 µmol/L])
Estimated glomerular filtration rate = 37 mL/min per 1.73 m² (>60 mL/min per 1.73 m²)
Serum urea nitrogen = 25 mg/dL (8-23 mg/dL) (SI: 8.9 mmol/L [2.9-8.2 mmol/L])
Plasma glucose = 75 mg/dL (70-99 mg/dL) (SI: 4.2 mmol/L [3.9-5.5 mmol/L])
Sodium = 140 mEq/L (136-142 mEq/L) (SI: 140 mmol/L [136-142 mmol/L])
Urinary albumin-to-creatinine ratio = 340 mg/g creat (30-300 mg/g creat)

He just completed 10-day use of a professional/blinded continuous glucose monitoring device and is here to discuss results (*see figure*). He reports no symptoms of hypoglycemia in the last month.

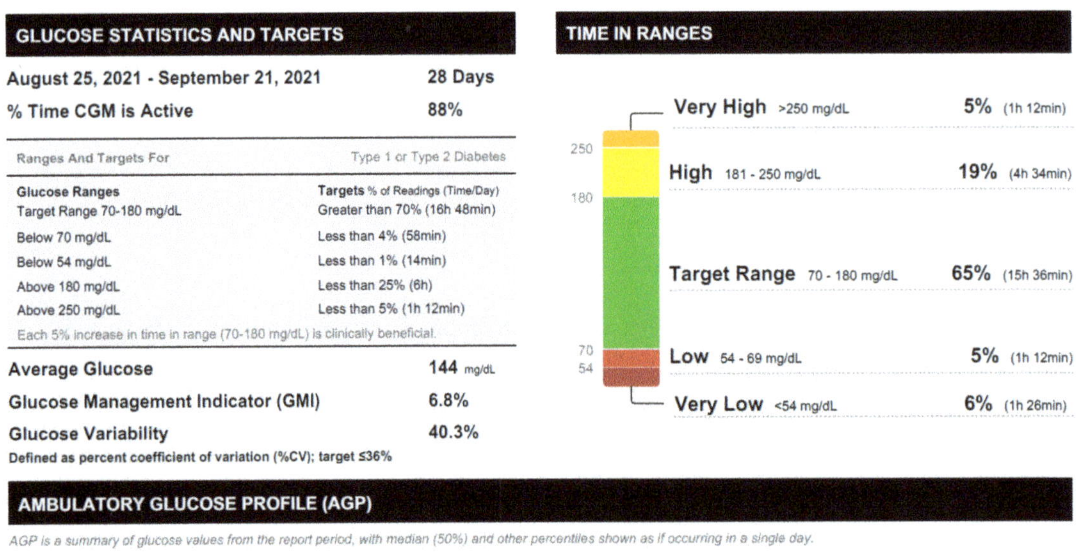

Which of the following is the best next step in this patient's management?

A. Reduce basal insulin by 20%
B. Reduce basal insulin by 20% and increase prandial insulin to 1 unit with each meal
C. Reduce basal insulin by 20%, reduce prandial insulin by 20%, and start a GLP-1 receptor agonist
D. Reduce basal insulin by 20%, reduce prandial insulin by 20%, and start an SGLT-2 inhibitor
E. Stop metformin

80 A 67-year-old woman with obesity, type 2 diabetes mellitus, hypertension, dyslipidemia, stage 3 chronic kidney insufficiency, osteopenia, and osteoarthritis is found to have bilateral adrenal enlargement during kidney ultrasonography.

On physical examination, her blood pressure is 142/85 mm Hg and pulse rate is 83 beats/min. Her height is 67 in (170.2 cm), and weight is 235 lb (106.8 kg) (BMI = 36.8 kg/m^2). She has abdominal obesity, a mild dorsocervical hump, and round facies. She has no plethora or bruises. Pale, thin striae are observed on the abdomen. There is no skin atrophy. Muscle strength is within normal limits.

Follow-up abdominal CT identifies bilateral adrenal gland nodules measuring up to 3 cm on the right side and 4.5 cm on the left side. Both nodules demonstrate a density less than 10 Hounsfield units (*see image, arrows*).

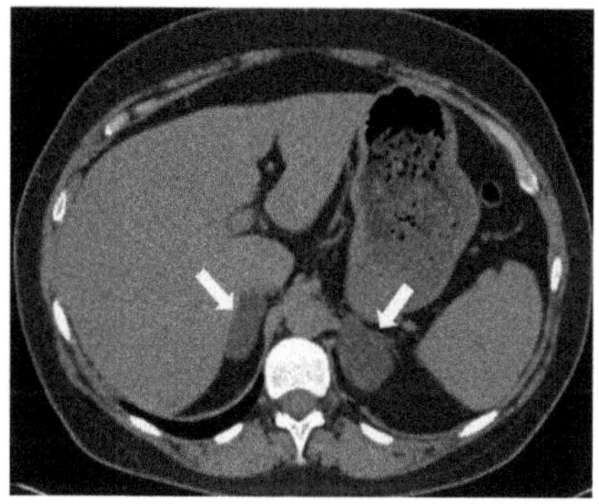

Laboratory test results (sample drawn at 8 AM):

- Serum cortisol = 12 µg/dL (5-25 µg/dL) (SI: 331 nmol/L [137.9-689.7 nmol/L])
- ACTH = 9 pg/mL (10-60 pg/mL) (SI: 2.0 pmol/L [2.2-13.2 pmol/L])
- Serum aldosterone = 5.8 ng/dL (4-21 ng/dL) (SI: 160.9 pmol/L [111.0-582.5 pmol/L])
- Plasma renin activity = 1.3 ng/mL per h (0.6-4.3 ng/mL per h)
- DHEA-S = 15 µg/dL (15-157 µg/dL) (SI: 0.41 µmol/L [0.41-4.25 µmol/L])

Following a 1-mg dexamethasone-suppression test, the morning serum cortisol concentration is 4.2 µg/dL (116 nmol/L) and the ACTH concentration is <5 pg/mL (<1.1 pmol/L). The urinary cortisol excretion is 50 µg/24 h (20-45 µg/24 h) (SI: 138 nmol/d [11-138 nmol/d]).

Which of the following is the best management approach for this patient?

A. Adrenal venous sampling
B. Bilateral adrenalectomy
C. Left adrenalectomy
D. Right adrenalectomy
E. Serum 17-hydroxyprogesterone measurement

81 A 38-year-old woman with a history of hepatitis C and vitamin D deficiency is referred for abnormal thyroid function test results. She takes vitamin D daily and started interferon alfa 4 months ago. She describes a 10-lb (4.5-kg) weight loss over the last month, fatigue, and palpitations.

On physical examination, her blood pressure is 148/68 mm Hg and pulse rate is 102 beats/min. Her thyroid gland is estimated to be around 20 g and is nontender. There are no palpable thyroid nodules or cervical adenopathy. She has a mild tremor in her hands bilaterally. The rest of her examination findings are normal.

Laboratory test results:

- TSH = <0.01 mIU/L (0.5-5.0 mIU/L)
- Free T_4 = 2.8 ng/dL (0.8-1.8 ng/dL) (SI: 36.04 pmol/L [10.30-23.17 pmol/L])
- Thyroid-stimulating immunoglobulin = 20% (≤120% of basal activity)
- TPO antibodies = 140 IU/mL (<2.0 IU/mL) (SI: 140 kIU/L [<2.0 kIU/L])
- Basic metabolic panel, normal

Which of the following is the best next step in this patient's management?

A. Perform radioiodine scan and uptake
B. Perform thyroid ultrasonography
C. Recommend total thyroidectomy
D. Start atenolol
E. Start methimazole

82 A 29-year-old woman with type 1 diabetes mellitus and mild nonproliferative diabetic retinopathy is in the 28th week of gestation. She calls the clinic because she feels unwell. Pregnancy to date has been uncomplicated, and while she recalls substantial morning sickness in the first trimester, she has been generally feeling fine. However, in the last 2 to 3 days, she has had nausea and dyspepsia. She tried a calcium carbonate antacid, but it did not help. This morning she reports bilious emesis.

Her morning glucose concentrations have been between 65 and 90 mg/dL (3.6 and 5.0 mmol/L), and postmeal glucose levels have been between 120 and 170 mg/dL (6.7 and 9.4 mmol/L). She uses a continuous glucose monitor that documents an average glucose concentration of 142 mg/dL (7.9 mmol/L) over the past 14 days, with 65% of the time spent in range (70-140 mg/dL [3.9-7.8 mmol/L]). She is on a basal-bolus insulin regimen. Her prepregnancy hemoglobin A_{1c} level was 6.8% (51 mmol/mol), and her glycemic control has generally been good. Insulin requirements have increased from a total daily dose of 0.5 units/kg before pregnancy to about 0.6 units/kg currently. She has no other relevant history. Besides insulin detemir and insulin aspart, her only other medication is a prenatal vitamin.

Glucose values from the last 6 days are shown (*see table*). The overall average value is 135 mg/dL (7.5 mmol/L).

Day	Prebreakfast	Postbreakfast	Prelunch	Postlunch	Predinner	Postdinner	Bedtime
0	162 mg/dL (SI: 9.0 mmol/L)	...	...	...	...	...	...
–1	104 mg/dL (SI: 5.8 mmol/L)	122 mg/dL (SI: 6.8 mmol/L)	132 mg/dL (SI: 7.3 mmol/L)	168 mg/dL (SI: 9.3 mmol/L)	143 mg/dL (SI: 7.9 mmol/L)	178 mg/dL (SI: 9.9 mmol/L)	149 mg/dL (SI: 8.3 mmol/L)
–2	115 mg/dL (SI: 6.4 mmol/L)	131 mg/dL (SI: 7.3 mmol/L)	125 mg/dL (SI: 6.9 mmol/L)	177 mg/dL (SI: 9.8 mmol/L)	152 mg/dL (SI: 8.4 mmol/L)	162 mg/dL (SI: 9.0 mmol/L)	131 mg/dL (SI: 7.3 mmol/L)
–3	98 mg/dL (SI: 5.4 mmol/L)	152 mg/dL (SI: 8.4 mmol/L)	144 mg/dL (SI: 8.0 mmol/L)	158 mg/dL (SI: 8.8 mmol/L)	95 mg/dL (SI: 5.3 mmol/L)	157 mg/dL (SI: 8.7 mmol/L)	164 mg/dL (SI: 9.1 mmol/L)
–4	93 mg/dL (SI: 5.2 mmol/L)	121 mg/dL (SI: 6.7 mmol/L)	133 mg/dL (SI: 7.4 mmol/L)	182 mg/dL (SI: 10.1 mmol/L)	167 mg/dL (SI: 9.3 mmol/L)	182 mg/dL (SI: 10.1 mmol/L)	124 mg/dL (SI: 6.9 mmol/L)
–5	102 mg/dL (SI: 5.7 mmol/L)	98 mg/dL (SI: 5.4 mmol/L)	111 mg/dL (SI: 6.2 mmol/L)	144 mg/dL (SI: 8.0 mmol/L)	98 mg/dL (SI: 5.4 mmol/L)	129 mg/dL (SI: 7.2 mmol/L)	101 mg/dL (SI: 5.6 mmol/L)

Which of the following is the most important recommendation now?

A. Check for blood ketones
B. Increase the correction factor to a more aggressive ratio
C. Increase the insulin-to-carbohydrate ratio
D. Measure serum amylase
E. Reduce the overnight basal insulin dose

83 A 30-year-old nonbinary individual whose sex assigned at birth was female is referred for gender-affirming chest surgery. Pronouns are they/them. They first became aware of incongruence of gender identity with sex assigned at birth at age 5 years. They did not further explore gender identity until adolescence when they saw pictures of androgynous individuals. Their identity is gender fluid. They are not interested in masculinizing hormone therapy, as they are bothered by the idea of hair growth. They note significant body dysphoria regarding their chest, so their primary goal is to proceed with chest surgery to align with an androgynous appearance. They bring a letter from their gender therapist regarding their diagnosis of gender dysphoria that supports chest surgery.

Which of the following is the best next step in this patient's management?

A. Follow-up visit in the next 6 months before referral for chest surgery
B. GnRH agonist therapy for a year before chest surgery
C. Referral for chest surgery
D. Referral for second letter of support for chest surgery
E. Testosterone therapy for a year before chest surgery

84 A 59-year-old woman with stage 3 chronic kidney disease is admitted to the hospital for hypocalcemia. She presented to the emergency department with paresthesias in her extremities, as well as muscle cramping. She is currently being treated for osteoporosis with denosumab, and her last injection was 10 days prior to presentation. She takes calcium citrate, 500 mg elemental calcium twice daily, and cholecalciferol, 2000 units daily, but she has not been taking these consistently. She also takes a proton-pump inhibitor.

The Chvostek sign is elicited on physical examination. Electrocardiography documents a QTc of 480 msec (<460 msec).

Laboratory test results on admission:

Serum calcium = 6.1 mg/dL (8.2-10.2 mg/dL) (SI: 1.5 mmol/L [2.1-2.6 mmol/L])
Serum phosphate = 2.4 mg/dL (2.3-4.7 mg/dL) (SI: 0.8 mmol/L [0.7-1.5 mmol/L])
Serum creatinine = 1.5 mg/dL (0.6-1.1 mg/dL) (SI: 132.6 µmol/L [53.0-97.2 µmol/L])
Glomerular filtration rate (estimated) = 39 mL/min per 1.73 m^2 (>60 mL/min per 1.73 m^2)
Serum intact PTH = 332 pg/mL (10-65 pg/mL) (SI: 332 ng/L [10-65 ng/L])
Serum 25-hydroxyvitamin D = 28 ng/mL (30-80 ng/mL [optimal]) (SI: 69.9 nmol/L [74.9-199.7 nmol/L])
Serum albumin = 3.7 g/dL (3.5-5.0 g/dL) (SI: 37 g/L [35-50 g/L])
Serum magnesium = 1.0 mg/dL (1.5-2.3 mg/dL) (SI: 0.4 mmol/L [0.6-0.9 mmol/L])

In addition to repleting this patient's magnesium, which of the following is the most appropriate next step in the management of her hypocalcemia?

A. Increase oral cholecalciferol intake
B. Increase oral elemental calcium intake
C. Start intravenous calcium therapy
D. Start oral calcitriol therapy
E. Start subcutaneous teriparatide therapy

85 A 34-year-old woman is evaluated during a routine prenatal visit when she is found to have elevated blood pressure of 170/90 mm Hg, pulse rate of 110 beats/min, and proteinuria. She is 34 weeks pregnant, and this is her third pregnancy. Her previous pregnancies were uneventful, and she has 2 healthy children, aged 7 and 5 years, both delivered via cesarean delivery. She has a 6-year history of anxiety, which is associated with tremors. For at least 2 years, she has had more frequent episodes of palpitations, associated with pallor, and feelings of impending doom. She reports that over the past month, these episodes have occurred frequently at night or whenever she lies down.

Her medical history includes hypothyroidism following thyroidectomy at a young age. She is adopted and does not have further information regarding the circumstances of this surgery. She takes levothyroxine regularly, and TSH has been monitored throughout pregnancy. Her TSH concentration is at goal for the third trimester.

Laboratory test results:

Plasma free metanephrine = 572 pg/mL (<99 pg/mL) (SI: 2.90 nmol/L [<0.50 nmol/L])
Plasma free normetanephrine = 203 pg/mL (<165 pg/mL) (SI: 1.11 nmol/L [<0.90 nmol/L])

Which of the following is the most essential next step in this patient's care?

A. Abdominal MRI
B. Abdominal ultrasonography
C. Emergent cesarean delivery
D. Initiation of doxazosin
E. Initiation of labetalol

86 A 74-year-old man with a history of gastroesophageal reflux disease and Schatzki ring presents for follow-up of a right thyroid nodule, which was diagnosed 5 years ago. Neck ultrasonography at that time demonstrated an isoechoic solid nodule measuring 4.8 × 3.9 × 3.8 cm. The patient underwent ultrasound-guided FNA biopsy with benign results.

Ultrasonography 3 years later revealed an increase in the nodule's size to 5.25 × 4.8 × 5.9 cm. The patient had no symptoms and underwent FNA biopsy again with benign results. Ongoing clinical surveillance was recommended.

Now the patient reports a "sticking" sensation in his neck when swallowing larger pills, a persistent cough for the last 3 months, and dyspnea with vigorous exercise. Schatzki ring has been managed with multiple dilatation procedures in the past, but he has not required a procedure since starting omeprazole 2 years ago. There is no dysphonia.

On physical examination, his blood pressure is 110/78 mm Hg and pulse rate is 69 beats/min. His height is 70 in (177.8 cm), and weight is 178 lb (80.9 kg) (BMI = 25.5 kg/m^2). Palpation of the thyroid gland reveals a large nodule replacing the right lobe with inferior extension to the clavicle. The left thyroid lobe is normal. There is no cervical lymphadenopathy. The rest of the examination findings are normal.

His TSH concentration is 2.0 mIU/L (0.5-5.0 mIU/L).

Repeated neck ultrasonography shows modest enlargement of the right thyroid nodule to 5.6 × 5.6 × 6.0 cm (26% increase in volume) without a change in sonographic appearance (*see image*).

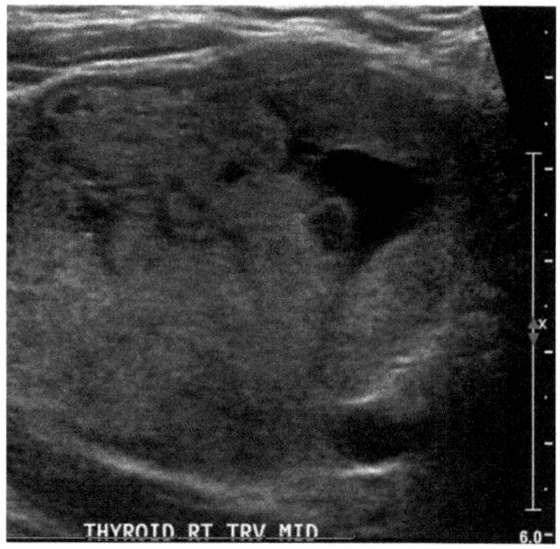

Which of the following is the most appropriate initial step in this patient's management?

A. CT imaging of the neck and chest
B. Flow-volume loop study
C. Neck ultrasonography in 12 months
D. Referral for total thyroidectomy
E. Referral for upper endoscopy

87 A 28-year-old woman is referred by her gynecologist for possible hypercortisolism. During the past year she has gained 30 lb (13.6 kg) and developed abdominal striae and facial hirsutism. Her menses have become irregular. She takes no medication. There is no known family history of endocrine disease.

On physical examination, her blood pressure is 140/98 mm Hg and pulse rate is 80 beats/min. Her height is 61.5 in (156.2 cm), and weight is 176 lb (80 kg) (BMI = 32.7 kg/m^2). She has thin skin, facial hirsutism, and purplish abdominal striae.

Laboratory test results:

Urinary free cortisol = 150 μg/24 h (4-50 μg/24 h) (SI: 414 nmol/d [11-138 nmol/d])
Serum cortisol after 1 mg dexamethasone administered the night before = 5.2 μg/dL (SI: 143.5 nmol/L)
Random plasma ACTH = 47 pg/mL (10-60 pg/mL) (SI: 10.3 pmol/L [2.2-13.2 pmol/L])

Pituitary MRI shows a 4-mm right-sided pituitary microadenoma.

In the pituitary adenoma cells, which of the following genes is most likely to have a pathogenic variant?

A. *AIP*
B. *GNAS*
C. *PRKAR1A*
D. *RET*
E. *USP8*

88 A 28-year-old woman with a history of irregular menses is seen in clinic for follow-up. She has had an appropriate evaluation of irregular menses, and laboratory test results are normal. Polycystic ovary syndrome has been diagnosed due to the presence of oligomenorrhea and hirsutism. She has no other medical concerns and takes no medications. Relevant family history includes type 2 diabetes mellitus and hypertension in her mother.

On physical examination, her height is 63 in (160 cm) and weight is 182 lb (82.7 kg) (BMI = 32.2 kg/m^2). Her blood pressure is 128/74 mm Hg, and pulse rate is 88 beats/min. She has a few narrow, white stretch marks on her abdomen and mild acanthosis nigricans. The rest of the examination findings are normal.

She is counseled about the risk of type 2 diabetes mellitus in women with polycystic ovary syndrome. She is not interested in pregnancy right away, but she will most likely consider it in the future.

Which of the following tests to assess for glucose intolerance should be recommended?

A. Hemoglobin A_{1c} measurement now
B. Fasting glucose measurement now
C. Oral glucose tolerance test (75 g) now
D. Oral glucose tolerance test (75 g) when she is pregnant (at gestational week 24)
E. Oral glucose tolerance test (1-hour with 50 g) when she is pregnant (at gestational week 24), followed by an oral glucose tolerance test (3-hour with 100 g) if needed

89 A 38-year-old man is referred by his oncologist for consideration of testosterone treatment. His medical history is notable for a left-sided stage IIIB seminoma that was treated with left orchidectomy, chemotherapy, and pelvic radiotherapy 5 years ago. He has 2 children, aged 12 and 8 years, and has no plans for future paternity. He reports low libido and erectile dysfunction. He has tried sildenafil, 50 mg, on several occasions without improvement of sexual dysfunction. He reports fatigue, low motivation, and occasionally low mood. Over the last 3 years, he has gained approximately 22 lb (10 kg). His dietary habits are poor, and he does not exercise.

On physical examination, his height is 73 in (185.4 cm) and weight is 229 lb (104.1 kg) (BMI = 30.2 kg/m^2). He has normal hair distribution, and his right testicle is 15 mL, without masses.

Current laboratory test results (8 AM, fasting):

Serum testosterone = 280 ng/dL (300-900 ng/dL) (SI: 9.7 nmol/L [10.4-31.2 nmol/L])
Repeat measurement 1 week later = 288 ng/dL (SI: 10.0 nmol/L)
LH = 32.0 mIU/mL (1.0-9.0 mIU/mL) (SI: 32.0 IU/L [1.0-9.0 IU/L])
FSH = 40.0 mIU/mL (1.0-13.0 mIU/mL) (SI: 40.0 IU/L [1.0-13.0 IU/L])

Which of the following is the best next step in addressing this patient's hypogonadism?

A. Clomiphene treatment
B. Free testosterone measurement
C. Optimization of lifestyle measures to lose weight plus an increase to the maximally tolerated dosage of the phosphodiesterase 5 inhibitor
D. Referral to psychiatrist for assessment and treatment of depression
E. Testosterone treatment

90 A 49-year-old woman has been referred for management of kidney stones. She underwent Roux-en-Y gastric bypass 5 years ago, which resulted in a stable 80-lb (36.4-kg) weight loss. She passed her first kidney stone 3 years ago and has since passed at least 6 others. During her last episode, which required an emergency department visit, noncontrast CT of the abdomen and pelvis identified a 3-mm left ureteral stone and a 6-mm stone in the right renal pelvis. Upon passage and collection of the left ureteral stone, biochemical analysis documented the composition to be predominantly calcium oxalate. She reports a normal diet. Although she consumes little dairy, she does take a calcium carbonate supplement, 500 mg 3 times daily.

Laboratory test results:

- Calcium = 9.4 mg/dL (8.2-10.2 mg/dL) (SI: 2.4 mmol/L [2.1-2.6 mmol/L])
- Albumin = 4.2 g/dL (3.5-5.0 g/dL) (SI: 42 g/L [35-50 g/L])
- Creatinine = 1.1 mg/dL (0.6-1.1 mg/dL) (SI: 97.2 µmol/L [53.0-97.2 µmol/L])
- Phosphate = 3.1 mg/dL (2.3-4.7 mg/dL) (SI: 1.0 mmol/L [0.7-1.5 mmol/L])
- 25-Hydroxyvitamin D = 34 ng/mL (30-80 ng/mL [optimal]) (SI: 84.9 nmol/L [74.9-199.7 nmol/L])
- 24-hour urine:
  - Volume = 1.5 L
  - Calcium = 178 mg/24 h (100-300 mg/24 h) (SI: 4.5 mmol/d [2.5-7.5 mmol/d])
  - Creatinine = 1.1 g/24 h (1.0-2.0 g/24 h) (SI: 9.7 mmol/d [8.8-17.7 mmol/d])
  - Oxalate = 56 mg/24 h (<40 mg/24 h) (SI: 638 mmol/d [<456 mmol/d])
  - Citrate = 278 mg/24 h (320-1240 mg/24 h) (SI: 14.5 mmol/d [16.7-64.5 mmol/d])
  - Sodium = 123 mEq/24 h (40-217 mEq/L) (SI: 123 mmol/d [40-217 mmol/d])
  - pH = 5.8

In addition to a low-oxalate and low-fat diet and increasing water intake to 2 L daily, which of the following is the best strategy to reduce this patient's risk of stone formation?

A. Change calcium supplement to calcium citrate, 630 mg twice daily
B. Prescribe potassium citrate, 20 mEq twice daily
C. Reduce animal protein intake
D. Reduce sodium intake to less than 2500 mg daily
E. Stop calcium supplements

91

A 34-year-old Hispanic woman is referred for abnormal thyroid blood test results. She has hypertension and dyslipidemia and takes amlodipine, 10 mg daily, and atorvastatin, 20 mg daily. In addition, she takes a prenatal vitamin daily.

On physical examination, her blood pressure is 132/78 mm Hg and pulse rate is 96 beats/min. There is no proptosis or diplopia. Her thyroid gland is not enlarged. Her heart has a regular rate and rhythm with no murmur. Lungs are clear to auscultation bilaterally. There is no tremor in her hands.

Laboratory test results:

- TSH = 2.2 mIU/L (0.5-5.0 mIU/L)
- Total T_4 = 17.6 µg/dL (5.5-12.5 µg/dL) (SI: 226.5 nmol/L [94.02-213.68 nmol/L])
- Free T_4 = 2.0 ng/dL (0.8-1.8 ng/dL) (SI: 25.74 pmol/L [10.30-23.17 pmol/L])
- Total T_3 = 162 ng/dL (70-200 ng/dL) (SI: 2.50 nmol/L [1.08-3.08 nmol/L])
- Free T_3 = 3.0 pg/mL (2.3-4.2 pg/mL) (SI: 4.60 pmol/L [3.53-6.45 pmol/L])
- Basic metabolic panel, normal

Which of the following is this patient's most likely diagnosis?

A. Biotin interference
B. Familial dysalbuminemic hyperthyroxinemia
C. Resistance to thyroid hormone
D. Thyroxine-binding globulin deficiency
E. TSH-secreting pituitary tumor

92

A 55-year-old White man with HIV infection, gastroesophageal reflux disease, and hypertension is referred for management of a lipid disorder. The patient reports that his cholesterol levels were normal until highly active antiretroviral therapy was initiated (which includes a protease inhibitor). Despite making dietary changes, he has seen no positive effect on his cholesterol profile. He does not drink alcohol, but he does smoke one-half pack of cigarettes daily. In addition to antiretroviral agents, he takes lisinopril, hydrochlorothiazide, and omeprazole. He has no family history of premature heart disease. He has never taken any cholesterol-lowering medications.

On physical examination, his blood pressure is 114/82 mm Hg and pulse rate is 85 beats/min. His height is 71 in (180 cm), and weight is 200 lb (91 kg) (BMI = 28 kg/m^2). He has no rashes, but lipoatrophy is noted in his cheeks and temporal area bilaterally. Lungs are clear to auscultation bilaterally. His heart sounds are normal and regular in rate and rhythm. He has increased abdominal fat. Bowel sounds are present, and his abdomen is nontender. He has no peripheral edema.

Laboratory test results:

Total cholesterol = 242 mg/dL (<200 mg/dL [optimal]) (SI: 6.27 mmol/L [<5.18 mmol/L])
HDL cholesterol = 34 mg/dL (>60 mg/dL [optimal]) (SI: 0.88 mmol/L [>1.55 mmol/L])
LDL cholesterol = 138 mg/dL (<100 mg/dL [optimal]) (SI: 3.57 mmol/L [<2.59 mmol/L])
Triglycerides = 350 mg/dL (<150 mmol/L [optimal]) (SI: 3.96 mmol/L [<1.70 mmol/L])

Given this patient's history and laboratory test results, which of the following medications would be best to start?

A. Atorvastatin
B. Fenofibrate
C. Lovastatin
D. Pravastatin
E. Simvastatin

93

A 57-year-old man presents for management of longstanding type 2 diabetes mellitus and Cushing syndrome. ACTH-independent hypercortisolism was recently diagnosed, and imaging documented bilateral adrenal macronodules (<10 Hounsfield units on noncontrast CT). Comorbidities include obesity, coronary artery disease status post coronary artery bypass grafting (x3), hypothyroidism, obstructive sleep apnea, hypertension, and hyperlipidemia. He also has a history of nonalcoholic fatty liver disease.

Current medications include once-daily insulin degludec; insulin lispro, 3 times daily with meals; metformin XR; and once-weekly dulaglutide. To manage his comorbidities, he is taking metoprolol, lisinopril, fenofibrate, atorvastatin, and levothyroxine.

He is informed that his hypercortisolism is related to the bilateral adrenal macronodules (right gland is larger than the left) and that right adrenalectomy would be the recommended treatment. The patient is very concerned about undergoing a surgical procedure. His primary care physician and cardiologist have also expressed concerns about his risk of adverse surgical outcomes. He has been referred by his local endocrinologist for a second opinion to discuss medical management.

On physical examination, his blood pressure is 148/84 mm Hg and pulse rate is 92 beats/min. His height is 71 in (180.3 cm), and weight is 315 lb (143.2 kg) (BMI = 43.9 kg/m^2). He has prominent abdominal adiposity. His face is slightly rounded in appearance, with moderate facial plethora. Acanthosis nigricans is noted in the skin folds of the neck. The rest of his examination findings are unremarkable.

Laboratory test results:

Hemoglobin A_{1c} = 9.2% (4.0%-5.6%) (77 mmol/mol [20-38 mmol/mol])
Creatinine = 1.2 mg/dL (0.7-1.3 mg/dL) (SI: 106.1 μmol/L [61.9-114.9 μmol/L])
Estimated glomerular filtration rate = >60 mL/min per 1.73 m^2 (>60 mL/min per 1.73 m^2)
Alanine aminotransferase = 72 U/L (10-40 U/L) (SI: 1.20 μkat/L [0.17-0.67 μkat/L])
Aspartate aminotransferase = 84 U/L (20-48 U/L) (SI: 1.40 μkat/L [0.33-0.80 μkat/L])

Which of the following should be initiated as the best next step in this patient's management?

A. Ketoconazole
B. Mifepristone
C. Mitotane
D. Osilodrostat
E. Pasireotide

94 30-year-old woman presents for follow-up of papillary thyroid carcinoma, which was initially detected after she sought medical attention for right neck fullness 4 months ago. She has no other medical problems. Neck ultrasonography revealed multiple thyroid nodules bilaterally, the largest of which was located in the right lobe and measured 3 × 2.9 × 2.1 cm. Calcified supraclavicular lymph nodes were noted on the right side. Ultrasound-guided FNA biopsy results of both the dominant right thyroid nodule and a right neck zone 4 (supraclavicular) lymph node were positive for papillary thyroid carcinoma. The patient underwent total thyroidectomy with bilateral central and right lateral neck dissection 4 weeks ago. Pathology demonstrated multifocal classic papillary thyroid carcinoma, and the largest tumor focus was 3.5 cm without extrathyroidal extension or vascular invasion. Surgical margins were negative. Overall, 13 of 16 central neck lymph nodes were positive for metastasis, and the largest tumor deposit was 1.1 cm. Six of 20 right lateral neck lymph nodes were positive, and the largest tumor deposit was 2.6 cm. No extranodal extension was noted.

The patient presents to discuss the next management steps. She reports feeling well overall but does note numbness of the skin under her chin. She currently takes levothyroxine, 150 mcg daily, on an empty stomach in the morning.

On physical examination, her blood pressure is 119/80 mm Hg and pulse rate is 95 beats/min. Her height is 66 in (167.6 cm), and weight is 152 lb (69.1 kg) (BMI = 24.5 kg/m^2). Healing anterior and right lateral neck scars are noted. There is no mass in the thyroid bed and no palpable cervical lymphadenopathy. The rest of the examination findings are normal.

Laboratory test results:

TSH = 4.5 mIU/L (0.5-5.0 mIU/L)
Thyroglobulin = 1.5 ng/mL (SI: <0.1 μg/L)
Thyroglobulin antibodies = <4 IU/mL (SI: <4 kIU/L)

In addition to increasing the patient's levothyroxine dosage, which of the following is the most appropriate next step?

Answer	Radioactive iodine, ^{131}I	Method of TSH stimulation
A.	30 mCi	Recombinant human TSH
B.	30 mCi	Thyroid hormone withdrawal
C.	100 mCi	Recombinant human TSH
D.	100 mCi	Thyroid hormone withdrawal
E.	200 mCi	Recombinant human TSH

95 A 78-year-old African American woman is hospitalized after falling and sustaining a left femoral neck fracture. She undergoes repair of her hip fracture 2 weeks later with no complications. She had surgical menopause at age 40 years and has not taken estrogen. She has a remote history of breast cancer treated with surgery and radiation therapy. She has not seen her primary care physician for the past several years due to difficulty with transportation. She has never had a bone density test performed. Her dietary calcium intake is approximately 600 mg daily, and she does not take any calcium or vitamin D supplements. Her mother fractured her right hip at a similar age.

On physical examination, she has tenderness and limited range of motion of the affected hip.

Laboratory test results:

Serum calcium = 9.2 mg/dL (8.2-10.2 mg/dL) (SI: 2.3 mmol/L [2.1-2.6 mmol/L])
Serum creatinine = 1.2 mg/dL (0.6-1.1 mg/dL) (SI: 106.1 μmol/L [53.0-97.2 μmol/L])
Glomerular filtration rate (estimated) = 55 mL/min per 1.73 m^2 (>60 mL/min per 1.73 m^2)
Serum 25-hydroxyvitamin D = 22 ng/mL (30-80 ng/mL [optimal]) (SI: 54.9 nmol/L [74.9-199.7 nmol/L])
Serum albumin = 4.0 g/dL (3.5-5.0 g/dL) (SI: 40 g/L [35-50 g/L])
Serum alkaline phosphatase = 150 U/L (50-120 U/L) (SI: 2.51 μkat/L [0.84-2.00 μkat/L])

In addition to counseling on fall prevention and adequate calcium and vitamin D supplementation, which of the following should be recommended now?

A. Administer denosumab injection
B. Administer zoledronic acid infusion
C. Start alendronate
D. Start raloxifene
E. Start teriparatide

96 An 80-year-old man with type 2 diabetes mellitus presents for follow-up. His medical history is notable for ischemic cardiomyopathy with left ventricular assist device implantation and stage 3 chronic kidney disease. Diabetes was diagnosed 20 years ago on the basis of routine screening. He was initially treated with oral medications. Because of kidney disease, insulin was initiated 15 years ago.

He is pleased to report a weight loss of 28 lb (12.7 kg), which he achieved through dietary modifications. Physical activity is limited, but he plans to increase his activity toward a goal of losing another 10 lb (4.5 kg). He reports no new symptoms, although he has had several hypoglycemic episodes requiring assistance.

He checks his glucose by fingerstick twice daily. Fasting glucose concentrations range from 75 to 95 mg/dL (4.2 to 5.3 mmol/L), and predinner concentrations range from 80 to 120 mg/dL (4.4 to 6.7 mmol/L). His current diabetes regimen consists of insulin glargine (U300), 52 units daily, and insulin aspart, 13 units taken twice daily with meals. Additional medications include aspirin, atorvastatin, carvedilol, iron sulfate, torsemide, and potassium chloride.

Laboratory test results:

Hemoglobin A_{1c} = 5.0% (4.0%-5.6%) (31 mmol/mol [20-38 mmol/mol]) (last measurement was 6.2% [44 mmol/mol])
Hemoglobin = 10.4 g/dL (13.8-17.2 g/dL) (SI: 104 g/L [138-172 g/L])
Platelet count = 88 × 10^3/µL (150-450 × 10^3/µL) (SI: 88 × 10^9/L [150-450 × 10^9/L])
White blood cell count = 6300/µL (4500-11,000/µL) (SI: 6.3 × 10^9/L [4.5-11.0 × 10^9/L])
Serum urea nitrogen = 41 mg/dL (8-23 mg/dL) (SI: 14.6 mmol/L [2.9-8.2 mmol/L])
Creatinine = 2.6 mg/dL (0.7-1.3 mg/dL) (SI: 229.8 µmol/L [61.9-114.9 µmol/L])
Estimated glomerular filtration rate = 22 mL/min per 1.73 m^2 (>60 mL/min per 1.73 m^2)

Which of the following options is the most important next step for the management of this patient's blood glucose?

A. Add an SGLT-2 inhibitor
B. Encourage physical activity
C. Prescribe a continuous glucose monitor
D. Reduce the insulin aspart dosage by 20%
E. Reduce the insulin glargine dosage by 20%

97 A 32-year-old woman is referred for treatment of hirsutism. After her last pregnancy, she switched from oral contraceptives to a progestin-eluting intrauterine device. She has not had any menses since its placement. Since weaning her infant 1 year ago, she has developed hair growth on her upper lip, chin, and neck and acne along her jaw line.

Menarche was at age 14 years, and oral contraceptives were initiated within that first year because of painful menses. Menses occurred monthly for the first year after menarche. She has either been on oral contraceptives, pregnant, or breastfeeding until this past year. She is not planning future pregnancies.

A combined oral contraceptive that she has tolerated in the past and previously improved acne is initiated. Two months later, she contacts the clinic because she is having spotting accompanied by cramping throughout the month. The acne and hair growth are not significantly changed.

Laboratory test results:

FSH, undetectable
Estradiol, undetectable
Prolactin = 9.7 ng/mL (4-30 ng/mL) (SI: 0.42 nmol/L [0.17-1.30 nmol/L])
TSH = 1.0 mIU/L (0.5-5.0 mIU/L)
DHEA-S = 281 μg/dL (31-228 μg/dL) (SI: 7.62 μmol/L [0.84-6.78 μmol/L])
Total testosterone = 35 ng/dL (8-60 ng/dL) (SI: 1.2 nmol/L [0.3-2.1 nmol/L])

Which of the following is the best next step in this patient's management?

A. Discontinue the oral contraceptive and initiate spironolactone, 100 mg daily
B. Perform pelvic ultrasonography
C. Remove the intrauterine device
D. Repeat hormone testing
E. Switch to a combined oral contraceptive with a different progestin

98 A 25-year-old woman with type 1 diabetes mellitus diagnosed at age 13 years presents for follow-up. She has recently been approved for insulin pump therapy and needs initial settings for the transition. She currently takes insulin glargine, 10 units in the morning and 15 units at bedtime, and uses an insulin-to-carbohydrate ratio of 1:12 for prandial insulin. She does not use a correction factor unless her blood glucose concentration is greater than 200 mg/dL (>11.1 mmol/L), in which case she administers 2 units. Over the last 30 days, she estimates she has used about 45 units of insulin daily (25 units basal and 20 units prandial). She notes occasional low glucose values at 2 AM despite values being 180 to 200 mg/dL (10.0-11.1 mmol/L) 3 hours earlier at bedtime. When she wakes in the morning at 6:30 AM, blood glucose values are typically 70 to 110 mg/dL (3.9-6.1 mmol/L). On days she does not eat breakfast, she notes glucose values rise by 30 mg/dL (1.7 mmol/L) by the time she arrives at work at 8 AM.

On physical examination, her height is 63 in (160 cm) and weight is 140 lb (63.6 kg) (BMI = 24.8 kg/m^2). Her blood pressure is 118/58 mm Hg, and pulse rate is 78 beats/min.

Laboratory test results (sample drawn while fasting):

Hemoglobin A_{1c} = 8.2% (4.0%-5.6%) (66 mmol/mol [20-38 mmol/mol])
Creatinine = 0.6 mg/dL (0.6-1.1 mg/dL) (SI: 53.0 μmol/L [53.0-97.2 μmol/L])
Serum urea nitrogen = 25 mg/dL (8-23 mg/dL) (SI: 8.9 mmol/L [2.9-8.2 mmol/L])
Plasma glucose = 78 mg/dL (70-99 mg/dL) (SI: 4.3 mmol/L [3.9-5.5 mmol/L])
Sodium = 140 mEq/L (136-142 mEq/L) (SI: 140 mmol/L [136-142 mmol/L])

Which of the following would be the best initial settings for this patient's new insulin pump?

Answer	Basal setting	Insulin-to-carbohydrate ratio	Correction factor
A.	12 AM to 12 AM: 1.0 unit/h	1:12	1:50
B.	12 AM to 3 AM: 0.6 units/h 3 AM to 8 AM: 0.8 units/h 8 AM to 12 AM: 0.7 units/h	1:12	1:50
C.	12 AM to 3 AM: 10.8 units/h 3 AM to 8 AM: 0.6 units/h 8 AM to 12 AM: 0.7 units/h	1:12	1:25
D.	12 AM to 12 AM: 0.7 units/h	1:18	1:50
E.	12 AM to 12 AM: 0.7 units/h	1:18	1:25

99 A 56-year-old man is noted to have a left adrenal mass on CT performed for evaluation of suspected right renal colic. Aside from a recent episode of depressed mood and difficulty sleeping following the death of his father, he is otherwise well. His only regular medication is amitriptyline, 25 mg nightly.

On physical examination, his height is 73 in (185.4 cm) and weight is 192 lb (87.3 kg) (BMI = 25.3 kg/m^2). His blood pressure is 152/82 mm Hg, and pulse rate is 76 beats/min and regular. The rest of the physical examination findings are unremarkable.

Laboratory test results:

Serum potassium = 3.7 mEq/L (3.5-5.0 mEq/L)
(SI: 3.7 mmol/L [3.5-5.0 mmol/L])
Plasma renin activity = 1.0 ng/mL per h (0.6-4.3 ng/mL per h)
Serum aldosterone = 8.2 ng/dL (4-21 ng/dL)
(SI: 227.5 pmol/L [111.0-582.5 pmol/L])
Cortisol following 1-mg dexamethasone-suppression test
= 2.4 µg/dL (SI: 66.2 nmol/L)
Plasma metanephrine = 72 pg/mL (<99 pg/mL)
(SI: 0.37 nmol/L [<0.50 nmol/L])
Plasma normetanephrine = 191 pg/mL (<165 pg/mL)
(SI: 1.04 nmol/L [<0.90 nmol/L])

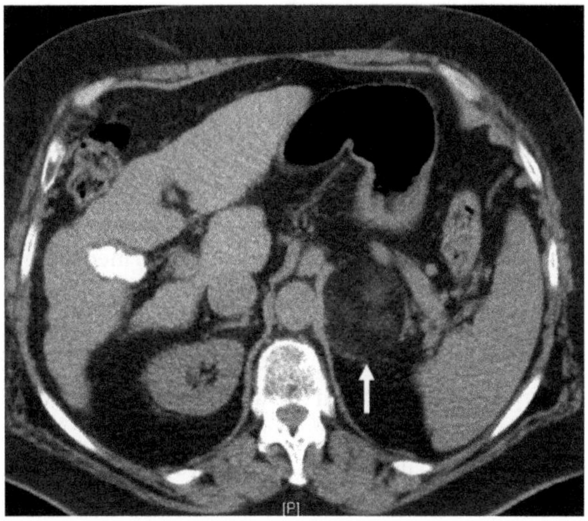

Unenhanced abdominal CT shows a 6-cm left adrenal mass (*see image, arrow*).

Which of the following is the most likely cause of the left adrenal mass?

A. Adrenal hemorrhage
B. Adrenal metastasis
C. Adrenal myelolipoma
D. Adrenocortical carcinoma
E. Pheochromocytoma

100 A 61-year-old man undergoes thyroid surgery for FNA biopsy–proven papillary thyroid cancer. At the time of surgery, the surgeon notices that the tumor is invading his trachea and his right sternocleidomastoid muscle. The surgeon is not able to remove all of the tumor from his trachea. The histopathology report reveals a 3-cm right papillary thyroid cancer with tall-cell features with capsular invasion, vascular invasion, and extrathyroidal extension, as well as metastases in 10 of 25 cervical lymph nodes. Six weeks after total thyroidectomy with central neck dissection, he receives 150 mCi of radioiodine treatment. The posttherapy scan is negative. Levothyroxine, 137 mcg daily, is initiated. He is now referred for further management 8 weeks after radioiodine treatment.

His medical history is notable for type 2 diabetes mellitus and hypertension. There is no family history of thyroid cancer. In addition to levothyroxine, he takes metformin, lisinopril, atorvastatin, and baby aspirin.

On physical examination, he has normal vital signs. There is a well-healed scar at the base of his neck with no palpable mass or cervical adenopathy. There is no lower-extremity edema.

Current laboratory test results:

TSH = 1.8 mIU/L (0.5-5.0 mIU/L)
Thyroglobulin = 35 ng/mL (3-42 ng/mL) (SI: 35 µg/L [3-42 µg/L]) (after surgery and radioactive iodine
treatment <1.0 ng/mL [SI: <1.0 µg/L])
Thyroglobulin antibodies, undetectable
Basic metabolic panel, normal

In addition to adjusting his levothyroxine dosage, which of the following is the best next step in this patient's management?

A. Add liothyronine
B. Perform neck ultrasonography
C. Perform PET/CT
D. Recommend another radioiodine treatment
E. Recommend external-beam radiation to the neck

101 A 36-year-old woman is referred for secondary amenorrhea in the context of recently diagnosed primary ovarian insufficiency. She has a history of a prolactinoma. The referring gynecologist and patient wonder whether her secondary amenorrhea is due to the prolactinoma rather than premature ovarian insufficiency. She is not currently trying to conceive.

She was first evaluated for secondary amenorrhea 2 years ago. At that time, a probable pituitary microadenoma was identified when imaging was performed after her prolactin concentration was documented to be 34.6 ng/mL (1.5 nmol/L) (repeated measurement = 40 ng/mL [1.7 nmol/L]). At first, her physician monitored her off medical therapy; menses returned spontaneously and were monthly. However, she began experiencing amenorrhea again, and dopamine agonist therapy was initiated. Last year, secondary amenorrhea developed while she was on cabergoline, and primary ovarian insufficiency was diagnosed based on the following laboratory test results:

FSH = 41.0 mIU/mL (2.0-12.0 mIU/mL) (SI: 41.0 IU/L [2.0-12.0 IU/L])
Estradiol = 34 pg/mL (10-180 pg/mL) (SI: 124.8 pmol/L [36.7-660.8 pmol/L])
Prolactin = 10 ng/mL (4-30 ng/mL) (SI: 0.43 nmol/L [0.17-1.30 nmol/L])

Menses have not returned in the past 9 months. She has no symptoms of weight loss, fatigue, or constipation.

Current laboratory test results:
FSH = 6.4 mIU/mL (2.0-12.0 mIU/mL) (SI: 6.4 IU/L [2.0-12.0 IU/L])
Prolactin = 35 ng/mL (4-30 ng/mL) (SI: 1.52 nmol/L [0.17-1.30 nmol/L])
TSH = 2.9 mIU/L (0.5-5.0 mIU/L)
TPO antibodies = 148.0 IU/L (≤1.75 IU/L)

Pelvic ultrasonography shows the thickness of the endometrial lining to be 11 mm with a dominant follicle/cyst on the right side.

Which of the following is the best next step in this patient's evaluation and management?

A. Evaluate for adrenal insufficiency
B. Increase the dosage of cabergoline
C. Initiate a 10-day course of progesterone to induce a withdrawal bleed
D. Prescribe a combined oral contraceptive
E. Prescribe transdermal estradiol

102 A 62-year-old woman with an 11-year history of type 2 diabetes mellitus presents for follow-up. Her diabetes is complicated by nonproliferative retinopathy and stage 3A chronic kidney disease, which have both been stable over the last 3 years. She currently takes insulin glargine, 50 units in the evening; metformin, 500 mg XR 1 tablet twice daily; and dulaglutide, 1.5 mg weekly. She reports her morning blood glucose values range from 85 to 112 mg/dL (4.7-6.2 mmol/L). She has no symptoms of hypoglycemia except when she is more active. She carries fruit snacks with her. She is excited to start pool aerobics and has a personal weight-loss goal of 10 lb (4.5 kg) over the next 6 months.

On physical examination, her height is 61 in (154.9 cm) and weight is 198 lb (90 kg) (BMI = 37.4 kg/m^2). Her blood pressure is 138/83 mm Hg, and pulse rate is 90 beats/min.

Laboratory test results (sample drawn while fasting):

Hemoglobin A_{1c} = 7.5% (4.0%-5.6%) (58 mmol/mol [20-38 mmol/mol]) (3 months ago it was 7.1% [54 mmol/mol])
Creatinine = 1.7 mg/dL (0.6-1.1 mg/dL) (SI: 150.3 µmol/L [53.0-97.2 µmol/L])
Estimated glomerular filtration rate = 32 mL/min per 1.73 m^2 (>60 mL/min per 1.73 m^2) (stable over the last year)
Serum urea nitrogen = 30 mg/dL (8-23 mg/dL) (SI: 10.7 mmol/L [2.9-8.2 mmol/L])
Plasma glucose = 80 mg/dL (70-99 mg/dL) (SI: 4.4 mmol/L [3.9-5.5 mmol/L])
Sodium = 139 mEq/L (136-142 mEq/L) (SI: 139 mmol/L [136-142 mmol/L])

Which of the following strategies is the best next step in this patient's management?

	Medication		
Answer	Metformin	Insulin glargine	Dulaglutide
A.	Continue	Continue current dosage	Titrate to maximum dosage tolerated
B.	Continue	Decrease dosage to 40 units	Titrate to maximum dosage tolerated
C.	Stop	Continue current dosage	Titrate to maximum dosage tolerated
D.	Stop	Increase dosage to 55 units	Continue current dosage
E.	Stop	Continue current dosage	Continue current dosage

103 A 28-year-old pregnant woman (G1P0) presents for evaluation and management of abnormal thyroid function test results. She is currently 8 weeks pregnant. At an appointment with her obstetrician last week, thyroid function tests were ordered because of a family history of hypothyroidism. She is unable to tolerate a prenatal vitamin because of significant pregnancy-related nausea and vomiting. Her medications include folic acid supplementation and ondansetron, as needed.

On physical examination, her blood pressure is 109/65 mm Hg and pulse rate is 86 beats/min. Her height is 70 in (177.8 cm), and weight is 160 lb (72.7 kg) (BMI = 23.0 kg/m^2). Thyroid examination findings are normal without goiter or palpable nodules. The rest of the examination findings are normal.

Laboratory test results:

TSH = 0.09 mIU/L (0.5-5.0 mIU/L)
Free T_4 = 1.22 ng/dL (0.8-1.8 ng/dL) (SI: 15.70 pmol/L [10.30-23.17 pmol/L])
Total T_3 = 140 ng/dL (70-200 ng/dL) (SI: 2.16 nmol/L [1.08-3.08 nmol/L])

In addition to ongoing monitoring of this patient's thyroid function, which of the following is the most appropriate treatment recommendation?

A. Methimazole
B. Potassium iodide supplementation
C. Propylthiouracil
D. Selenium supplementation
E. No additional treatment is needed

104 A 36-year-old man presents for evaluation of a several-year history of postprandial symptoms. He underwent laparoscopic Roux-en-Y gastric bypass 5 years ago, done primarily to treat severe gastroesophageal reflux and Barrett esophagus. He weighed approximately 235.5 lb (107 kg) at the time of surgery and reached a nadir weight of 141 lb (64.1 kg), which he has maintained for the last 2 years.

The patient describes symptoms of tachycardia, shaking, sweats, and difficulty concentrating that occur within 60 to 90 minutes of eating. These symptoms tend to happen about twice a week, typically in the evenings. He has had 1 seizure. When the seizure occurred, his continuous glucose monitor documented a glucose concentration of 15 mg/dL (0.8 mmol/L). He carries glucagon and glucose tablets. He is becoming more fearful because his awareness of symptoms seems to be decreasing.

He adheres to the postbariatric diet program, including separating eating and drinking, avoiding carbonated beverages, and limiting simple carbohydrates. He has tried acarbose, calcium-channel blockers, and a GLP-1 receptor agonist without much improvement in the frequency or severity of symptoms. Overall, he feels quite fatigued and is having difficulty functioning at work.

He currently takes 1 multivitamin with minerals twice daily; vitamin D_3, 2000 units once daily; and vitamin B_{12}, 1000 mcg subcutaneously once monthly.

Cholelithiasis was recently diagnosed after he presented to the emergency department with abdominal pain and bloating, and he plans to undergo cholecystectomy in the near future.

On physical examination, he appears anxious. His height is 70.1 in (178 cm), and weight is 141 lb (64.1 kg) (BMI = 20.2 kg/m^2).

Laboratory test results:

Hemoglobin = 13.1 g/dL (13.8-17.2 g/dL) (SI: 131 g/L [138-172 g/L])
Mean corpuscular volume = 99 μm^3 (80-100 μm^3) (SI: 99 fL [80-100 fL])
AST = 72 U/L (20-48 U/L) (SI: 1.20 μkat/L [0.33-0.80 μkat/L])
ALT = 55 U/L (10-40 U/L) (SI: 0.92 μkat/L [0.17-0.67 μkat/L])
Vitamin B_{12}, normal

Results of a standard, nonliquid mixed-meal study before this visit (120 minutes after the meal [symptomatic]):

Plasma glucose = 41 mg/dL (SI: 2.3 mmol/L)
Insulin = 72 μIU/mL (SI: 500.0 pmol/L)
C-peptide = 8.3 ng/mL (SI: 2.7 nmol/L)

Which of the following is the best next step in this patient's management?

A. Administer a short-acting somatostatin analogue before each meal
B. Proceed with a 72-hour fast
C. Refer to surgery for gastric bypass reversal
D. Screen for excess alcohol use
E. Start empiric treatment for small intestinal bacterial overgrowth

105

At a visit with his primary care physician, a 70-year-old man describes a 1-year history of muscle weakness that has progressed to the point that he is having mild difficulty walking and standing up from a seated position. Results of a complete blood count, complete metabolic profile, thyroid function tests, and creatine kinase measurement are normal except for an elevated alkaline phosphatase concentration of 211 U/L (3.52 μkat/L). The patient is referred to a physical therapist and instructed to return in 3 months for repeated measurement of alkaline phosphatase. Five weeks later, he experiences progressive right hip pain located to his groin. Due to the progressive pain, he reports to the emergency department where hip CT identifies a possible right femoral neck insufficiency fracture. Hip MRI confirms the diagnosis. He is referred to an orthopedic surgeon who recommends off-loading and rest.

The patient is then referred for evaluation of the insufficiency fracture.

DXA bone density scan:

L1-4 spine T-score = −1.7
Left femoral neck T-score = −1.0
Left total hip T-score = −1.2

Laboratory test results:

Calcium = 9.2 mg/dL (8.2-10.2 mg/dL) (SI: 2.3 mmol/L [2.1-2.6 mmol/L])
Albumin = 3.8 g/dL (3.5-5.0 g/dL) (SI: 38 g/L [35-50 g/L])
Intact PTH = 56 pg/mL (10-65 pg/mL) (SI: 56 ng/L [10-65 ng/L])
Creatinine = 0.8 mg/dL (0.7-1.3 mg/dL) (SI: 70.7 μmol/L [61.9-114.9 μmol/L])
Phosphate = 1.1 mg/dL (2.3-4.7 mg/dL) (SI: 0.4 mmol/L [0.7-1.5 mmol/L])

Magnesium = 2.2 mg/dL (1.5-2.3 mg/dL) (SI: 0.9 mmol/L [0.6-0.9 mmol/L])
25-Hydroxyvitamin D = 23 ng/mL (30-80 ng/mL [optimal]) (SI: 57.4 nmol/L [74.9-199.7 nmol/L])

Repeat laboratory testing:
Calcium = 9.6 mg/dL (SI: 2.4 mmol/L)
Albumin = 4.0 g/dL (SI: 40 g/L)
Creatinine = 0.9 mg/dL (SI: 79.6 μmol/L)
Phosphate = 0.9 mg/dL (SI: 0.3 mmol/L)

Which of the following is the best next step in this patient's management?

A. Measure 1,25-dihydroxyvitamin D
B. Measure serum FGF-23
C. Order fasting second-morning urine for phosphate and creatinine measurements
D. Prescribe alendronate, 70 mg weekly
E. Prescribe potassium phosphate/sodium phosphate, 250 mg 4 times daily

106 A 64-year-old man is admitted to the hospital with acute, severe COVID-19. He has an 8-year history of type 2 diabetes mellitus treated with metformin and an SGLT-2 inhibitor, dyslipidemia treated with a statin, hypertension treated with an ACE inhibitor, and obesity (BMI = 31 kg/m^2). Two months ago, his primary care physician prescribed topical testosterone treatment when he presented with erectile dysfunction. Before starting testosterone therapy, his serum total testosterone concentration was 290 ng/dL (10.0 nmol/L). Testosterone treatment was stopped at hospital admission.

On hospital day 5, he develops respiratory failure due to superimposed bacterial pneumonia and is admitted to the intensive care unit for mechanical ventilation. On hospital day 15, while still on mechanical ventilation, the intensive care unit team requests a morning serum testosterone measurement, which is 90 ng/dL (3.1 nmol/L). Current treatment includes glucocorticoids, intravenous antibiotics, and insulin infusion. The intensive care unit team is concerned that his low serum testosterone level may impede respiratory muscle function and thus delay weaning from mechanical ventilation.

Which of the following is the best next step in this patient's endocrine management?

A. Full panel to assess pituitary function
B. Intramuscular testosterone treatment
C. Measurement of free testosterone, SHBG, and gonadotropins
D. Repeat serum testosterone measurement after recovery from acute illness
E. Topical testosterone treatment

107 A 37-year-old Asian American man with hypothyroidism presents for a routine annual follow-up appointment. He is in good health and has no concerns. He takes levothyroxine, 125 mcg daily, on an empty stomach. His family history is notable for hypertension in his father and type 2 diabetes mellitus in his maternal grandmother. He exercises twice weekly. He has no history of tobacco or illicit substance use, and he consumes 3 to 4 alcoholic beverages per week.

On physical examination, his blood pressure is 126/78 mm Hg and pulse rate is 78 beats/min. His height is 69 in (175.3 cm), and weight is 155 lb (70 kg) (BMI = 22.9 kg/m^2).

Laboratory test results (done 1 year ago):
Total cholesterol = 176 mg/dL (<200 mg/dL [optimal]) (SI: 4.56 mmol/L [<5.18 mmol/L])
Triglycerides = 166 mg/dL (<150 mg/dL [optimal]) (SI: 1.88 mmol/L [<1.70 mmol/L])
HDL cholesterol = 42 mg/dL (>60 mg/dL [optimal]) (SI: 1.09 mmol/L [>1.55 mmol/L])
LDL cholesterol = 114 mg/dL (<100 mg/dL [optimal]) (SI: 2.95 mmol/L [<2.59 mmol/L])

His TSH concentration measured this week is 1.2 mIU/L (0.5-5.0 mIU/L).

Which of the following evaluations is the best next step?

A. Free T_4 measurement
B. Hemoglobin A_{1c} measurement
C. High-sensitivity C-reactive protein
D. Lipoprotein(a) measurement
E. Repeat fasting lipid panel

108 A 26-year-old man is referred for evaluation of hypercalcemia. He has had multiple episodes of kidney stones over the past several years. His dietary calcium intake is approximately 600 mg daily, and he does not take any calcium or vitamin D supplements. He has no history of fragility fractures or thyroid disease. His mother has osteoporosis, and his brother has nephrolithiasis.

Physical examination findings, including vital signs, are unremarkable.

Laboratory test results:

Serum calcium = 11.2 mg/dL (8.2-10.2 mg/dL) (SI: 2.8 mmol/L [2.1-2.6 mmol/L])
Serum phosphate = 3.4 mg/dL (2.3-4.7 mg/dL) (SI: 1.1 mmol/L [0.7-1.5 mmol/L])
Serum creatinine = 1.1 mg/dL (0.7-1.3 mg/dL) (SI: 97.2 μmol/L [61.9-114.9 μmol/L])
Serum intact PTH = 16 pg/mL (10-65 pg/mL) (SI: 16 ng/L [10-65 ng/L])
Serum 25-hydroxyvitamin D = 32 ng/mL (30-80 ng/mL [optimal]) (SI: 79.9 nmol/L [74.9-199.7 nmol/L])
Serum 1,25-dihydroxyvitamin D = 95 pg/mL (16-65 pg/mL) (SI: 247 pmol/L [41.6-169.0 pmol/L])
Serum albumin = 4.2 g/dL (3.5-5.0 g/dL) (SI: 42 g/L [35-50 g/L])
Urinary calcium = 310 mg/24 h (100-300 mg/24 h) (SI: 7.8 mmol/d [2.5-7.5 mmol/d])
Urinary creatinine = 1.0 g/24 h (1.0-2.0 g/24 h) (SI: 8.8 mmol/d [8.8-17.7 mmol/d])

A pathogenic variant in which of the following genes most likely explains this patient's clinical presentation?

A. *CASR*
B. *CYP24A1*
C. *MEN1*
D. *RET*
E. *VDR*

109 A 28-year-old woman is evaluated for infertility. She has irregular menses that occur every 2 to 3 months. She stopped oral contraceptives 1 year ago to try and conceive. After excluding other conditions and documenting elevated total and free testosterone, polycystic ovary syndrome is diagnosed. Metformin is prescribed, and her menses become more regular, now occurring about every 28 days. She would like to know the best way to confirm whether she is ovulating.

Which of the following is the best indicator of ovulation for this patient?

A. Basal body temperature
B. Day 3 FSH and estradiol measurements
C. Day 21 progesterone measurement
D. Home ovulation predictor kit
E. Presence of Mittelschmerz

110 At an appointment in an outpatient clinic, a 66-year-old woman is noted to have a blood pressure of 200/110 mm Hg and pulse rate of 98 beats/min. She reports chest tightness and heart pounding; she is sent to the local emergency department and is admitted to the hospital for evaluation.

She has a longstanding history of hypertension, but her blood pressure control has been more difficult in recent years; she currently takes 4 antihypertensive agents: lisinopril, 40 mg daily; hydrochlorothiazide, 25 mg daily;

clonidine, 0.2 mg 3 times daily; and amlodipine, 10 mg daily. Additional comorbidities include obesity, type 2 diabetes mellitus, sleep apnea, dyslipidemia, gastroesophageal reflux disease, and anxiety.

Laboratory test results:

Plasma free metanephrine = 118 pg/mL (<99 pg/mL) (SI: 0.6 nmol/L [<0.50 nmol/L])
Plasma free normetanephrine = 220 pg/mL (<165 pg/mL) (SI: 1.2 nmol/L [<0.90 nmol/L])

Her kidney function and serum electrolytes are normal. Abdominal CT shows normal adrenal glands. The patient is referred to endocrinology after hospital discharge.

Which of the following is the best next step in this patient's evaluation?

A. Chromogranin A measurement
B. CT of the chest and neck
C. 24-Hour urinary metanephrine measurement
D. MIBG scan
E. Repeated plasma metanephrine measurement

111 A 79-year-old woman with a history of gastroesophageal reflux, hypertension, and hyperlipidemia consults with her primary care physician regarding several weeks of numbness of her lips and fingers. She does not smoke cigarettes or drink alcohol, reports no recent changes in her diet, and describes no discomfort. She does not take any supplements and consumes 3 servings of dairy daily. Gastroesophageal reflux was diagnosed 2 years ago, at which time she was prescribed omeprazole. She has been without gastroesophageal reflux symptoms since that time. Hypertension was diagnosed 6 months ago, and she is treated with hydrochlorothiazide. She also takes atorvastatin. Serum calcium, creatinine, and alkaline phosphatase concentrations were normal 6 months ago. DXA performed 2 years ago documented osteopenia.

On physical examination, her temperature is 98.2°F (36.8°C), blood pressure is 123/69 mm Hg, and pulse rate is 72 beats/min. Examination findings are unremarkable, including absence of the Chvostek sign.

Laboratory test results:

Calcium = 7.8 mg/dL (8.2-10.2 mg/dL) (SI: 2.0 mmol/L [2.1-2.6 mmol/L])
Albumin = 3.8 g/dL (3.5-5.0 g/dL) (SI: 38 g/L [35-50 g/L])
Creatinine = 1.0 mg/dL (0.6-1.1 mg/dL) (SI: 88.4 µmol/L [53.0-97.2 µmol/L])
Intact PTH = 32 pg/mL (10-65 pg/mL) (SI: 32 ng/L [10-65 ng/L])
Phosphate = 2.9 mg/dL (2.3-4.7 mg/dL) (SI: 0.9 mmol/L [0.7-1.5 mmol/L])
Magnesium = 0.7 mg/dL (1.5-2.3 mg/dL) (SI: 0.3 mmol/L [0.6-0.9 mmol/L])
25-Hydroxyvitamin D = 28 ng/mL (30-80 ng/mL [optimal]) (SI: 69.9 nmol/L [74.9-199.7 nmol/L])

In addition to prescribing calcium and magnesium supplements, which of the following is the best next step?

A. Ask about a family history of calcium and magnesium disorders
B. Discontinue omeprazole
C. Order brain MRI
D. Order 24-hour urine for calcium, magnesium, and creatinine measurements
E. Prescribe calcitriol

112 A 47-year-old man with a history of acromegaly due to a 2.1-cm pituitary macroadenoma has undergone debulking surgery. Pathology confirms a densely granulated adenoma with positive immunostaining for GH (negative for prolactin). Postoperative MRI shows a good surgical result, with a residual adenoma in the left cavernous sinus.

Laboratory test results (before medical therapy):

Measurement	Preoperatively	6 months after surgery	Reference ranges
IGF-1	835 ng/mL (SI: 109.4 nmol/L)	490 ng/mL (SI: 64.2 nmol/L)	91-246 ng/mL (SI: 11.9-32.2 nmol/L)
GH	13.9 ng/mL (SI: 13.9 μg/L)	2.8 ng/mL (SI: 2.8 μg/L)	0.01-3.61 ng/mL (SI: 0.01-3.61 μg/L)

Lanreotide depot, 90 mg every 4 weeks, is prescribed, and the dosage is later increased to 120 mg every 4 weeks.

Laboratory test results after 6 months of lanreotide depot, 120 mg every 4 weeks:
GH = 2.1 ng/mL (0.01-3.61 ng/mL) (SI: 2.1 μg/L [0.01-3.61 μg/L])
IGF-1 = 310 ng/mL (91-246 ng/mL) (SI: 40.6 nmol/L [11.9-32.2 nmol/L])
Prolactin = 9 ng/mL (4-23 ng/mL) (SI: 0.39 nmol/L [0.17-1.00 nmol/L])

At this visit, he is concerned about lower back pain. He takes losartan, 100 mg daily, for hypertension, and metformin, 850 mg twice daily. His blood pressure is 136/92 mm Hg, and pulse rate is 88 beats/min. His height is 70 in (178 cm), and weight is 230 lb (104.5 kg) (BMI = 33 kg/m^2).

Liver enzyme concentrations are normal, and his hemoglobin A_{1c} concentration is 6.5% (4.0%-5.6%) (48 mmol/mol [20-38 mmol/mol]).

Which of the following is the best next step in this patient's management?

A. Add cabergoline
B. Add pegvisomant
C. Refer for radiotherapy
D. Switch to octreotide
E. Switch to pasireotide

113 A 55-year-old man presents for a weight management assessment. He is motivated to lose weight, but he has struggled to make sustainable improvements to his dietary habits. He is experiencing lower-extremity mechanical joint pain and has trouble performing activities of daily such as bending, stooping, and maintaining self-hygiene.

The patient is on a limited income and cites this as the most significant barrier to making good food choices. He relies on the local food pantry for most of his meals. He has met with a dietitian in the past but found it difficult to adhere to the recommendations because of cost. Although he does not have access to an exercise facility, he tries to be as active as possible.

His current medication regimen consists of bupropion, 150 mg daily, and levothyroxine, 150 mcg daily.

On physical examination, his height is 64 in (163 cm) and weight is 342 lb (155 kg) (BMI = 58 kg/m^2). He has no facial rounding or supraclavicular fullness. His weight is primarily distributed centrally, and there is no peripheral edema. He has a large, firm thyroid gland on examination.

Laboratory test results:
Fasting glucose = 110 mg/dL (70-99 mg/dL) (SI: 6.1 mmol/L [3.9-5.5 mmol/L])
TSH = 6.2 mIU/L (0.5-5.0 mIU/L)

Which of the following is the best next step in this patient's management?

A. Increase the levothyroxine dosage to 175 mcg daily
B. Prescribe a GLP-1 receptor agonist to help with weight loss and glycemic control
C. Prescribe a physical activity regimen consisting of at least 150 minutes of moderate-intensity exercise per week
D. Recommend a meal replacement program
E. Set up frequent visits with the local health coach

114 A 68-year-old man with a 15-year history of type 2 diabetes mellitus presents for follow-up. His diabetes is complicated by peripheral neuropathy and progression to stage 3b chronic kidney disease within the last year. He currently takes metformin, 500 mg XR twice daily, and glimepiride, 2 mg daily. He reports a recent emergency department visit for hypoglycemia and states that his blood glucose values typically range from 70 to 230 mg/dL (3.9 to 12.8 mmol/L).

On physical examination, his blood pressure is 149/87 mm Hg and pulse rate is 87 beats/min. His height is 69 in (175.3 cm), and weight is 209 lb (95 kg) (BMI = 30.9 kg/m^2).

Laboratory test results (sample drawn while fasting):

Hemoglobin A_{1c} = 8.5% (4.0%-5.6%) (69 mmol/mol [20-38 mmol/mol])
Creatinine = 2.1 mg/dL (0.7-1.3 mg/dL) (SI: 185.6 µmol/L [61.9-114.9 µmol/L])
Estimated glomerular filtration rate = 33 mL/min per 1.73 m^2 (>60 mL/min per 1.73 m^2)
Serum urea nitrogen = 50 mg/dL (8-23 mg/dL) (SI: 17.9 mmol/L [2.9-8.2 mmol/L])
Plasma glucose = 77 mg/dL (70-99 mg/dL) (SI: 4.3 mmol/L [3.9-5.5 mmol/L])
Sodium = 137 mEq/L (136-142 mEq/L) (SI: 137 mmol/L [136-142 mmol/L])
Urinary albumin-to-creatinine ratio = 427 mg/g creat (<30 mg/g creat)

Which of the following is the best next step to achieve the most beneficial glycemic effect?

Answer	Oral medications	Basal insulin
A.	• Stop metformin • Continue glimepiride	Start 14 units daily
B.	• Stop metformin • Escalate glimepiride dosage	Start 14 units daily
C.	• Continue metformin • Stop glimepiride	Start 14 units daily
D.	• Continue metformin • Escalate glimepiride dosage • Start empagliflozin	None
E.	• Continue metformin • Stop glimepiride • Start empagliflozin	Start 14 units daily

115 A 43-year-old premenopausal woman is referred for management of type 1 osteogenesis imperfecta. She was diagnosed at age 2 years and has sustained a few long bone fractures, the most recent being a fracture of her right distal radius after falling on a concrete floor at age 13 years. DXA shows a lowest Z-score of –2.6 in the lumbar spine, with stable bone mineral density overall compared with measurements 2 years ago. She has good dietary calcium intake and takes a daily vitamin D supplement. She has never received pharmacologic therapy for her bone health.

On physical examination, she has blue-gray discoloration of her sclerae and mild scoliosis.

Laboratory testing documents normal results from a basic metabolic panel and measurements of alkaline phosphatase and serum 25-hydroxyvitamin D.

Which of the following is the best recommendation now?

A. Repeat DXA scan at age 65 years
B. Repeat DXA scan in 2 years
C. Start alendronate
D. Start denosumab
E. Start teriparatide

116 A 28-year-old Asian man started experiencing muscle weakness last night. When he woke in the morning, he had difficulty walking and his girlfriend brought him to urgent care. He has also noticed palpitations and diarrhea over the last week. Laboratory tests in urgent care document a potassium concentration of 2.2 mEq/L (2.2 mmol/L) and a normal complete blood cell count. He receives 20 mEq of potassium chloride and is transferred to the emergency department for admission and further workup.

In the emergency department, he appears anxious. His blood pressure is 138/86 mm Hg, and pulse rate is 110 beats/min. There is no proptosis. His thyroid gland is twice normal size and firm with no nodularity. There is no cervical adenopathy. There is a tremor in his outstretched hands. Neurologic examination reveals lower-extremity weakness. The rest of the physical examination findings are unremarkable.

Laboratory test results on arrival to the emergency department:

Sodium = 138 mEq/L (136-142 mEq/L) (SI: 138 mmol/L [136-142 mmol/L])
Potassium = 2.4 mEq/L (3.5-5.0 mEq/L) (SI: 2.4 mmol/L [3.5-5.0 mmol/L])
Bicarbonate = 24 mEq/L (21-28 mEq/L) (SI: 24 mmol/L [21-28 mmol/L])
Creatinine = 1.0 mg/dL (0.7-1.3 mg/dL) (SI: 88.4 μmol/L [61.9-114.9 μmol/L])
Calcium = 8.6 mg/dL (8.2-10.2 mg/dL) (SI: 2.2 mmol/L [2.1-2.6 mmol/L])
Phosphate = 2.3 mg/dL (2.3-4.7 mg/dL) (SI: 0.7 mmol/L [0.7-1.5 mmol/L])
Magnesium = 1.5 mg/dL (1.5-2.3 mg/dL) (SI: 0.6 mmol/L [0.6-0.9 mmol/L])
TSH = <0.01 mIU/L (0.5-5.5 mIU/L)
Free T_4 = 2.8 ng/dL (0.8-1.8 ng/dL) (SI: 36.01 pmol/L [10.30-23.17 pmol/L])

Electrocardiography shows sinus tachycardia at a rate of 116 beats/min.

In addition to careful potassium supplementation, which of the following is the most appropriate next step in this patient's management?

A. β-Adrenergic blocker
B. Immunoglobulin therapy
C. Methimazole
D. Prednisone
E. Radioiodine treatment

117 A 26-year-old Black woman presents for a follow-up appointment for type 1 diabetes mellitus without known complications. Diabetes was diagnosed 12 years ago. Apart from at the time of diagnosis, diabetic ketoacidosis requiring hospitalization occurred once, 3 years ago, due to an intercurrent illness. Her main concern is how to improve glycemic control, and she expresses interest in insulin pump therapy.

She recalls having good glycemic control until she went to college, but over the last 6 years, her hemoglobin A_{1c} level has consistently ranged between 9.0% and 12.0% (75 and 108 mmol/mol). She is on a basal-bolus insulin regimen with insulin glargine and insulin glulisine. Two years ago, she initiated continuous glucose monitoring, and it demonstrates 80% usage with an average glucose value of 262 mg/dL (14.5 mmol/L). Her hemoglobin A_{1c} level on point-of-care testing is 11.2% (99 mmol/mol). She admits to nonadherence to her treatment regimen and misses basal insulin injections 2 to 3 times per week and bolus insulin injections 2 to 3 times per week. She attributes this difficulty to a hectic work and school schedule. She has no notable medical history, and her only additional medication is an oral contraceptive pill.

Which of the following is the best next step to help improve this patient's glycemic control?

A. Change insulin regimen to premixed NPH/regular (70/30) twice daily
B. Change insulin glargine to insulin degludec
C. Prescribe hybrid closed-loop therapy
D. Refer her to a diabetes educator
E. Refer her to a psychologist

118 A 69-year-old man was diagnosed with multiple myeloma last month. He also has a medical history of hypertension, type 2 diabetes mellitus, and carotid stenosis. Other than laboratory values confirming a monoclonal gammopathy, biochemical findings from his evaluation at the time of diagnosis were normal. The patient was referred to a hematologist, and bortezomib was prescribed last week. Despite his new diagnosis, he reports no symptoms other than mild fatigue.

His primary care physician orders routine laboratory testing:

Sodium = 135 mEq/L (136-142 mEq/L) (SI: 135 mmol/L [136-142 mmol/L])
Potassium = 3.5 mEq/L (3.5-5.0 mEq/L) (SI: 3.5 mmol/L [3.5-5.0 mmol/L])
Chloride = 108 mEq/L (96-106 mEq/L) (SI: 108 mmol/L [96-106 mmol/L])
Carbon dioxide = 27 mEq/L (22-28 mEq/L) (SI: 27 mmol/L [22-28 mmol/L])
Anion gap = 0 mEq/L (3-11 mEq/L) (SI: 0 mmol/L [3-11 mmol/L])
Serum urea nitrogen = 19 mg/dL (8-23 mg/dL) (SI: 6.8 mmol/L [2.9-8.2 mmol/L])
Creatinine = 1.2 mg/dL (0.7-1.3 mg/dL) (SI: 106.1 μmol/L [61.9-114.9 μmol/L])
Glucose = 101 mg/dL (70-99 mg/dL) (SI: 5.6 mmol/L [3.9-5.5 mmol/L])
Calcium = 10.9 mg/dL (8.2-10.2 mg/dL) (SI: 2.8 mmol/L [2.1-2.6 mmol/L])
Albumin = 3.7 g/dL (3.5-5.0 g/dL) (SI: 37 g/L [35-50 g/L])
Protein (total) = 9.2 g/dL (6.3-7.9 g/dL) (SI: 92 g/L [63-79 g/L])

After reviewing the laboratory values, the patient's primary care physician contacts him regarding the hypercalcemia. The patient reports that he is not taking calcium supplements or calcium-containing antacids and does not consume much dairy. He has no polyuria, polydipsia, or abdominal pain.

Which of the following should be measured next?

A. 1,25-Dihydroxyvitamin D
B. 24-Hour urine for calcium and creatinine
C. Intact PTH
D. Ionized calcium
E. Phosphate

119 A 34-year-old woman is concerned that she might have hormonal problems underlying her inability to lose weight. She reports progressively gaining weight over the past 1 to 2 years, despite active efforts to eat healthier and walk for 30 minutes 3 times a week. She has a history of irregular menses and mild acne, and polycystic ovary syndrome has been diagnosed. Her only medication is an oral contraceptive pill.

On physical examination, her blood pressure is 140/86 mm Hg and pulse rate is 78 beats/min. Her height is 64 in (162.5 cm), and weight is 180 lb (81.8 kg) (BMI = 30.9 kg/m^2). Excess adiposity is distributed predominantly centrally. Muscle strength is normal. She has lentiginous lesions around her mouth, including on her lips. She also has dark pink striae on her abdomen and inner upper arms.

Laboratory test results (sample drawn at 8 AM):

Blood glucose = 121 mg/dL (70-99 mg/dL) (SI: 6.7 nmol/L [3.9-5.5 mmol/L])
Serum creatinine, normal
Electrolytes, normal
Testosterone, normal
Serum cortisol = 28 μg/dL (5-25 μg/dL) (SI: 772.5 nmol/L [137.9-689.7 nmol/L])
ACTH = 8 pg/mL (10-60 pg/mL) (SI: 1.8 pmol/L [2.2-13.2 pmol/L])

Which of the following is the most appropriate next step in this patient's evaluation?

A. Abdominal CT
B. 24-Hour urinary cortisol and creatinine measurements
C. Overnight 1-mg dexamethasone-suppression test
D. Pituitary-directed MRI
E. Serum DHEA-S measurement

120 A 73-year-old woman with a 9-year history of type 2 diabetes mellitus complicated by recurrent yeast infections presents for follow-up. She had a cerebrovascular accident 2 years ago, but she has no residual weakness, is very active, and walks without issues. She currently takes metformin, 1000 mg twice daily, and semaglutide, 1 mg weekly (just increased 1 month ago). At-home blood pressure measurements are in the range of 110 to 135 mm Hg (systolic) and 62 to 78 mm Hg (diastolic). Additional medications are lisinopril, 40 mg daily, and chlorthalidone, 25 mg every morning. She is very pleased that she has lost 8 lb (3.6 kg) since initiating semaglutide. She has no symptoms of dizziness upon standing and no fall history.

On physical examination, her blood pressure is 111/63 mm Hg and pulse rate is 79 beats/min. Her height is 63 in (160 cm), and weight is 150 lb (68.2 kg) (BMI = 26.6 kg/m^2).

Laboratory test results (sample drawn while fasting):

Hemoglobin A_{1c} = 7.3% (4.0%-5.6%) (56 mmol/mol [20-38 mmol/mol])
Creatinine = 0.8 mg/dL (0.6-1.1 mg/dL) (SI: 70.7 µmol/L [53.0-97.2 µmol/L])
Serum urea nitrogen = 20 mg/dL (8-23 mg/dL) (SI: 7.1 mmol/L [2.9-8.2 mmol/L])
Plasma glucose = 112 mg/dL (70-99 mg/dL) (SI: 6.2 mmol/L [3.9-5.5 mmol/L])
Sodium = 141 mEq/L (136-142 mEq/L) (SI: 141 mmol/L [136-142 mmol/L])

Which of the following is the best next step in this patient's management?

A. Add amlodipine
B. Add dapagliflozin
C. Continue current therapy but change lisinopril dosing to bedtime
D. Continue current therapy but switch chlorthalidone administration to bedtime
E. Reduce the lisinopril dosage to 20 mg daily

ANSWERS

ENDOCRINE SELF-ASSESSMENT PROGRAM 2023

Part II

1 **ANSWER: D) Zoledronic acid, 5 mg intravenously 6 months after her last denosumab injection**

Data published over the past 5 years support the importance of selecting the correct sequence of osteoporosis medications. Denosumab is a potent antiresorptive agent that has much shorter period of biologic action (about 6 months) compared with the much longer period of action of bisphosphonates (5 to 10 years). The US FDA approved denosumab in 2009, but in 2017 there were reports of a high risk of vertebral fractures after stopping the medication. A post hoc analysis of the pivotal FREEDOM trial and the extension study reported that the risk of vertebral fractures is nearly 6-fold higher in patients who discontinue denosumab than in those who do not. Because of this, drug holidays or delays in administration (Answer E) are not appropriate with denosumab, unlike with bisphosphonates.

In a patient for whom it becomes necessary to transition to another osteoporosis medication, sequencing to an anabolic medication such as teriparatide or abaloparatide (Answer A) leads to increased bone resorption and decreased bone density that most likely also increases fracture risk. In the DATA-SWITCH trial, 2 years of denosumab followed by teriparatide resulted in a significant decline in spine and hip bone density within 6 to 12 months of starting teriparatide. The mechanism of bone density decline remains unclear, but it may be due to the accumulation of immature but inactive osteoclasts during denosumab treatment that become active with anabolic therapy and/or a decrease in the osteoblast product osteoprotegerin that favors osteoclast formation.

Several studies have examined the effects on bone density when denosumab therapy is followed with zoledronic acid. In 1 study, zoledronic acid was administered after the last denosumab injection either 6 months later, 9 months later, or when bone turnover markers had significantly increased. In all groups, spine bone mineral density decreased approximately 3% to 5%. The European Calcified Tissue Society (ECTS) published a set of recommendations in 2020 recommending that patients who had received denosumab for more than 2 and a half years should switch to zoledronic acid administered 6 months after the last denosumab injection (Answer D).

Although alendronate (Answer B) is a reasonable option, ECTS recommends alendronate for patients who have been treated with denosumab for *less than* 2 and a half years.

Since the patient is at higher risk for fractures, raloxifene (Answer C) would not be the best option given its more modest fracture-reducing effects.

Educational Objective

Manage the transition from denosumab to another osteoporosis medication.

Reference(s)

Cummings SR, Ferrari S, Eastell R, et al. Vertebral fractures after discontinuation of denosumab: a post hoc analysis of the randomized placebo-controlled FREEDOM trial and its extension. *J Bone Miner Res.* 2018;33(2):190-198. PMID: 29105841

Leder BZ, Tsai JN, Uihlein AV, et al. Denosumab and teriparatide transitions in postmenopausal osteoporosis (the DATA-Switch study): extension of a randomised controlled trial. *Lancet.* 2015;386(9999):1147-1155. PMID: 26144908

Anastasilakis AD, Papapoulos SE, Polyzos SA, Appelman-Dijkstra NM, Makras P. Zoledronate for the prevention of bone loss in women discontinuing denosumab treatment. A prospective 2-year clinical trial. *J Bone Miner Res.* 2019;34(12):2220-2228. PMID: 31433518

Tsourdi E, Zillikens MC, Meier C, et al. Fracture risk and management of discontinuation of denosumab therapy: a systematic review and position statement by ECTS. *J Clin Endocrinol Metab.* 2020 [online ahead of print] PMID: 33103722

Reid IR, Horne AM, Mihov B, Gamble GD. Bone loss after denosumab: only partial protection with zolendronate. *Calcif Tissue Int.* 2017;101(4):371-374. PMID: 28500448

2 **ANSWER: D) Measurement of plasma metanephrines**

The discovery of an adrenal mass in a patient undergoing evaluation for suspected bronchogenic carcinoma raises concerns of metastatic spread of the primary tumor, which has potential ramifications for disease staging. However, adrenal incidentalomas are common in the general population and are identified on 4% to 7% of abdominal CT or MRI scans in patients older than 40 years. Many of these are truly incidental and are not associated with endocrine dysfunction.

Adrenal tumors can be broadly classified into 5 main categories:

1. Adrenal adenomas and nodular hyperplasia
2. Other benign lesions (eg, myelolipoma, cyst, hematoma, ganglioneuroma)
3. Adrenocortical carcinoma
4. Pheochromocytoma
5. Other malignant tumors (eg, metastasis, lymphoma, sarcoma)

Although the case mix varies considerably among series, at a population level it has been estimated that 8% to 9% of adrenal incidentalomas are malignant, with metastases predominating in this subgroup. However, even if the latter is strongly suspected, it is important to adopt a systematic approach to assessment.

With modern imaging techniques (triple-phase CT, in-phase and out-of-phase MRI), most adrenal incidentalomas are readily classified as benign adrenal adenomas. In this case, the lesion is less than 4 cm in diameter, but the density on unenhanced CT is 35 Hounsfield units (HU), which is above the threshold (<10 HU) that would allow the mass to be confidently diagnosed as an adenoma (assuming a homogeneous appearance). At first glance, the triple-phase study report appears to provide reassurance with absolute washout values (78.6%; calculated as: [early postintravenous phase HU – delayed-phase HU] / [early post-intravenous phase HU – noncontrast HU] × 100) and relative washout values (52.4%; calculated as: [early postintravenous phase HU – delayed-phase HU] / [early postintravenous phase HU] × 100]) that are typically seen with adrenal adenomas (≥60% and ≥40% respectively). Importantly, other pathologies may display washout characteristics that overlap those of lipid-poor adenomas, including pheochromocytomas and hypervascular metastases (eg, renal cell carcinoma, hepatocellular carcinoma). In addition, in this case, the degree of enhancement following contrast injection is particularly marked, with the arterial phase value 1 minute after contrast exceeding 100 HU. Taken together, these findings mandate screening for pheochromocytoma, and hence measuring plasma metanephrines (Answer D) is the most appropriate next step in this patient's management.

Although a tissue diagnosis will most likely be needed to guide treatment, biopsy of either the lung lesion (Answer B) or the adrenal mass (Answer A) is not advisable until a pheochromocytoma has been excluded to avoid precipitating a catecholamine crisis. If biopsy is deemed necessary before laboratory results are available, then prior α-adrenoceptor blockade is required.

The possibility that the patient has Cushing syndrome might be suggested by several clinical features (multiple bruises on the upper and lower limbs, type 2 diabetes, hypertension). In this setting, several etiologies would need to be considered: (1) small cell lung cancer with ectopic ACTH secretion; (2) cortisol-secreting adrenocortical carcinoma; and (3) ACTH-secreting pheochromocytoma. Accordingly, screening for autonomous hypercortisolism, including with dexamethasone-suppression testing (Answer E) and, if confirmed, establishing whether it is ACTH-dependent (Answer C) may need to be considered. However, in this case, long-term treatment with prednisolone for polymyalgia rheumatica is a more likely explanation for the clinical manifestations of glucocorticoid excess.

Another important reason for delaying dexamethasone-suppression testing until a pheochromocytoma has been excluded is the small but well-described risk of inducing a catecholamine crisis with glucocorticoid therapy, although previous case reports suggest this is only likely to be a problem with dosages greater than the 1 mg used in the overnight dexamethasone-suppression test.

Educational Objective

Exclude pheochromocytoma in any patient with an indeterminate adrenal mass, even if another cause (eg, metastasis) is suspected, and describe the variability in pheochromocytoma appearance on contrast-enhanced CT.

Reference(s)

Fassnacht M, Arlt W, Bancos I, et al. Management of adrenal incidentalomas: European Society of Endocrinology clinical practice guideline in collaboration with the European Network for the Study of Adrenal Tumors. *Eur J Endocrinol.* 2016;175(2):G1-G34. PMID: 27390021

Bancos I, Prete A. Approach to the patient with adrenal incidentaloma. *J Clin Endocrinol Metab.* 2021;106(11):3331-3353. PMID: 34260734

Canu L, Van Hemert JAW, Kerstens MN, et al. CT characteristics of pheochromocytoma: relevance for the evaluation of adrenal incidentaloma. *J Clin Endocrinol Metab.* 2019;104(2):312-318. PMID: 30383267

Goroshi M, Jadhav SS, Sarathi V, et al. Radiological differentiation of phaeochromocytoma from other malignant adrenal masses: important of wash-in characteristics on multiphase CECT. *Endocr Connect.* 2019;8(7):898-905. PMID: 31252396

3 **ANSWER: C) Primary hypogonadism masked by ill health before liver transplant**

Major stress from any acute or chronic illness can suppress the hypothalamic-pituitary-gonadal (HPG) axis. The degree of HPG-axis suppression is usually proportional to the severity and duration of the offending illness. However, individual susceptibility may differ, and factors such as increasing age or preexisting comorbidities (eg, obesity) may increase the risk of HPG-axis suppression caused by an intercurrent illness. While acute stress can cause immediate and direct Leydig-cell suppression, when the stress is prolonged, gonadotropins become suppressed, further decreasing testosterone concentrations. Therefore, patients with HPG-axis suppression in the context of severe chronic disease typically present with low serum testosterone and low or inappropriately normal LH concentrations. The exact mechanisms underlying chronic stress-induced hypogonadotropic hypogonadism are not fully understood and may include inhibition of GnRH release via opioid-, dopaminergic-, glucocorticoid-, or inflammation-related pathways. Usually, HPG-axis suppression is functional and, in contrast to organic hypogonadism due to structural disease of the HPG axis, is expected to be reversible following resolution of the underlying illness. In men with decompensated liver cirrhosis, low testosterone is common (occurring in 60%-90% of men), and gonadotropins are typically low or low-normal, as with any other severe illness. Low testosterone is an excellent marker of poor health in men with cirrhosis and predicts mortality even independently of established prognostic parameters, such as the model for end-stage liver disease (MELD) score or serum sodium concentration. However, in this patient, the biochemical severity of the pretransplant hypogonadotropic hypogonadism was unusual (pretransplant testosterone concentrations in cirrhotic men are typically 145 to 260 ng/dL [5.0-9.0 nmol/L]). Unfortunately, a thorough assessment of his gonadal status was not performed before transplant. In most men with functional hypogonadotropic hypogonadism due to ill health before liver transplant, the HPG axis recovers after a successful transplant restores general health, although this recovery may take several months. Of note, whether testosterone treatment before liver transplant provides clinically meaningful health benefits has not been established; the largest randomized controlled trial to date included 101 men with established cirrhosis and a serum total testosterone concentration less than 346 ng/dL (<12 nmol/L) (or free testosterone concentration <6.6 ng/dL [<0.23 nmol/L]). Over 12 months, compared with placebo, testosterone treatment increased lean appendicular mass (the primary outcome) by 1.7 kg, increased total lean mass by 4.7 kg, reduced fat mass, increased bone density and hemoglobin, but had no effect on mortality.

Interestingly, at evaluation now, 18 months after this patient's successful transplant, his testosterone concentration is still repeatedly very low, but gonadotropins are now clearly elevated. Moreover, he has clinical features suggesting genuine organic hypogonadism. The best explanation for these findings is that he had preexisting genuine primary hypogonadism that was masked by ill health before his liver transplant (Answer C). Ill health before transplant led to hypothalamic-pituitary suppression causing functional central hypogonadism superimposed on, and hence masking, his underlying genuine primary hypogonadism due to previous alcohol and orchitis. Primary hypogonadism has now been unmasked as his general health has improved. This patient had no contraindication to testosterone or desire for paternity, and testosterone replacement was initiated. Testosterone treatment led to improved libido and energy, thus enabling him to lose weight and improve his glycemic control.

While the dynamics of HPG axis recovery after liver transplant (or recovery from other chronic disease suppressing the HPG axis) have not been studied prospectively in detail, it is possible that modestly raised gonadotropins could precede eventual testosterone recovery, representing a transient biochemical picture resembling primary hypogonadism (a potential explanation not listed among the answers listed in the vignette). However, the persistently markedly high gonadotropins and low testosterone over 8 weeks 18 months after liver transplant, as well as the history of mumps orchitis as a plausible etiology for his primary hypogonadism (with asymmetric testicular size), make this possibility less likely. However, as was done in this man, documenting persistent primary hypogonadism over time is important before committing to lifelong testosterone replacement, especially in the early months after liver transplant.

Weight gain (Answer A) is associated with central suppression of the HPG axis, and obesity typically presents with functional hypogonadotropic hypogonadism (which can be reversible with weight loss) but not with primary hypogonadism. Moreover, his serum testosterone is disproportionally low relative to his modest obesity.

Likewise, suboptimally controlled diabetes mellitus (Answer B) can be associated with central suppression of the HPG axis, and patients present with hypogonadotropic, not primary, hypogonadism. His hemoglobin A_{1c} level was only modestly elevated, suggesting that his glucose levels were not sufficiently high to cause HPG-axis suppression.

While tacrolimus (Answer E) has been associated with damage to the seminiferous tubules in rodent models in some studies, there are no preclinical or human data reporting that tacrolimus affects Leydig-cell function.

Sertoli-cell–only syndrome (Answer D) is a mostly idiopathic condition (although some patients have microdeletions in the Y chromosome), and the diagnosis is typically made in men aged 20 to 40 years who present with infertility. Affected men have very low or absent spermatogenesis. While histologic findings can vary, typically only Sertoli cells line the seminiferous tubules and germ cells, and spermatozoa are usually absent. In some cases, sperm can be recovered during testicular sperm extraction. Affected men present with elevated FSH, but Leydig-cell function is not affected, and hence serum testosterone and LH are typically normal.

Educational Objective

Explain how ill health can lead to hypothalamic-pituitary suppression, hence masking genuine primary hypogonadism.

Reference(s)

Sinclair M, Grossmann M, Gow PJ, Angus PW. Testosterone in men with advanced liver disease: abnormalities and implications. *J Gastroenterol Hepatol.* 2015;30(2):244-251. PMID: 25087838

Spratt DI, Cox P, Orav J, Moloney J, Bigos T. Reproductive axis suppression in acute illness is related to disease severity. *J Clin Endocrinol Metab.* 1993;76(6):1548-1554. PMID: 8501163

Woolf PD, Hamill RW, McDonald JV, Lee LA, Kelly M. Transient hypogonadotropic hypogonadism caused by critical illness. *J Clin Endocrinol Metab.* 1985;60(3):444-450. PMID: 3919042

Sinclair M, Grossmann M, Hoermann R, Angus PW, Gow PJ. Testosterone therapy increases muscle mass in men with cirrhosis and low testosterone: a randomised controlled trial. *J Hepatol.* 2016;65(5):906-913. PMID: 27312945

4 ANSWER: E) Heterozygous familial hypercholesterolemia

Familial hypercholesterolemia (FH) (Answer E) is an autosomal dominant disorder characterized by elevations in LDL cholesterol. The most common pathogenic variants causing this disease occur in the genes encoding the LDL receptor, apolipoprotein B, and PCSK9. Affected individuals inherit 1 abnormal allele, which leads to heterozygous FH. Individuals who inherit 2 abnormal alleles have homozygous FH (if the pathogenic variants are identical), compound heterozygous FH (2 different pathogenic variants in the same gene), or double heterozygous FH (2 pathogenic variants in 2 different genes). In the general population, heterozygous FH has a prevalence of 1 in 200 to 1 in 500, and homozygous FH has a prevalence of 1 in 160,000 to 1 in 300,000.

Features that characterize FH include extensor tendon xanthomas, a family history of premature atherosclerotic cardiovascular disease, and elevated LDL-cholesterol concentrations. LDL-cholesterol cutoffs to diagnose heterozygous FH and homozygous FH are greater than 190 mg/dL (>4.92 mmol/L) and greater than 400 mg/dL (>10.36 mmol/L), respectively. Several diagnostic tools are available such as the Dutch Lipid Clinic Network Score and the Make Early Diagnosis to Prevent Early Death criteria. Identifying affected individuals early is crucial to prevent atherosclerotic events and to perform cascade screening. Treatment is usually combination therapy, with statins being the preferred initial agent. Almost all affected individuals need at least 2 medications to achieve adequate LDL-cholesterol lowering. The patient described in this vignette has physical examination findings, family history, and LDL-cholesterol levels consistent with heterozygous FH. Inherited disorders of lipid metabolism are shown in the *table.*

Familial hypobetalipoproteinemia (Answer D) is a codominant inherited disorder characterized by low concentrations of LDL cholesterol (<fifth percentile). It is caused by pathogenic variants in the gene encoding apolipoprotein B, which lead to production of a truncated apolipoprotein B protein, or by loss-of-function pathogenic variants in the gene encoding PCSK9. The prevalence of familial hypobetalipoproteinemia is thought to be 1 in 1000 to 1 in 3000. Clinically, when this condition is caused by a pathogenic variant in the apolipoprotein B gene, individuals are asymptomatic, but they are at increased risk for fatty liver disease. Hepatic function tests and abdominal ultrasonography should be performed regularly because of an increased risk of developing cirrhosis. Affected patients should be counseled on adhering to a low-fat diet and avoiding factors that increase the risk of liver disease. Individuals with familial hypobetalipoproteinemia due to a *PCSK9* pathogenic variant are also asymptomatic, and they are at decreased risk of cardiovascular disease. This finding, in addition to the findings in the Dallas Heart study (less coronary heart disease in patients with loss-of-function pathogenic variants in *PCSK9*), contributed to the discovery of PCSK9 inhibitors.

Table. Inherited Disorders of Lipid Metabolism

Disorder	Prevalence	Inheritance	Gene(s)	Lipid profile	Clinical findings
Familial hypercholesterolemia (heterozygous)	1 in 200 to 1 in 500	Autosomal dominant	*LDLR, PCSK9, APOB*	LDL-C >190 mg/dL (SI: >4.92 mmol/L)	Extensor tendon xanthomas, corneal arcus, premature coronary heart disease
Familial hypercholesterolemia (homozygous)	1 in 160,000 to 1 in 300,000	Autosomal dominant	*LDLR, PCSK9, APOB*	LDL-C >400 mg/dL (SI: >10.36 mmol/L)	Extensor tendon xanthomas; severe, premature, atherosclerotic cardiovascular disease
Familial combined hyperlipidemia	1 in 100	Polygenic	Polygenic	ApoB >120 mg/dL (SI: >1.2 g/L) Elevations in LDL-C and/or triglycerides	Premature coronary heart
Familial chylomicronemia syndrome	1 in 1,000,000	Autosomal recessive	*LPL* (most common), *APOC2, APOA5, LMF1, GPIHBP1*	Triglycerides >1000 mg/dL (SI: >11.30 mmol/L)	Eruptive xanthomas, lipemia retinalis, pancreatitis, hepatosplenomegaly
Familial dysbetalipoproteinemia	1 in 150 to 1 in 10,000	Autosomal dominant (10%) or autosomal recessive (90%)	*APOE*	Total cholesterol and triglycerides >90th percentile	Eruptive xanthomas, palmar crease xanthomas, tendon xanthomas, premature cardiovascular disease; second metabolic stressor
Familial hypobetalipoproteinemia	1 in 1000 to 1 in 3000	Autosomal codominant	*APOB, PCSK9*	LDL-C <5th percentile	Asymptomatic, fatty liver, cirrhosis, decreased risk of cardiovascular disease

Abbreviations: ApoB, apolipoprotein B; LDL-C, low-density lipoprotein cholesterol.

Familial chylomicronemia syndrome (Answer A) is an autosomal recessive disorder. Most cases are caused by pathogenic variants in the gene encoding lipoprotein lipase, but pathogenic variants in genes encoding apolipoprotein C2, lipase maturation factor 1, and glycosylphosphatidylinositol-anchored HDL-binding protein 1 are also responsible for this disease. Familial chylomicronemia syndrome has a prevalence of 1 in 1,000,000, and the hallmark of this condition is severe hypertriglyceridemia (>1000 mg/dL [>11.3 mmol/L]), which conveys an increased risk of developing pancreatitis. The cornerstone of management is limiting fat intake to less than 5% of total calories. Triglyceride-lowering medications do not effectively treat familial chylomicronemia syndrome.

Familial dysbetalipoproteinemia (Answer C) is due to pathogenic variants in the gene encoding apolipoprotein E. The condition can be inherited either in an autosomal recessive manner (90% of cases) or autosomal dominant manner (10% of cases). Patients with the recessive form have 2 *E2* alleles; however, to develop familial dysbetalipoproteinemia, an individual also needs a secondary risk factor such as insulin resistance, metabolic syndrome, or obesity. The prevalence of familial dysbetalipoproteinemia varies from 1 in 150 to 1 in 10,000 in the general population. Clinical features include eruptive xanthomas, palmar crease xanthomas (a pathognomonic sign for this disease), and tendon xanthomas. Affected patients have increased total cholesterol and triglycerides, and they are at risk for premature cardiovascular disease. Treatment includes a low-fat and low-carbohydrate diet and medications such as statins and fibrates.

Familial combined hyperlipidemia (Answer B) is a polygenic disorder characterized by elevations of apolipoprotein B and triglycerides in at least 2 family members and the presence of premature cardiovascular disease. It is the most common inherited form of dyslipidemia, occurring in 1 in 100 persons. There are no specific physical examination findings associated with this condition. Pharmacologic treatment options include statins and fibrates.

Educational Objective

Diagnose heterozygous familial hypercholesterolemia.

Reference(s)

McGowan MP, Dehkordi SH, Moriarty PM, Duell PB. Diagnosis and treatment of heterozygous familial hypercholesterolemia. *J Am Heart Assoc.* 2019;8(24):e013225. PMID: 31838973

Hooper AJ, Burnett JR. Update on primary hypobetalipoproteinemia. *Curr Atheroscler Rep.* 2014;16(7):423. PMID: 24781598

Goldberg RB, Chait A. A comprehensive update on the chylomicronemia syndrome. *Front Endocrinol (Lausanne).* 2020;11:593931. PMID: 33193106

Koopal C, Marais DA, Westerink J, Visseren FLJ. Autosomal dominant familial dysbetalipoproteinemia: a pathophysiological framework and practical approach to diagnosis and therapy. *J Clin Lipidol.* 2017;11(1):12-23. PMID: 28391878

Brahm AJ, Hegele RA. Combined hyperlipidemia: familial but not (usually) monogenic. *Curr Opin Lipidol.* 2016;27(2):131-140. PMID: 26709473

5 ANSWER: E) Provide reassurance and continue current therapies

Worsening of retinopathy is often observed when abrupt improvements in glycemic control occur in women preparing for pregnancy, during pregnancy, in patients receiving insulin- or non–insulin-based treatments, or in patients who have undergone bariatric surgery. Risk factors include suboptimal glycemic control and hypertension. Worsening microvascular complications may manifest before the patient sees any of the long-term benefits of optimizing glycemic control. The exact mechanism of this phenomenon remains unclear, and there are numerous hypotheses. If worsening retinopathy occurs, patient counseling and reassurance are recommended (Answer E), as well as close follow-up with ophthalmology to ensure stabilization and appropriate treatment.

The landmark Diabetes Control and Complications Trial (DCCT) documented the frequency, the importance of, and the risk factors for early worsening of diabetic retinopathy allocated to intensive insulin treatment vs conventional treatment in patients with type 1 diabetes who had none-to-moderate nonproliferative diabetic retinopathy. At the 6-month and/or 12-month visit, early worsening was observed in significantly more patients assigned to receive intensive treatment (13.1%) vs conventional treatment (7.6%) ($P < .001$).

Because of the risk of worsening diabetic retinopathy in patients with longstanding, suboptimally controlled diabetes in particular, it is best to tighten glycemic control over a prolonged period, with a step-wise approach to intensification. Depending on the circumstances, more frequent dilated eye examination should be considered in certain patients when aggressive improvements in glycemic control cannot be avoided (eg, pregnancy). For patients such as the one in this vignette who are motivated to rapidly improve their glycemic control, the provider should explain why the goal is to proceed slowly and should include ophthalmology in the process early.

While ACE and angiotensin receptor blocker therapy has been reported to reduce the risk of diabetic retinopathy, this patient is already taking an ACE inhibitor and currently has well-controlled blood pressure. Accordingly, increasing the lisinopril dosage (Answer D) or adding losartan (Answer B) is not appropriate now. Moreover, combination ACE/angiotensin receptor blocker therapy is not recommended. In the ONTARGET study (Ongoing Telmisartan Alone and in Combination with Ramipril Global Endpoint Trial), the combination of the 2 drugs was associated with more adverse events without an increased benefit. For these reasons, addition of losartan is incorrect.

Regarding fibrates (Answer A) and/or statin therapy and the risk of diabetic retinopathy in patients with diabetes, the data are too weak to conclude there are clear benefits, and no properly powered studies definitively demonstrate benefits. A systematic review identified 8 randomized controlled trials with limited methodologic quality that assessed the effects of fibrates and/or statins on diabetic retinopathy. Based on these findings, the effects of statins for this purpose are uncertain. Fibrates seemed to reduce the incidence of macular edema (low certainty evidence) without increasing adverse events (low- to very low-certainty evidence). Most limited data are derived from patients with type 2 diabetes. Presently, there is not strong evidence to initiate fibrate therapy to treat retinopathy in patients with type 1 diabetes, and it is not indicated in this patient whose triglyceride level is only mildly elevated.

While some data describe benefits of fenofibrate on retinopathy (Effects of Long-Term Fenofibrate Therapy on Cardiovascular Events in 9795 People with Type 2 Diabetes [FIELD] and Effects of Medical Therapies on Retinopathy Progression in Type 2 Diabetes [ACCORD]), these studies were conducted in patients with type 2 diabetes. In the FIELD study, fenofibrate (200 mg daily) reduced the requirements for laser therapy and prevented disease progression in patients with preexisting diabetic retinopathy. In the ACCORD eye study, fenofibrate

(160 mg daily) with simvastatin (compared with simvastatin alone) resulted in a 40% reduction in the odds of retinopathy progressing over 4 years. The relevancy of these findings for younger patients and for those with type 1 diabetes remains uncertain.

Given that this patient currently has very well-controlled diabetes, switching to insulin pump therapy (Answer C), while perhaps a good consideration down the road, is not warranted and would certainly not improve the acute worsening of her diabetic retinopathy in the near-term.

Educational Objective

Explain how clinically significant, acute improvements in glycemic control may increase the risk of developing or worsening microvascular complications, including retinopathy.

Reference(s)

Bain SC, Klufas MA, Ho A, Matthews DR. Worsening of diabetic retinopathy with rapid improvement in systemic glucose control: a review. *Diabetes Obes Metab.* 2019;21(3):454-466. PMID: 30226298

Hooymans JM, Ballegooie EV, Schweitzer NM, Doorebos H, Reitsma WD, Slutter WJ. Worsening of diabetic retinopathy with strict control of blood sugar. *Lancet.* 1982;2(8295):438. PMID: 6124825

Early worsening of diabetic retinopathy in the Diabetes Control and Complications Trial. *Arch Ophthalmol.* 1998;116(7):874-886. PMID: 9682700

ONTARGET Investigators; Yusuf S, Teo KK, et al. Telmisartan, ramipril, or both in patients at high risk for vascular events. *N Engl J Med.* 2008;358(15):1547-1559. PMID: 18378520

Mozetic V, Pacheco RL, de Oliveira Cruz Latorraca C, Riera R. Statins and/or fibrates for diabetic retinopathy: a systematic review and meta-analysis. *Diabetol Metab Syndr.* 2019;11:92. PMID: 31719846

Wang B, Wang F, Zhang Y, et al. Effects of RAS inhibitors on diabetic retinopathy: a systematic review and meta-analysis. *Lancet Diabetes Endocrinol.* 2015;3(4):263-274. PMID: 25660574

Keech AC, Mitchell P, Summanen PA, et al. Effect of fenofibrate on the need for laser treatment for diabetic retinopathy (FIELD study): a randomised controlled trial. *Lancet.* 2007;370(9600):1687-1697. PMID: 17988728

ACCORD Study Group; ACCORD Eye Study Group; Chew EY, et al. Effects of medical therapies on retinopathy progression in type 2 diabetes. *N Engl J Med.* 2010;363(3):233-244. PMID: 20587587

6 ANSWER: C) Macimorelin-stimulation test after stopping amitriptyline

Traumatic brain injury (TBI) is a frequent cause of disability. While the highest prevalence of TBI is observed in young male patients, TBI can occur at any age. TBI is recognized as a common cause of hypopituitarism, which may manifest clinically several years after the traumatic event. Typically, MRI of the pituitary gland does not show any obvious abnormality. Another often unrecognized cause of hypopituitarism with normal appearance on MRI is subarachnoid hemorrhage.

While hypopituitarism can be transient in the first few months after the acute event, it is generally believed that hypopituitarism is permanent if it is diagnosed more than 1 year after the event. While TBI-induced hypopituitarism can vary in presentation, GH is the most commonly affected anterior pituitary hormone (with prevalence up to 25% in some studies), followed by gonadotropins, TSH, and ACTH. This patient has normal morning cortisol and free T_4 levels and is still menstruating. Therefore, her pituitary function is otherwise normal, but GH deficiency cannot be completely ruled out by a normal IGF-1 concentration (thus, Answer E is incorrect). Indeed, up to 25% of women and up to 50% of men with proven GH deficiency have normal levels of serum IGF-1. The only way to rule out GH deficiency in such patients is to perform a GH-stimulation test. While insulin-induced hypoglycemia test (not offered as an option here) is considered the gold standard to diagnose GH deficiency, it is not done in many centers because of the need for close medical supervision. Additionally, it has some contraindications (older age, history of seizure, and history of coronary artery disease). Most GH-stimulation tests are significantly affected by BMI. This is particularly true for the glucagon-stimulation test (Answer B). Current guidelines define the GH cutoff for glucagon-stimulation testing as 3 ng/mL (3 µg/L) in patients with a BMI less than 25 kg/m^2 and 1 ng/mL (1 µg/L) in patients with a BMI greater than 30 kg/m^2. The cutoff is in a nonspecific range between 1 and 3 ng/mL (1 and 3 µg/L) for patients with a BMI between 25 and 30 kg/m^2, like the patient described in this vignette. Therefore, the interpretation of the test results would be challenging. Additionally, the glucagon-stimulation test is long (4 hours) and potentially unpleasant (nausea and vomiting may occur).

Arginine (Answer A) is a very poor GH stimulant in adults, and it should not be used by itself (regardless of whether the patient is on any medication). Arginine can be used in conjunction with GHRH, with cutoffs that are well established and BMI-dependent, but GHRH is not available in the United States, and this combination was not offered as an option in this vignette. Losartan would not affect GH response to arginine.

IGFBP-3 (Answer D) is a GH-dependent protein that binds IGF-1. Despite this, it is not helpful in the diagnosis of adult GH deficiency.

Macimorelin (Answer C), an orally absorbed nonpeptidic ghrelin receptor agonist, is a powerful stimulus of GH secretion. It can be used for GH-stimulation testing at the dose of 0.5 mg/kg. This test is relatively short (90 minutes) and well tolerated. Additionally, recent data suggest that the FDA-proposed GH cutoff (2.8 ng/mL [2.8 µg/L]) is not affected by BMI, at least up to 36 kg/m^2. Attention must be paid to drugs that increase the QT interval, as cases of QT-interval elongation have been observed during the macimorelin test. If possible, such medications (eg, amitriptyline in this case) should be discontinued before the test. If this is not possible, electrocardiography should be performed before the macimorelin test. One week after stopping amitriptyline, this patient underwent macimorelin testing, which showed a normal peak GH value (7.6 ng/mL [7.6 µg/L]), thus ruling out GH deficiency.

Educational Objective

Diagnose GH deficiency in an overweight patient.

Reference(s)

Yuen KCJ, Biller BMK, Radovick S, et al. American Association of Clinical Endocrinologists and American College of Endocrinology guidelines for management of growth hormone deficiency in adults and patients transitioning from pediatric to adult care. *Endocr Pract.* 2019;25(11):1191-1232. PMID: 31760824

Garcia JM, Biller BMK, Korbonits M, et al. Macimorelin as a diagnostic test for adult GH deficiency. *J Clin Endocrinol Metab.* 2018;103(8):3083-3093. PMID: 29860473

Garcia JM, Biller BMK, Korbonits M, et al. Sensitivity and specificity of the macimorelin test for diagnosis of AGHD. *Endocr Connect.* 2021;10(1):76-83. PMID: 33320108

Corneli G, Di Somma C, Prodam F, et al. Cut-off limits of the GH response to GHRH plus arginine test and IGF-I levels for the diagnosis of GH deficiency in late adolescents and young adults. *Eur J Endocrinol.* 2007;157(6):701-708. PMID: 18057376

Tan CL, Alavi SA, Baldeweg SE, et al. The screening and management of pituitary dysfunction following traumatic brain injury in adults: British Neurotrauma Group guidance. *J Neurol Neurosurg Psychiatry.* 2017;88(11):971-981. PMID: 28860331

7 ANSWER: A) Discontinue basal insulin and monitor blood glucose values only

Roux-en-Y gastric bypass can produce excellent outcomes for patients with type 2 diabetes. The STAMPEDE trial showed significant improvement in glycemic control 5 years after bariatric surgery (sleeve gastrectomy or Roux-en-Y gastric bypass) when compared with standard medical management. Improvements in glycemic control occur early after gastric bypass surgery, often in the immediate postoperative period before any weight loss has been achieved. As patients lose weight, blood glucose control tends to improve further. Most patients reach their nadir weight 12 to 18 months after gastric bypass surgery, while maximum improvement in hemoglobin A_{1c} occurs about 12 months after surgery.

Adjusting diabetes medications in the postoperative period is largely dependent on the results of blood glucose monitoring. In this particular patient who has experienced greatly improved glycemic control and ongoing weight loss, the most appropriate step is to discontinue treatment for diabetes and continue monitoring blood glucose values (Answer A). Nothing in the clinical vignette suggests that she has type 1 diabetes or is insulinopenic.

Several mechanisms account for improved glycemic control following bariatric surgery. Calorie restriction, as occurs immediately in the postoperative period, improves hepatic insulin sensitivity. A hypocaloric diet similar to that seen after Roux-en-Y gastric bypass in patients with type 2 diabetes improves endogenous glucose production and β-cell function. In the longer term, factors related to bile-acid metabolism, incretin hormones, intestinal nutrient sensitivity, and other forms of intestinal adaptation have all been postulated to influence diabetes remission.

The likelihood of achieving remission of type 2 diabetes after bariatric surgery is dependent on the degree of weight loss achieved, preoperative duration of diabetes, and presurgical treatment. The latter is relevant if the patient is taking high doses of insulin, suggesting limited β-cell reserve. Scoring systems can help predict the likelihood of diabetes remission following Roux-en-Y gastric bypass. For example, the externally validated DiaRem clinical predictive score uses 4 preoperative clinical variables (age, hemoglobin A_{1c}, other diabetes medications, and treatment with insulin) to predict the probability of diabetes remission after Roux-en-Y gastric bypass. An alternative scoring system (which has not been externally validated) called the Diabetes Surgical Score uses BMI, C-peptide concentration, type 2 diabetes duration, and patient age to construct a multidimensional 10-point scale along which greater scores indicate a better chance of diabetes remission. Using a scoring system may predict the likelihood of diabetes remission after Roux-en-Y gastric bypass with moderate accuracy, and it can help guide shared decision-making when a patient with diabetes is contemplating bariatric surgery.

Continuing insulin (Answers C, D, and E), even at a reduced dosage, would put the patient at risk of developing hypoglycemia, as she is anticipated to lose more weight and improve glycemic control further. If she does eventually develop elevated blood glucose concentrations, metformin could be reintroduced (Answer B), but it is not necessary now. The patient should continue to monitor blood glucose levels periodically to determine if the addition of pharmacotherapy is warranted.

Educational Objective

Guide the cessation of antidiabetes medications after bariatric surgery in a patient in the active weight-loss phase.

Reference(s)

Schauer PR, Bhatt DL, Kirwan JP. Bariatric surgery or intensive medical therapy for diabetes - 5-year outcomes. *N Engl J Med.* 2017;376(7):641-651. PMID: 28199805

Sathananthan M, Shah M, Edens KL, et al. Six and 12 weeks of caloric restriction increases β cell function and lowers fasting and postprandial glucose concentrations in people with type 2 diabetes. *J Nutr.* 2015;145(9):2046-2051. PMID: 26246321

Laferrere B, Teixeira J, McGinty J, et al. Effect of weight loss by gastric bypass surgery versus hypocaloric diet on glucose and incretin levels in patients with type 2 diabetes. *J Clin Endocrinol Metab.* 2008;93(7):2479-2485. PMID: 18430778

Hamza N, Abbas MH, Darwish A, Shafeek Z, New J, Ammori BJ. Predictors of remission of type 2 diabetes mellitus after laparoscopic gastric banding and bypass. *Surg Obes Relat Dis.* 2011;7(6):691-696. PMID: 20688578

8 ANSWER: C) Prescribe risedronate

Aromatase inhibitors reduce breast cancer recurrence and are used in premenopausal women who have undergone oophorectomy or are prescribed GnRH agonist therapy, as well as in postmenopausal women. These medications have profound adverse effects, including reduced bone density and increased fracture risk. Aromatase inhibitors block the conversion of the precursor testosterone to estrogen. As in menopause, a decline in circulating estrogens increases osteoclastogenesis and augments osteoblast apoptosis, leading to an overall decrease in bone mineral density.

Bisphosphonates reduce bone loss in postmenopausal women treated with aromatase inhibitors. Since the effects of aromatase inhibitors are so profound, the threshold for treating low bone mass is lower. Thus, recommending no therapy (Answer E) is incorrect. Two expert consensus guidelines have been published that recommend, in addition to calcium and vitamin D supplementation, prescribing a bisphosphonate for postmenopausal women taking an aromatase inhibitor who have a spine or hip T-score less than –2.0. Thus, the best next step in managing this patient's osteopenia is prescribing risedronate (Answer C).

Denosumab (Answer A) is an option as well, but given the cost and consequences of missed doses, this is not the initial best option.

Due to the theoretical risk of osteosarcoma, teriparatide (Answer D) would be contraindicated for this patient because she has received external-beam radiation that unavoidably targets the rib cage. There also remains theoretical concern that anabolic therapy, by increasing bone turnover and proliferative factors in the bone marrow that may fuel bone metastasis cancer growth, may activate dormant breast cancer cells in bone.

Raloxifene (Answer B) would also not be recommended because this selective estrogen receptor modulator has not been well studied in combination with aromatase inhibitors in women with breast cancer.

Educational Objective

Manage low bone mass in a woman with breast cancer who is being treated with an aromatase inhibitor.

Reference(s)

Eastell R, Hannon RA, Cuzick J, Dowsett M, Clack G, Adams JE, ATAC Trialists' Group. Effect of an aromatase inhibitor on BMD and bone turnover markers: 2-year results of the anastrozole, tamoxifen, alone or in combination (ATAC) trial (18233230). *J Bone Miner Res.* 2006;21(8):1215-1223. PMID: 16869719

Markopoulos C, Tzoracoleftherakis E, Polychronis A, et al. Management of anastrozole-induced bone loss in breast cancer patients with oral risedronate: results from the ARBI prospective clinical trial. *Breast Cancer Res.* 2010;12(2):R24. PMID: 20398352

Greenspan SL, Brufsky A, Lembersky BC, et al. Risedronate prevents bone loss in breast cancer survivors: a 2-year, randomized, double-blind, placebo-controlled clinical trial. *J Clin Oncol.* 2008;26(16):2644-2652. PMID: 18427147

Van Poznak C, Hannon RA, Mackey JR, et al. Prevention of aromatase inhibitor-induced bone loss using risedronate: the SABRE trial. *J Clin Oncol.* 2010;28(6):967-975. PMID: 20065185

Reid DM, Doughty J, Eastell R, et al. Guidance for the management of breast cancer treatment-induced bone loss: a consensus position statement from a UK Expert Group. *Cancer Treat Rev.* 2008;34(Suppl 1):S3-S18. PMID: 18515009

Hadji P, Aapro MS, Body J-J, et al. Management of aromatase inhibitor-associated bone loss (AIBL) in postmenopausal women with hormone sensitive breast cancer: joint position statement of the IOF, CABS, ECTS, IEG, ESCEO IMS, and SIOG. *J Bone Oncol.* 2017;7:1-12. PMID: 28413771

9 ANSWER: A) Change the correction factor to 1:70

Patients with type 1 diabetes typically require a total daily insulin dose of 0.4 to 1.0 unit/kg (most commonly 0.5 to 0.7 units/kg). If endogenous function is still present at the time of diagnosis, initial insulin requirements may be low but increase over time with ongoing destruction of the β-islet cells. Patients who are very active and/or are at their ideal body weight typically require less insulin than patients with a BMI greater than 25 kg/m^2. Insulin requirements are also often increased during puberty and illness. Persons with a lower BMI or optimized BMI are often very sensitive and responsive to insulin, and thus may be at high risk for hypoglycemia with even small amounts of excess insulin compared with needs, such as illustrated in this vignette.

Recent American Diabetes Association guidelines continue to highlight that most patients with type 1 diabetes should be treated with multiple daily injections of prandial and basal insulin or continuous subcutaneous insulin infusion and that patients with type 1 diabetes should receive education on how to match prandial insulin doses to carbohydrate intake, premeal blood glucose, and anticipated physical activity. Basal insulin suppresses glucose production in the liver while insulin with food consumption stimulates peripheral glucose uptake and inhibits hepatic glucose output. The International Society for Pediatric and Adolescent Diabetes and the American Diabetes Association recommend that basal insulin account for 30% to 50% of the total daily insulin dose. However, as more data become available from partial hybrid closed-loop systems, it is apparent that basal insulin commonly accounts for closer to 30% and that "overbasalization" is a frequent issue.

When initiating insulin, traditional teaching is to start at 0.5 unit/kg with 50% of the total daily dose of insulin as basal and 50% as prandial. The calculated total daily insulin dose is used to determine the sensitivity or to predict how much glucose will drop with administration of 1 unit of insulin. This is commonly referred to as insulin sensitivity or the correction factor. Insulin sensitivity is calculated as: 1500 to 2200 mg/dL / total daily dose (most commonly 1500-1800 mg/dL). The *American Diabetes Association/JDRF Type 1 Diabetes Sourcebook* provides detailed information on intensification of therapy to meet individualized needs.

In this patient's case, the clinician must recognize his sensitivity to insulin given his low BMI (19.4 kg/m^2) and also his increased activity as an athlete. His predicted total daily insulin dose is:

0.5 unit/kg × 61.2 kg = 30 units

He currently takes only 10 units of basal insulin, so reducing the basal insulin dose (Answer E) is incorrect, especially because in the fasting state, his glucose concentration is stable and does not decline. To estimate an insulin-to-carbohydrate ratio, the following formula can be used: 450 to 500/total daily dose of insulin. However, this formula is based on little evidence, and in practice carbohydrate rates are often selected conservatively and then titrated by clinical effect. If this calculation is performed using his current total daily dose, then 450 to 500 / 25 indicates 1 unit per 18 to 20 g carbohydrate, which is appropriate. Thus, changing his insulin-to-carbohydrate ratio (Answer B) is not the best step. However, his predicted sensitivity or correction is estimated at 60 to 72 (using 1500/25 or 1800/25). Given his recurrent hypoglycemia during the day, the best next step is to change the correction factor to 1:70 (Answer A).

Given his overall low insulin requirements and sensitivity, recognizing that he may benefit from an insulin delivery device that allows for 0.5 units of insulin to be dispensed is also important. His correctional scale may be even better optimized by administering 0.5 unit per 35 mg/dL glucose instead of 1 unit per 18 mg/dL glucose; this can be achieved by using junior insulin pens, junior insulin syringes, "smart pens," and insulin pumps, all of which allow for this microdelivery.

Changing his correctional goal to 150 mg/dL before exercise or adjusting mealtime insulin to 1 less than the predicted dose needed for carbohydrate intake before activity may also help him avoid hypoglycemia, but neither strategy was a choice. Neither "feeding" the insulin on board by eating a snack every 2 hours (Answer C) nor counseling against exercise (Answer D) is the best way to avoid hypoglycemia when the appropriate change would be to adjust the amount of insulin administered.

Educational Objective

Identify patients who are sensitive to insulin and calculate their correction/sensitivity to insulin.

Reference(s)

American Diabetes Association. 9. Pharmacologic approaches to glycemic treatment: standards of medical care in diabetes-2021. *Diabetes Care.* 2021;44(Suppl 1):S111-S124. PMID: 33298420

Rasmussen VF, Vestergaard ET, Schwandt A, et al. Proportion of basal to total insulin dose is associated with metabolic control, body mass index, and treatment modality in children with type 1 diabetes-a cross-sectional study with data from the International SWEET Registry. *J Pediatr.* 2019;215:216-222.e1. PMID: 31345576

Peters A, Laffel L, Chiang JL. *American Diabetes Association/JDRF Type 1 Diabetes Sourcebook.* 1st ed. American Diabetes Association. 2013.

Hirsch IB. Type 1 diabetes mellitus and the use of flexible insulin regimens. *Am Fam Physician.* 1999;60(8):2343-2352. PMID: 10593324

10 **ANSWER: B) Measure progesterone by liquid chromatography–tandem mass spectrometry**

Congenital adrenal hyperplasia (CAH) due to 21-hydroxylase deficiency is one of the most common autosomal recessive diseases. More severe enzyme deficiency results in classic CAH with adrenal insufficiency and ambiguous genitalia in females. Nonclassic CAH, which is not associated with adrenal insufficiency, is more common than classic CAH. In the US White population, the prevalence of nonclassic CAH may be as high as 1 in 200. Nonclassic CAH can present with symptoms similar to those of polycystic ovary syndrome, as in this vignette (eg, menstrual irregularity, hirsutism, and/or infertility). Increased androgen production results from an increase in adrenal gland stimulation needed to maintain normal glucocorticoid and mineralocorticoid production when 21-hydroxylase conversion of 17 hydroxyprogesterone to 11-deoxycortisol is impaired.

The management of hirsutism in adult women with nonclassic CAH is the same as management of hirsutism in women without CAH. Glucocorticoids are not recommended to manage hirsutism because women are more likely to experience weight gain and even glucose intolerance at the dosages needed to suppress androgens. Although reduced fertility rates are reported in women with CAH, this is in part due to fewer women trying to conceive, as pregnancy rates can be as high as 60% to 80%. Only 10% to 25% of women with CAH try to conceive. Numerous factors contribute to decreased desire to conceive, such as anatomical considerations (eg, vaginal stenosis, suboptimal surgical reconstruction) and anxiety regarding body image and sexual function. Two retrospective studies found that most pregnancies in this patient population occurred prior to the mother's diagnosis of nonclassic CAH. Hydrocortisone treatment was used to improve fertility in 23% of participants who became pregnant in 1 study and in 42% of participants in another study. These 2 studies also reported fewer miscarriage rates in those receiving hydrocortisone, although a different study reported no difference in miscarriage rates but a shorter time to conception with hydrocortisone. Therefore, glucocorticoid treatment is not necessary for women with nonclassic CAH to conceive, but it might be considered for women with nonclassic CAH who present with infertility, as in this case.

Glucocorticoid replacement in nonclassic CAH prevents the increased release of ACTH to more effectively decrease 17-hydroxyprogesterone, androgen, and progesterone concentrations that interfere with ovulation and implantation. In women with classic CAH, longer-acting glucocorticoids such as prednisone or prednisolone might be prescribed at night, especially if patients are trying to conceive. Longer-acting glucocorticoids help to lower follicular-phase progesterone (ideally <0.6 ng/mL [<2 nmol/L]), which has been shown to increase the likelihood of pregnancy. Luteal-phase progesterone (Answer C) can indicate ovulatory cycles when the concentration is greater than 3 ng/mL (>9.5 nmol/L), but its measurement would not be useful in this case when embryo transfer is being planned.

When sex steroid values are not consistent with patient symptoms, measurement by liquid chromatography–tandem mass spectrometry (LC-MS/MS) (Answer B) should be considered. Steroid hormone structural similarity reduces specificity of immunoassays when cross-reactivity with hormones structurally related to the hormone being measured leads to falsely elevated measurements. LC-MS/MS has very high specificity and the ability to discriminate among steroid hormones. Immunoassays, however, have the advantage of shorter time for preparation and results, which is better for evaluating patients before fertility treatments.

In this case, progesterone continued to rise despite higher doses of prednisolone that should have suppressed morning ACTH and stimulation of adrenal progesterone production. The high 17-hydroxyprogesterone concentrations increase the possibility of cross-reactivity, falsely increasing the immunoassay results, and this was confirmed by LC-MS/MS. The concentration of progesterone retested by LC-MS/MS was found to be 1.1 ng/mL (3.5 nmol/L). Her prednisolone dosage was increased to 10 mg daily and the subsequent progesterone concentration by LC-MS/MS was 0.55 ng/mL (1.7 nmol/L). 17-Hydroxyprogesterone does not need to be normalized when treating adults with CAH, regardless of whether they are trying to conceive, as this tends to lead to glucocorticoid overtreatment. Thus, increasing the prednisolone dosage to further decrease 17-hydroxyprogesterone (Answer A) is not appropriate.

Switching glucocorticoid to dexamethasone (Answer E) in women with CAH can prevent virilization of a female fetus because it is not inactivated by placental 11β-hydroxysteroid dehydrogenase type II and can suppress fetal ACTH and potentially decrease the likelihood that genital surgery will be needed. However, treatment is recommended only in the context of research trials because of the controversy regarding the potential treatment of unaffected fetuses before knowing the sex and genotype of the fetus and the unknown long-term effects of high-dosage dexamethasone. For suppression of progesterone, prednisolone would be a better choice because it is less likely to cause adverse effects and would not affect the fetus, as it is inactivated by the placenta.

Educational Objective

Identify pregnancy goals and treatment considerations, including challenges in assay interpretation in women with nonclassic congenital adrenal hyperplasia.

Reference(s)

Speiser P, Azziz R, Baskin L, et al; Endocrine Society. Congenital adrenal hyperplasia due to steroid 21-hydroxylase deficiency: an Endocrine Society clinical practice guideline. *J Clin Endocrinol Metab.* 2010;95(9):4133-4160. PMID: 20823466

Carmina E, Dewailly D, Escobar-Morreale HF, et al. Non-classic congenital adrenal hyperplasia due to 21-hydroxylase deficiency revisited: an update with a special focus on adolescent and adult women. *Hum Reprod Update.* 2017;23(5):580-599. PMID: 28582566

Moran C, Azziz R, Weintrob N, Witchel SF, et al. Reproductive outcome of women with 21-hydroxylase-deficient nonclassic adrenal hyperplasia. *J Clin Endocrinol Metab.* 2006;91(9):3451-3456. PMID: 16822826

Bidet M, Bellanné-Chantelot C, Galand-Portier MB, et al. Fertility in women with nonclassical congenital adrenal hyperplasia due to 21-hydroxylase deficiency. *J Clin Endocrinol Metab.* 2010;95(3):1182-1190. PMID: 20080854

Eyal O, Ayalon-Dangur I, Segev-Becker A, et al. Pregnancy in women with nonclassic congenital adrenal hyperplasia: time to conceive and outcome. *Clin Endocrinol (Oxf).* 2017;87(5):552-556. PMID: 28731586

Schiffer L, Adaway JE, Baranowski ES, Arlt W, Keevil BG. A novel high-throughput assay for the measurement of salivary progesterone by liquid chromatography tandem mass spectrometry. *Ann Clinical Biochem.* 2018;56(1):64-71. PMID: 29792048

11 ANSWER: E) Discontinue lisinopril when conception is confirmed; initiate extended-release nifedipine

ACE inhibitors and angiotensin receptor blockers are clearly contraindicated during the second and third trimesters of pregnancy due to the occurrence of a fetopathy characterized by underdeveloped calvarium, renal dysplasia, pulmonary hypoplasia, intrauterine growth restriction, and/or oligohydramnios. However, ACE inhibitors are prescribed in up to 40% of reproductive-aged women who are treated for hypertension, per one NHANES survey. To address the question of whether first-trimester exposure to ACE inhibitors results in congenital malformations, Bateman et al examined a cohort of more than 1 million pregnancies linked to liveborn neonates from Medicaid claims between 2000 and 2010, of which 4107 were exposed to ACE inhibitors during the first trimester. After controlling for confounders, there was no increased risk of congenital malformations. In the absence of a well-controlled trial, this is the largest study to address this question. Thus, the 2022 American Diabetes Association standards of medical care suggest that ACE inhibitors, angiotensin receptor blockers, and statins be stopped at conception. Lisinopril does not need to be discontinued until conception is confirmed (thus, Answers A, B, and C are incorrect). In women of reproductive age, ACE inhibitors and angiotensin receptor blockers should be used after having a discussion regarding risks and benefits, particularly if contraceptives are not being used.

Antihypertensive medications that are considered safe and effective in pregnancy include labetalol, methyldopa, long-acting nifedipine, diltiazem, clonidine, and prazosin. Of these, it appears that the former 3 are most preferred by authors for management of chronic hypertension. Atenolol (Answers B and D) is specifically discouraged because of demonstrated adverse neonatal effects, including bradycardia and hypoglycemia. Diuretics are generally not preferred because of reduced placental blood flow. Of the listed choices, the best strategy for this patient is to discontinue lisinopril at conception and prescribe extended-release nifedipine (Answer E).

A clinical point is that blood pressure is normally lower during pregnancy. While there are few randomized controlled trials regarding the use of antihypertensive agents in pregnant individuals who have diabetes, the target blood pressure is 110-135/85 mm Hg in pregnant women who have diabetes and chronic hypertension to prevent severe maternal hypertension and to minimize impaired fetal growth.

Educational Objective

Advise patients with preexisting diabetes mellitus and hypertension regarding treatment during pregnancy.

Reference(s)

American Diabetes Association Professional Practice Committee; American Diabetes Association. Professional Practice Committee; et al. 15. Management of diabetes in pregnancy: standards of medical care in diabetes-2022. *Diabetes Care.* 2022;45(Supplement_1):S232–S243 PMID: 34964864

Bateman BT, Patorno E, Desai RJ, et al. Angiotensin-converting enzyme inhibitors and the risk of congenital malformations. *Obstet Gynecol.* 2017;129(1):174-184. PMID: 27926639

12 ANSWER: D) Primary adrenal insufficiency due to tuberculosis

This patient has symptoms (abdominal pain, nausea, vomiting, and weight loss) and electrolyte abnormalities (hyponatremia, hyperkalemia) suggestive of adrenal insufficiency. Adrenal insufficiency must be promptly suspected in any patient with a similar clinical presentation. Failure to recognize and treat decompensated adrenal insufficiency can be fatal. Without a preestablished diagnosis, adrenal insufficiency may be missed because its clinical features are nonspecific. This patient's initial evaluation focused on her gastrointestinal symptoms and included abdominal imaging before hormonal testing. She has bilateral calcification of her adrenal glands. The differential diagnosis for adrenal calcifications includes tuberculosis, histoplasmosis, old hemorrhage, pheochromocytoma, adrenal cortical carcinoma, neuroblastoma, teratoma, and metastasis. This patient, who presents with bilateral adrenal calcifications, suspected adrenal insufficiency, electrolyte abnormalities, and history of frequent travel to India, had a positive test for tuberculosis (Answer D). The tuberculostatic drug rifampicin is a CYP3A4 inducer, and it increases the metabolism of hydrocortisone. Consequently, in patients treated with rifampin, higher than physiological dosages of hydrocortisone are necessary.

Adrenal cortical carcinoma (Answer A) and pheochromocytoma (Answer B) are usually unilateral. Approximately 60% of adrenal carcinomas produce cortical hormones in excess (most often cortisol and androgens), and pheochromocytomas produce catecholamines. Both tumors can cause hypertension; this patient had low-normal blood pressure.

Bilateral adrenal hemorrhage (Answer C) can present with adrenal insufficiency and calcifications. Risk factors for adrenal hemorrhage include anticoagulant/antithrombotic therapy, thromboembolic disease, hypercoagulable disorders, physical trauma, and sepsis, particularly meningococcemia (Waterhouse-Friderichsen syndrome), none of which were present in this patient.

Long-term use of opioids can cause secondary adrenal insufficiency (Answer E), and the risk increases with higher dosages. Oxycodone, 5 mg (morphine equivalent dose = 7.5) taken sporadically has a low likelihood of causing adrenal insufficiency. Hyponatremia can occur in secondary and tertiary adrenal insufficiency and is caused by inappropriate increase in vasopressin secretion or action due to cortisol deficiency. However, hyperkalemia is not present because aldosterone synthesis remains normal, as it is regulated via the renin-angiotensin system.

Educational Objective

Identify causes of adrenal calcifications in a patient with adrenal insufficiency.

Reference(s)

Consul N, Venkatesan AM, Blair KJ, et al. Calcified adrenal lesions: pattern recognition approach on computed tomography with pathologic correlation. *J Comput Assist Tomogr.* 2020;44(2):178-187. PMID: 32195796

Hahner S, Ross RJ, Arlt W, et al. Adrenal insufficiency. *Nat Rev Dis Primers.* 2021;7(1):19. PMID: 33707469

13 **ANSWER: C) Obtain comprehensive metabolic panel**

This patient has the sensation of a neck lump, and neck ultrasonography has revealed a hypoechoic lesion below her left thyroid lobe. She also has a history of kidney stones. These findings should raise the possibility of a parathyroid adenoma rather than a thyroid nodule. Parathyroid adenomas can cause primary hyperparathyroidism, which leads to hypercalcemia. Therefore, a comprehensive metabolic panel (Answer C) should be ordered.

Parathyroid glands are located behind the thyroid gland, and they regulate the serum calcium concentration. Commonly, there are 2 superior parathyroid glands and 2 inferior parathyroid glands, but sometimes individuals have supernumerary glands or fewer than 4 parathyroid glands. The superior parathyroid glands are derived from the fourth pharyngeal pouch and are located near the posterolateral aspect of the superior pole of the thyroid. The inferior parathyroid glands are derived from the third pharyngeal pouch and are located near the inferior poles of the thyroid gland or thymus. A recent meta-analysis revealed that up to 16% of parathyroid glands are in an ectopic location such as the mediastinum, retropharyngeal/paraesophageal space, carotid sheath, and within the thyroid gland. The most common finding in a patient with a parathyroid adenoma is the presence of hypercalcemia in the context of primary hyperparathyroidism.

A normal parathyroid gland measures 5 × 3 × 1 mm, weighs approximately 40 to 50 mg, and is rarely identified by imaging. Neck ultrasonography can identify a parathyroid adenoma larger than 1 cm, although the accuracy of neck ultrasonography depends on examiner skill and experience. Parathyroid adenomas typically appear well circumscribed, oval- or bean-shaped, and homogeneously hypoechoic with respect to normal thyroid tissue. Neck ultrasonography can also identify an echogenic thyroid capsule separating the thyroid from the parathyroid gland. Parathyroid adenomas have high cellularity and low content of fatty tissue, which explains the hypoechogenicity. Furthermore, use of color Doppler is fundamental in identifying parathyroid adenomas because of possible detection of a feeding artery (branch of the inferior thyroid artery) that enters the adenoma by one of its poles and distributes toward the periphery. This pattern is also called "vascular arch," and it can help distinguish an adenoma from an enlarged lymph node in which the vascularity is usually in the hilum.

Preoperative localization of parathyroid adenomas is essential for minimally invasive parathyroid surgery, which has become the preferred surgical intervention. In addition to neck ultrasonography, other imaging modalities can be used to identify parathyroid adenomas such as parathyroid scintigraphy (sestamibi SPECT/CT), neck CT, and neck MRI. In recent years, 4-dimensional CT has emerged to localize parathyroid adenomas preoperatively in patients with primary hyperparathyroidism. In a recent single-institution retrospective study, the use of parathyroid 4-dimensional CT was superior to sestamibi SPECT/CT in preoperative localization of parathyroid adenomas in patients with primary hyperparathyroidism. The diagnostic performance did not improve with the combination of these 2 imaging modalities compared with the performance of parathyroid 4-dimensional CT alone.

This patient's thyroid gland seems homogeneous and does not have characteristics of Hashimoto thyroiditis. Therefore, measurement of TPO antibodies (Answer B) is not indicated. The patient's neck lump sensation cannot be explained by this thyroid ultrasonography finding and this is a common scenario in clinical practice. Furthermore, FNA biopsy is not routinely performed for parathyroid adenomas.

An ^{123}I thyroid scan (Answer E) is usually performed in patients with suppressed TSH, but this patient's TSH concentration is within the reference range.

Serum thyroglobulin (Answer A) is measured in the follow-up of patients with thyroid cancer or in patients with thyrotoxicosis to delineate the cause. However, this patient has neither of these indications.

In this vignette, neck CT (Answer D) would not provide more information about the hypoechoic lesion than could be ascertained with neck ultrasonography.

Educational Objective

Identify the characteristics of a parathyroid adenoma on neck ultrasonography.

Reference(s)

Taterra D, Wong LM, Vikse J, et al. The prevalence and anatomy of parathyroid glands: a meta-analysis with implications for parathyroid surgery. *Langenbecks Arch Surg.* 2019;404(1):63-70. PMID: 30762091

Rickes S, Sitzy J, Neye H, Ocran KW, Wermke W. High-resolution ultrasound in combination with color-Doppler sonography for preoperative localization of parathyroid adenomas in patients with primary hyperparathyroidism. *Ultraschall Med.* 2003;24(2):85-89. PMID: 12698372

Ulanovski D, Feinmesser R, Cohen M, Sulkes J, Dudkiewicz M, Shpitzer T. Preoperative evaluation of patients with parathyroid adenoma: role of high-resolution ultrasonography. *Head Neck.* 2002;24(1):1-5. PMID: 11774396

Yeh R, Tay Y-KD, Tabacco G, et al. Diagnostic performance of 4D CT and sestamibi SPECT/CT in localizing parathyroid adenomas in primary hyperparathyroidism. *Radiology.* 2019;291(2):469-476. PMID: 30835187

14 ANSWER: C) Switch to denosumab

This postmenopausal woman has severe osteoporosis (very low T-scores and a right hip fragility fracture) in the setting of prior gastrointestinal intolerance to an oral bisphosphonate. Her regimen was recently switched to abaloparatide, a PTHrP analogue used as an osteoanabolic agent in the treatment of osteoporosis, and she has developed dizziness, with orthostasis documented on physical examination. In a clinical trial of women with postmenopausal osteoporosis, the incidence of dizziness was higher in the abaloparatide group (10%) than in the placebo group (6%). The prescribing information for abaloparatide states that orthostatic hypotension may occur with abaloparatide and lists this as one of the warnings and precautions for this medication. This adverse effect typically occurs with the first few doses and within 4 hours of injection. Associated symptoms may include dizziness, palpitations, tachycardia, and/or nausea. For the first several doses, abaloparatide should be administered in a setting where the patient can sit or lie down if necessary. It is recommended to instruct patients to sit or lie down if symptoms develop after dose administration. In addition, it may be helpful to administer the dose at bedtime. Of note, orthostatic hypotension is also one of the possible short-term adverse effects of teriparatide (PTH 1-34) use.

Because this patient's dizziness has not resolved after 2 months of abaloparatide therapy, it would be best to switch her regimen to another agent to decrease her fall risk and improve her quality of life. Therefore, continuing abaloparatide (Answer A) is not the best choice. Simply discontinuing abaloparatide (Answer B) would not be appropriate, as her severe osteoporosis needs to be treated.

Raloxifene (Answer D) is a selective estrogen receptor modulator approved for the treatment of postmenopausal osteoporosis. However, it is considered a second-line agent because it only decreases the risk of vertebral fractures and has no effect on hip or other nonvertebral fracture risk. Switching to this agent would not be the best choice in this patient who is at high risk of future fracture, especially given her recent right hip fracture and low T-score in the left femoral neck. Similar to estrogen, safety concerns with raloxifene include an increased risk of venous thromboembolism.

Switching to zoledronic acid (Answer E), an intravenous bisphosphonate, would not be the best choice in this case given the patient's impaired kidney function. Zoledronic acid is contraindicated in the setting of chronic kidney disease with an estimated glomerular filtration rate less than 35 mL/min per 1.73 m^2.

Switching to denosumab (Answer C), which is a potent antiresorptive agent that is not excreted by the kidneys, would be the most appropriate recommendation for this patient. Denosumab is a fully human monoclonal antibody to the receptor activator of nuclear factor kappaB ligand (RANKL). By blocking the binding of RANKL to RANK, it reduces osteoclast formation, function, and survival, which results in decreased bone resorption and increased bone density. Denosumab is administered by subcutaneous injection once every 6 months. Because of emerging concerns about an increased risk of vertebral fracture after discontinuation of denosumab, a "drug holiday" would not be appropriate, and the need for indefinite administration of denosumab or switching to an alternative therapy, if possible, should be discussed with patients before its initiation. It is important to remember that denosumab may induce significant hypocalcemia in patients with kidney impairment; ensuring that patients maintain an adequate amount of calcium and vitamin D supplementation is critical to avoid this complication, especially with conditions that predispose to hypocalcemia such as chronic kidney disease or malabsorption syndromes. Denosumab should not be given to patients with preexisting hypocalcemia until it is corrected.

Romosozumab, a monoclonal antibody to sclerostin, is another approved treatment for postmenopausal osteoporosis, but it was not given as an option in this vignette. Romosozumab has a black box warning of the potential risk of myocardial infarction, stroke, and cardiovascular death and should not be initiated in patients who have had a myocardial infarction or stroke within the preceding year.

Educational Objective

Identify dizziness/hypotension as a possible adverse effect of abaloparatide therapy and recommend the most appropriate intervention.

Reference(s)

Miller PD, Hattersley G, Riis BJ, et al; ACTIVE Study Investigators. Effect of abaloparatide vs placebo on new vertebral fractures in postmenopausal women with osteoporosis: a randomized clinical trial [published correction appears in *JAMA.* 2017;317(4):442]. *JAMA.* 2016;316(7):722-733. PMID: 27533157

Bone HG, Wagman RB, Brandi ML, et al. 10 years of denosumab treatment in postmenopausal women with osteoporosis: results from the phase 3 randomised FREEDOM trial and open-label extension. *Lancet Diabetes Endocrinol.* 2017;5(7):513-523. PMID: 28546097

15 **ANSWER: D) Measurement of serum cortisol**

This patient presented with pituitary apoplexy in the setting of a previously diagnosed pituitary adenoma. T1-weighted MRI shows a bright mass compressing the optic chiasm, with a fluid-fluid level typical of recent hemorrhage. Pituitary apoplexy is an uncommon clinical syndrome secondary to abrupt hemorrhage or infarction of preexisting pituitary adenomas. Because pituitary apoplexy is the presenting event for most patients with this condition, it is difficult to determine its exact incidence in patients with pituitary adenomas. Pituitary apoplexy is estimated to be a complication for 1% to 10% of pituitary adenomas, especially nonfunctioning tumors. While it has been associated with many triggering factors, such as nonpituitary surgery, diabetic ketoacidosis, use of anticoagulation, COVID-19 infections, hypertensive crisis, and flying, the only convincing triggering event seems to be performance of pituitary dynamic testing. Additionally, patients with familial isolated pituitary adenoma syndrome due to pathogenic variants in the *AIP* gene seem to develop pituitary apoplexy more frequently than patients with sporadic adenomas, possibly due to rapid tumor growth.

The cardinal symptom of pituitary apoplexy is severe headache, typically of sudden onset, sometimes associated with visual disturbances or ocular nerve palsy. Treatment of apoplexy is not necessarily surgical, as cranial nerve palsy and headaches may resolve without surgical intervention. However, surgery is indicated when the patient has loss of consciousness or a significant visual field defect, as in this vignette.

While it is debated whether surgery must be done urgently or can be postponed for few days, the urgent issue in affected patients is the assessment (and treatment, if needed) of adrenal insufficiency. In this case, the patient has normal vital signs, and therefore there is time to assess his adrenal function by measuring serum cortisol (Answer D). Should the cortisol concentration be frankly low or nondiagnostic and/or should his vital signs deteriorate, intravenous glucocorticoids can be administered (Answer B). However, doing this as a first step would be incorrect, as it would prevent accurate assessment of his current adrenal function.

Intervening surgically (Answer E) before assessing the function of the hypothalamic-pituitary-adrenal axis would be incorrect.

Measuring prolactin after dilution (Answer C) is not needed in this case. Dilution is necessary to rule out the "hook effect," an event that occurs when the antigen concentration is so high that it overwhelms the assay, causing falsely low results. This typically happens in patients with giant prolactinomas. In this case, the patient's adenoma is not secreting prolactin, as the prolactin concentration was only borderline-elevated 5 years prior to this event, despite a sizable adenoma (2 cm) (consistent with hyperprolactinemia due to stalk compression). While low prolactin has been reported as being predictive of permanent hypopituitarism in patients with pituitary apoplexy, this is not the most urgent issue to address in this case.

Finally, optical coherence tomography (Answer A) can identify retinal nerve fiber layer loss in the eyes of patients with chiasmatic compression. While this test has a prognostic value in predicting visual outcomes after decompressive surgery, it would not be needed at this point, as the patient presented with obvious surgical indication (bitemporal hemianopsia). Therefore, optical coherence tomography would not be the most appropriate next step in this patient.

Educational Objective

Recommend the appropriate order of action in the management of pituitary apoplexy.

Reference(s)

Briet C, Salenave S, Bonneville JF, Laws ER, Chanson P. Pituitary apoplexy. *Endocr Rev.* 2015;36(6):622-645. PMID: 26414232

Abbara A, Clarke S, Eng PC, et al. Clinical and biochemical characteristics of patients presenting with pituitary apoplexy. *Endocr Connect.* 2018;7(10):1058-1066. PMID: 30139818

Baldeweg SE, Vanderpump M, Drake W, et al; Society for Endocrinology Clinical Committee. Society for Endocrinology Endocrine Emergency Guidance: emergency management of pituitary apoplexy in adult patients. *Endocr Connect.* 2016;5(5):G12-G15. PMID: 27935817

16 **ANSWER: D) Obtain and initiate a new supply of her existing insulin therapies**

Clinicians must recognize situations where the compromising of insulin therapy may be the etiology of suboptimal glycemic control. This is particularly true for patients not on insulin pump therapy for whom infusion set issues are a dominant reason. In this patient, an acute issue with her insulin supply should be suspected as the cause of unexpected decompensation in glycemic control. Thus, the most appropriate intervention is to obtain and initiate a new supply of her existing insulin therapies (Answer D) and observe the subsequent glycemic control. If an insulin supply issue is to blame, improvement in glycemia should be observed shortly after initiating a new supply of insulin.

Reasons for compromised insulin therapy include expired insulin (eg, patients trying to exhaust their insulin supply past the expiration date rather than throw it away) and exposure to extreme heat or cold (eg, left in car). Once the insulin product is punctured via needle, it is considered open. The insulin product can then be stored in the refrigerator or at room temperature; however, regardless of where it is stored, the expiration date specified by the manufacture still applies. The expiration date after opening of an insulin product is generally 30 days, but it can be shorter or longer for some insulins. This is an important matter to review with patients. In this vignette, given the patient's daily dose of 22 units of insulin glargine, the vial of insulin glargine could theoretically last 45 days, well beyond the manufacturer's stated limit of 28 days. Asking the patient whether she discards the insulin supply at 30 days, even if there is still insulin remaining in the vial, would be important. However, in this case, the patient's insulin supply was compromised by the boyfriend who was injecting water into the insulin vials to make her think the insulin was still in sufficient supply while he was using the money allocated for insulin prescription refills to purchase narcotics.

Checking other markers of glycemic control, such as glycated serum protein (fructosamine [Answer C], or 1,5-anhydroglucitol [Answer B]), can help identify inadequate glycemic control and the need for therapeutic adjustment in situations where the hemoglobin A_{1c} value may not be accurate. Fructosamine reflects the level of glycated serum proteins (mostly albumin). It has a shorter half-life of 2 to 3 weeks, whereas the half-life of hemoglobin A_{1c} is dependent on the lifecycle of a mature red blood cell in the circulation (100 to 120 days in a healthy individual). Thus, fructosamine measurement represents a shorter period of preceding blood glucose levels, and it responds more quickly to treatment (changes in blood glucose control) than does hemoglobin A_{1c}. Likewise, 1,5-anhydroglucitol can help identify suboptimal glycemic control in situations where the hemoglobin A_{1c} may not be accurate. 1,5-Anhydroglucitol is a validated marker of short-term glycemic control; blood concentrations of 1,5-anhydroglucitol decrease during hyperglycemia. It is a metabolically inert polyol that competes with glucose for reabsorption in the kidneys. Compared with hemoglobin A_{1c} or fructosamine, 1,5-anhydroglucitol more accurately reflects rapid changes in glycemia. In this case, there is no reason to suspect that hemoglobin A_{1c} is inaccurate, so assessing these additional markers is not warranted.

Referring this patient to counseling (Answer E) is not the most appropriate intervention, as she has had longstanding good glycemic control and has not historically expressed concerns of being overwhelmed with diabetes management.

GLP-1 receptor agonists (Answer A) are not approved for use in patients with type 1 diabetes. While some benefit could be expected and has been reported with liraglutide therapy, it would not be the best intervention at this time, even if off-label use were considered.

Educational Objective

Identify reasons for abrupt worsening of glycemic control in patients with longstanding optimally controlled diabetes when nonadherence is not the suspected etiology.

Reference(s)

Dungan KM. 1,5-anhydroglucitol (GlycoMark) as a marker of short-term glycemic control and glycemic excursions. *Expert Rev Mol Diagn.* 2008;8(1):9-19. PMID: 18088226

Radin MS. Pitfalls in hemoglobin A1c measurement: when results may be misleading. *J Gen Intern Med.* 2014;29(2):388-394. PMID: 24002631

Johnson RN, Metcalf PA, Baker JR. Fructosamine: a new approach to the estimation of serum glycosylprotein. An index of diabetic control. *Clin Chim Acta.* 1983;127(1):87-95. PMID: 6825313

Mathieu C, Zinman B, Hemmingsson JU, et al; ADJUNCT ONE Investigators. Efficacy and safety of liraglutide added to insulin treatment in type 1 diabetes: the ADJUNCT ONE Treat-To-Target Randomized Trial. *Diabetes Care.* 2016;39(10):1702-1710. PMID: 27506222

Ahrén B, Hirsch IB, Pieber TR, et al; ADJUNCT TWO Investigators. Efficacy and safety of liraglutide added to capped insulin treatment in subjects with type 1 diabetes: The ADJUNCT TWO Randomized Trial. *Diabetes Care.* 2016;39(10):1693-1701. PMID: 27493132

17 ANSWER: C) Measure serum free T_4

Mitotane is a steroidogenesis inhibitor and adrenolytic agent that is used in the medical treatment of adrenocortical cancer. The ideal therapeutic concentration of mitotane ranges from 14 to 20 mg/L. Mitotane leads to adrenal insufficiency with the need for glucocorticoid replacement at higher dosages (expected range of 30 to 100 mg hydrocortisone daily) compared with those typically required for primary adrenal insufficiency. Mitotane may in some cases affect mineralocorticoid synthesis and replacement with fludrocortisone is also needed. Other endocrine adverse effects can occur in the context of mitotane treatment. Partial central hypothyroidism has been observed with low free T_4, normal free T_3 and TSH, and impaired TSH response to thyrotropin-releasing hormone. In vitro studies using murine thyrotrope cell lines have demonstrated that this is not a laboratory artifact. Mitotane concentrations in the therapeutic range inhibit TSH secretion, block TSH response to thyrotropin-releasing hormone, and reduce cell viability. Given this patient's unexplained hyponatremia, possible symptoms of hypothyroidism (constipation and fatigue), and ongoing treatment with mitotane, diagnostic testing to evaluate for central hypothyroidism is needed by measuring serum free T_4 (Answer C). Mitotane therapy has been associated with other endocrine adverse effects, including hypercholesterolemia and male hypogonadism. Mitotane increases serum concentrations of most binding globulins, including SHBG, and is associated with a reduction in free testosterone levels. Mitotane is also a strong inhibitor of 5α-reductase activity.

There is no clinical indication to discontinue prednisone and restart intravenous hydrocortisone (Answer A) given that the patient is tolerating oral medications following resolution of her acute adrenal crisis.

Increasing the prednisone dosage (Answer B) is also not indicated. The patient is receiving higher than usual physiologic glucocorticoid replacement and split daily dosing to account for the increase in cortisol metabolism induced by mitotane. No symptoms are present that suggest insufficient glucocorticoid replacement, and orthostatic vital signs are normal.

Measuring serum tissue transglutaminase antibodies (Answer D) is not indicated given the absence of symptoms suggestive of celiac disease.

Performing CT of the abdomen and pelvis with contrast (Answer E) or another abdominal imaging study (ie, MRI) should be done at regular intervals to assess for disease progression, but imaging is not needed now and is unlikely to provide an explanation for the patient's symptoms and hyponatremia.

Educational Objective

Identify central hypothyroidism as a possible complication of mitotane treatment.

Reference(s)

Russo M, Scollo C, Pellegriti G, et al. Mitotane treatment in patients with adrenocortical cancer causes central hypothyroidism. *Clin Endocrinol (Oxf).* 2016;84(4):614-619. PMID: 26221968

18 ANSWER: B) Monomelic amyotrophy

This patient has well-controlled type 1 diabetes and slowly progressive neurologic (motor) symptoms in an upper extremity. This is not consistent with treatment-induced neuropathy of diabetes (Answer E), a small fiber neuropathy that can present with severe treatment-resistant pain and/or autonomic dysfunction. Treatment-induced neuropathy of diabetes presents acutely in patients who have rapid improvement in blood glucose (over 8 weeks) and reduction in hemoglobin A_{1c} of 2% or more in 3 months. This patient does not have a history of rapidly improving glycemic control, and he also does not have pain.

Myasthenia gravis (Answer C) is an autoimmune disease of neuromuscular transmission. About 60% of patients with myasthenia gravis present between ages 20 and 40 years. Affected patients can present with ocular symptoms (diplopia, ptosis), bulbar symptoms (dysphagia or dysphonia), limb involvement (weakness), and isolated respiratory involvement. Myasthenia gravis is less likely in this patient because of isolated limb weakness, as this is an uncommon finding and occurs in less than 5% of cases. The patient in this vignette did have serologic testing for acetylcholine receptor and muscle-specific tyrosine kinase antibodies, both of which were not elevated. Although seronegative myasthenia gravis is still possible, it is unlikely.

Stiff-person syndrome (Answer D) is a progressive disease that leads to muscle stiffness, rigidity, and spasm. It is thought to be an autoimmune process that affects GABAergic pathways. Affected individuals are usually between ages 20 and 50 years and often have an autoimmune condition. About 30% of affected individuals have type 1 diabetes; however, only 0.01% of persons with type 1 diabetes present with stiff-person syndrome. The patient in this vignette does not have stiffness or rigidity, making stiff-person syndrome unlikely.

Carpal tunnel syndrome (Answer A) is caused by median nerve (origin: brachial plexus C5-T1) compression as it courses through the carpal tunnel. Diabetes is a risk factor for carpal tunnel syndrome, and it should be considered in this patient. However, his lack of sensory abnormalities and predominant motor findings make this diagnosis less likely. Patients with carpal tunnel syndrome typically have pain and paresthesias (less commonly weakness) in the median nerve distribution, which includes sensory innervation to the thumb, index, middle, and half of the ring finger. It also includes motor innervation to thenar musculature.

This patient's presentation is most consistent with focal (ie, monomelic) amyotrophy (Answer B). The clinical presentation is focal atrophy and weakness, usually including 1 arm and hand, and lower extremities are rarely affected. A form of monomelic amyotrophy known as Hirayama disease is more common in individuals of East Asian origin and is rarely seen in western countries. Symptoms progress over 1 to 5 years and then stabilize. Cervical spine MRI is the imaging modality of choice, and it typically shows flattening of the spine in the neutral position and anterior displacement of dura in the flexed position. Repeated ischemia of the spinal cord, due to anterior displacement of dura during flexion, is thought to be the etiology of symptoms. There is no cure for this condition; a cervical brace might help stabilize neck, and physical and occupational therapy may be required. Surgery is rarely advised due to unclear benefit. This patient had MRI of the cervical spine and was noted to have characteristic findings of monomelic amyotrophy.

Educational Objective

Evaluate focal neuropathy in a patient with type 1 diabetes mellitus.

Reference(s)

Liao M-F, Chang H-S, Chang K-H, et al. Correlations of clinical, neuroimaging, and electrophysiological features in Hirayama disease. *Medicine (Baltimore).* 2016;95(28):e4210. PMID: 27428223

Al-Hashel JY, Abdelnabi EA, Ismail II. Monomelic amyotrophy (Hirayama disease): a rare case report and literature review. *Case Rep Neurol.* 2020;12(3):291-298. PMID: 33082767

19

ANSWER: C) Liddle syndrome

This man has hypertension with unprovoked hypokalemic alkalosis, low plasma renin, and low aldosterone. Both genetic and acquired causes are recognized:

Genetic:

- Activating pathogenic variants in the mineralocorticoid receptor gene
- Apparent mineralocorticoid excess
- CYP11B1 deficiency
- CYP17A1 deficiency
- Glucocorticoid resistance
- Liddle syndrome

Acquired:

- Deoxycorticosterone-secreting tumor
- High-salt diet
- Licorice or grapefruit juice
- Low renin hypertension
- Nonsteroidal antiinflammatory drugs/cyclooxygenase 2 inhibitors
- Severe hypercortisolism

In a young patient with a strongly suggestive family history (early-onset hypertension with premature cardiovascular disease), an inherited basis should be considered once dietary and medication confounders have been excluded. In this case, an autosomal dominant mode of inheritance is suggested, which potentially points to 2 disorders: (1) an activating pathogenic variant in the mineralocorticoid receptor gene and (2) Liddle syndrome.

To date, a single kindred has been reported with a heterozygous gain-of-function variant in the *NR3C2* gene (encoding the mineralocorticoid receptor) in a 15-year-old boy and 7 family members with early-onset severe hypertension, suppressed renin, low aldosterone, and mild hypokalemia. The reported variant was shown to induce a conformational change that stabilized complexes of the mutant mineralocorticoid receptor with aldosterone, progesterone, and spironolactone, predisposing to exacerbation of hypertension in pregnancy and during treatment with spironolactone.

Liddle syndrome (Answer C), a monogenic form of low-renin hypertension with autosomal dominant transmission, is caused by germline gain-of-function pathogenic variants in the *SCNN1A*, *SCNN1B*, and *SCNN1G* genes, which encode the α, β, and γ subunits of the epithelial sodium channel, respectively. More than 30 different causal variants in more than 70 families have been identified. Liddle syndrome typically presents with early-onset hypertension, although milder clinical phenotypes have been reported (including normokalemic). Liddle syndrome is therefore more likely to explain the early-onset hypertension with low renin and low aldosterone in this kindred.

Congenital adrenal hyperplasia may rarely be associated with hypertension in patients with *CYP17A1* (encoding 17α-hydroxylase and 17,20-lyase) or *CYP11B1* (encoding 11β-hydroxylase) pathogenic variants. Biallelic variants in the *CYP17A1* gene are associated with reduced 17α-hydroxylation of progesterone and pregnenolone, with consequent impaired generation of DHEA and androstenedione (leading to 46,XY pseudohermaphroditism [with female external genitalia] or 46,XX primary amenorrhea with delayed sexual development). Excess progesterone is directed towards overproduction of deoxycorticosterone and corticosterone that stimulate the mineralocorticoid receptor. Presentation is typically in childhood/adolescence. 11β-Hydroxylase deficiency leads to impaired conversion of deoxycorticosterone and deoxycortisol to corticosterone and cortisol, respectively, with resultant hypertension and virilization and precocious puberty. Presentation is usually at a young age (infancy and early childhood). Accordingly, congenital adrenal hyperplasia due to 11β-hydroxylase deficiency (Answer A) is not consistent with the clinical presentation in this case.

The syndrome of apparent mineralocorticoid excess (Answer E) is a rare form of severe juvenile hypertension, which is usually inherited in an autosomal recessive manner. It is caused by impaired function of the enzyme 11β-hydroxysteroid dehydrogenase type 2 (11β-HSD2) (encoded by the *HSD11B2* gene), which is critically required to inactivate cortisol through conversion to cortisone. Defective 11β-HSD2 function results in unregulated and excessive stimulation of the mineralocorticoid receptor by cortisol, with accompanying low plasma renin and low plasma aldosterone. In its classic form, it is characterized by low birth weight, failure to thrive, onset of severe hypertension in early childhood, hypercalciuria, and nephrocalcinosis. A late-onset form has been described in adults with compound heterozygous variants who have a milder phenotype. Chronic excessive ingestion of licorice (containing glycyrrhetinic acid and its metabolite glycyrrhizic acid) or grapefruit juice has been reported to produce a clinical picture that mimics apparent mineralocorticoid excess by inducing an acquired deficiency of 11β-HSD2. The clinical presentation and apparent mode of inheritance in this case are not suggestive of apparent mineralocorticoid excess.

Glucocorticoid resistance syndrome (Answer B) is an autosomal recessive disorder caused by point variants or deletions in the *NR3C1* gene, which encodes the glucocorticoid receptor. End-organ insensitivity to glucocorticoid action leads to compensatory ACTH hypersecretion with increased production of cortisol, adrenal androgens, and precursors with mineralocorticoid activity (eg, deoxycorticosterone, deoxycortisol). The development of low-renin hypertension is also a likely consequence of saturation of 11β-HSD2 function. Features of glucocorticoid insufficiency are usually evident and affected children may manifest precocious puberty. Twenty-four–hour urinary free cortisol levels are elevated. Glucocorticoid resistance syndrome is therefore unlikely in this patient.

Unlike other causes of monogenic hypertension, pseudohypoaldosteronism type 2 (Gordon syndrome) (Answer D) is associated with hyperkalemia. Pathogenic variants in several genes (*WNK1*, *WNK4*, *KLHL3*, and *CUL3*) have been implicated in its pathogenesis through increased trafficking of the sodium-chloride cotransporter to the apical membrane of the distal convoluted tubule, with resultant increased reabsorption of luminal sodium chloride. This in turn leads to reduced sodium absorption more distally with accompanying decreased potassium and hydrogen ion secretion, resulting in hyperkalemia and metabolic acidosis. The clinical and biochemical phenotype of pseudohypoaldosteronism type 2 does not therefore fit with this patient's presentation.

Educational Objective

Differentiate among aldosterone-independent causes of mineralocorticoid excess.

Reference(s)

Khandelwal P, Deinum J. Monogenic forms of low-renin hypertension: clinical and molecular insights. *Pediatr Nephrol.* 2022;37(7):1495-1509. PMID: 34414500

Monticone S, Losano I, Tetti M, Buffolo F, Veglio F, Mulatero P. Diagnostic approach to low-renin hypertension. *Clin Endocrinol (Oxf).* 2018;89(4):385-396. PMID: 29758100

20 ANSWER: C) Start hydrocortisone

Subarachnoid hemorrhage (SAH) with negative initial neurovascular imaging (sometimes referred to as "angiogram negative" or "nonaneurysmal" SAH) is well recognized and has been reported in up to 10% of cases in some large series. The role of further imaging after initial negative angiography is still debated, with several studies failing to show additional diagnostic value, particularly in certain subtypes (eg, perimesencephalic SAH).

Hyponatremia is a common complication following SAH. It has been observed in up to 50% of all patients admitted to the neurocritical care unit with nontraumatic SAH, with 10% to 15% developing more marked hyponatremia (sodium <130 mEq/L [<130 mmol/L]). It may be multifactorial in origin, although 2 conditions feature prominently in clinical algorithms for management of hyponatremia complicating SAH: syndrome of inappropriate antidiuretic hormone secretion (SIADH) and cerebral salt-wasting syndrome. Clinically, both conditions are characterized by hyponatremia with elevated (inappropriate) urinary sodium excretion and absence of edema. Whereas cerebral salt-wasting is associated with hypovolemia and polyuria, patients with SIADH are euvolemic or even slightly hypervolemic and typically have low to modest urine output. However, this distinction can be blurred in patients who have received significant volumes of sodium chloride-containing intravenous infusions as part of the initial management of SAH.

Importantly, several groups have highlighted the possibility of acute hypocortisolism developing in the aftermath of SAH (presumed to be secondary to pituitary injury) and manifesting with hyponatremia. In one prospective study, 49 of 100 patients with acute nontraumatic aneurysmal SAH developed hyponatremia. Of the 40 patients who presented biochemically as having SIADH, 4 were found to have acute glucocorticoid deficiency, and treatment with intravenous hydrocortisone rapidly restored the plasma sodium concentration to normal in this subgroup.

In this patient, several of the criteria required to diagnose SIADH have been met:

- Clinical euvolemia
- Hypoosmolar hyponatremia
- Less than maximally dilute urine (osmolality >100 mOsm/kg [>100 mmol/kg])
- Inappropriate urinary sodium excretion (>30 mEq/L [>30 mmol/L])
- Normal kidney function

However, thyroid function tests show a picture that is potentially consistent with central hypothyroidism, plasma glucose is borderline low, and blood pressure is 110/70 mm Hg despite likely active fluid management in the context of SAH. All point to possible hypocortisolism. Thus, while awaiting results of hypothalamic-pituitary-adrenal axis assessment, hydrocortisone replacement (Answer C) should be started. Unusually in this case, careful reevaluation of the initial imaging revealed that the patient had developed pituitary apoplexy with subarachnoid extension in a previously undiagnosed pituitary adenoma.

The use of fluid restriction (Answer A), intravenous hypertonic sodium chloride (Answer B), and tolvaptan (arginine vasopressin V2 receptor [AVPR2] antagonist) (Answer E) may all feature in the management of SIADH, although additional considerations (eg, requirement to avoid dehydration) must be taken into account in the context of SAH. This is a particular concern with AVPR2 antagonist therapy, where unregulated aquaresis can result in dehydration and overexuberant correction of hyponatremia, with the attendant risk of osmotic demyelination. However, in this case, a diagnosis of SIADH cannot be made until hypocortisolism has been formally excluded or corrected.

Levothyroxine replacement (Answer D) may be required in due course, especially in this patient in whom pituitary apoplexy has occurred. Levothyroxine should not be commenced until hypocortisolism has been corrected, as the accompanying increase in metabolism coupled with enhanced cortisol clearance can predispose to an adrenal crisis when adrenal reserve is diminished. Consideration should also be given to the possibility of confounding nonthyroidal illness changes in any acutely unwell patient.

Educational Objective

Describe how hypocortisolism can complicate subarachnoid hemorrhage and how pituitary apoplexy may mimic subarachnoid hemorrhage.

Reference(s)

Hannon MJ, Behan LA, O'Brien MMC, et al. Hyponatremia following mild/moderate subarachnoid hemorrhage is due to SIAD and glucocorticoid deficiency and not cerebral salt wasting. *J Clin Endocrinol Metab.* 2014;99(1):291-298. PMID: 24248182

Briet C, Salenave S, Bonneville J-F, Laws ER, Chanson P. Pituitary apoplexy. *Endocr Rev.* 2015;36(6):622-645. PMID: 26414232

Sergides IG, Minhas PA, Antoun N, Pickard JD. Pituitary apoplexy can mimic subarachnoid haemorrhage clinically and radiologically. *Emerg Med J.* 2007;24(4):308. PMID: 17384396

21 ANSWER: C) Roll the insulin bottle between his hands until it is uniformly cloudy, then inject usual dose

In the last 25 years, numerous basal insulin choices have become available in the form of long-acting insulin analogues, which have a "flatter" activity profile and longer duration of action than original NPH insulin. In patients with type 1 diabetes, these analogues may better reduce hypoglycemia, promote less weight gain, and improve hemoglobin A_{1c} more than human insulins. More modest advantages of insulin analogues have been observed in clinical trials of patients with type 2 diabetes, and these benefits are even less well defined in clinical practice. Insulin analogues are more expensive than NPH insulin. NPH insulin may be a cost-effective choice for patients with limited resources and is currently available without a prescription at some stores for about $25 dollars per vial.

When converting from analogue insulin (most commonly given once daily) to NPH insulin, it is important to instruct the patient on the differences between the insulins. Analogue insulins appear clear, but NPH insulin is a suspension and thus appears cloudy. Patients using analogue insulins are often instructed that a cloudy appearance may indicate contamination and that it should not be used if it has this appearance. Because NPH insulin is expected to be cloudy, returning the bottle to the pharmacy (Answer B) is not necessary. Using proper technique for preparing NPH insulin is important, as it can affect its potency. The appropriate technique is to instruct the patient to roll the NPH insulin bottle until it is uniformly cloudy, then inject (Answer C). However, excess agitation, such as shaking the bottle (Answer D), should also be avoided to prevent loss of potency, clumping, frosting, or precipitation. Insulin may be stored at room temperature for periods specified by the manufacturer, typically up to 28 days. However, patients should be instructed to review duration of storage for individual insulin at room temperature once in use and to avoid extreme temperatures (<36°F or >86°F [<2°C or >30°C]). Using insulin at room temperature limits local irritation at the injection site, which may occur when insulin is cold. Thus, storing an open insulin bottle in the refrigerator between uses (Answer E) is incorrect.

Compared with analogue basal insulin, NPH insulin has a shorter duration of action and thus is given twice daily. In addition, most patients transitioning to NPH insulin require a dosage increase of approximately 20%. This patient's dosage was appropriately adjusted. As described above, the morning hyperglycemia is most likely due to the insulin not being properly suspended before injection. The first step should be to instruct the patient in the correct preparation of NPH. Increasing the evening NPH insulin dose by 8 units (Answer A) is not the best answer, especially if he is still not preparing the insulin correctly before use.

Educational Objective

Guide patients on appropriate preparation and storage of NPH insulin.

Reference(s)

American Diabetes Association. 9. Pharmacologic approaches to glycemic treatment: standards of medical care in diabetes-2021. *Diabetes Care.* 2021;44(Suppl 1):S111-S124. PMID: 33298420

American Diabetes Association. Insulin administration. *Diabetes Care.* 2002;24(11):1984-1987. PMID: 11679469

Cowart K. Overbasalization: addressing hesitancy in treatment intensification beyond basal insulin. *Clin Diabetes.* 2020;38(3):304-310. PMID: 32699482

22 **ANSWER: D) Levothyroxine**

Thyroid hormones regulate cholesterol synthesis through different mechanisms. Thyroid hormone induces cholesterol synthesis by prompting the hepatic expression of hydroxymethylglutaryl coenzyme A reductase; increasing the expression of LDL-cholesterol receptors in fibroblasts, liver, and other tissues; and controlling intestinal absorption of cholesterol via the Niemann-Pick C1-like 1 protein. In the setting of hypothyroidism, the decrease in LDL-cholesterol receptors and increased intestinal absorption of cholesterol outweigh the effect on LDL-cholesterol synthesis leading to high LDL-cholesterol levels. Lipoprotein lipase activity is lower in the setting of hypothyroidism, which leads to decreased clearance of triglyceride-rich lipoproteins and hypertriglyceridemia. HDL cholesterol is either normal or slightly increased in the setting of hypothyroidism, as the concentration of cholesteryl ester transfer protein is decreased. Lipid abnormalities caused by hypothyroidism can be corrected with levothyroxine therapy (Answer D). Twelve weeks after starting levothyroxine, this patient's repeated TSH measurement was 6.0 mIU/L, and her triglyceride concentration was 134 mg/dL (1.51 mmol/L). This patient was also asked to lower her fat and carbohydrate intake. In this case, starting a pharmacologic agent that lowers triglycerides (such as a fibrate, fish oil, or a statin) should be delayed given that she is asymptomatic and specifically has no abdominal pain.

Fenofibrate (Answer B) induces the expression of peroxisome proliferator–activated receptor α, which increases the expression of lipoprotein lipase. This class of medication is the first choice when treating primary hypertriglyceridemia. However, in this patient, the correct approach is to first treat her hypothyroidism. If, despite correcting her TSH, her triglycerides are still elevated (>500 mg/dL [>5.65 mmol/L]), then starting a fibrate would be the correct approach.

PCSK9 inhibitors (Answer E) are approved to lower LDL cholesterol in patients with clinical atherosclerotic cardiovascular disease or familial hypercholesterolemia whose LDL-cholesterol concentration is not at goal. PCSK9 inhibitors are not approved for triglyceride lowering.

Statins (Answer A) lower triglycerides by 15% to 30%, with higher-intensity statins leading to greater triglyceride reduction. Starting statin therapy in patients with hypertriglyceridemia is reasonable; however, this patient needs correction of hypothyroidism first.

Icosapent ethyl (Answer C) is a type of omega-3 fatty acid that lowers triglycerides by decreasing VLDL synthesis, enhancing clearance of VLDL particles and enhancing the activity of lipoprotein lipase. Because of pill burden and cost, this medication is usually second-line therapy when treating hypertriglyceridemia.

Bile-acid sequestrants are contraindicated, as this medication class raises triglycerides.

Educational Objective

Manage hypertriglyceridemia secondary to overt hypothyroidism.

Reference(s)

Pearce EN. Update in lipid alterations in subclinical hypothyroidism. *J Clin Endocrinol Metab.* 2012;97(2):326-333. PMID: 22205712

Simha V. Management of hypertriglyceridemia. *BMJ.* 2020;371;m3109. PMID: 33046451

Berglund L, Brunzell JD, Goldberg AC, et al; Endocrine Society. Evaluation and treatment of hypertriglyceridemia: an Endocrine Society clinical practice guideline. *J Clin Endocrinol Metab.* 2012;97(9):2969-2989. PMID: 22962670

Kotwal A, Cortes T, Genere N, et al. Treatment of thyroid dysfunction and serum lipids: a systematic review and meta-analysis. *J Clin Endocrinol Metab.* 2020;105(12):dgaa672. PMID: 32954428

23 ANSWER: E) Wean analgesic medications, especially opioids

This patient presents with clinical and biochemical evidence of hypogonadotropic hypogonadism and secondary adrenal failure. While obesity has been associated with hypogonadotropic hypogonadism, men with class 1 obesity (BMI 30 to <35 kg/m^2) or class 2 obesity (BMI 35 to <40 kg/m^2) primarily exhibit modest reductions in total testosterone concentrations due to obesity-associated reductions in SHBG. Free testosterone (if measured by gold standard equilibrium dialysis) has typically been reported to be normal. Moreover, men with class 1 or 2 obesity often present with nonspecific androgen deficiency-like symptoms; whether these symptoms (eg, fatigue, low libido) are causally associated with reductions in serum testosterone or are due to associated comorbidities (eg, sleep apnea, depression) is not clear. The clinical and biochemical severity of this man's hypogonadism is therefore not explained by his relatively modest obesity, and his hypogonadism is unlikely to improve with weight-loss measures (Answer D). Moreover, obesity would not explain his secondary adrenal failure.

While men who abuse anabolic steroids may present with low concentrations of serum testosterone and gonadotropins, they often display evidence of exogenous androgenization (eg, muscular physique, truncal acne, small testes) and a tendency to have polycythemia, rather than the mild anemia seen in this case, which is suggestive of genuine hypogonadism. In addition, secondary adrenal failure is not a typical feature of anabolic steroid abuse. Whether it is ethical to order anabolic steroid testing without informing the patient (Answer B) is highly debatable. Anabolic steroid testing is not standardized across laboratories, and diagnostic precision is uncertain. Patients can easily avoid detection by temporarily pausing anabolic steroid use or by providing someone else's urine sample. In clinical practice, the best "diagnostic test" for anabolic steroid abuse remains to ask the patient directly.

Hypogonadotropic hypogonadism due to pituitary pathology is usually evident on pituitary MRI, unless it is caused by a microprolactinoma. The normal prolactin level and normal pituitary MRI findings essentially rule out pituitary pathology, and repeating pituitary MRI in 6 months (Answer A) is not indicated.

Patients with congenital hypogonadotropic hypogonadism due to a pathogenic variant present with failure of pubertal progression (high-pitched voice, tall stature, and small testes) and, in some cases, anosmia. The clinical picture in this vignette is not consistent with congenital hypogonadotropic hypogonadism and genetic testing (Answer C) is not indicated.

The most likely explanation for this man's hypogonadotropic hypogonadism and associated secondary adrenal failure is exposure to opioids (Answer E). Opioids inhibit pulsatile GnRH secretion from the hypothalamus. They also reduce the pituitary response to GnRH, consequently causing reduced LH and, to a lesser degree, reducing FSH secretion from the anterior pituitary, which in turn leads to decreased testosterone secretion from the testes. Low serum testosterone is common in men using opioids. In a recent meta-analysis and systematic review of 15 studies with 3250 participants (99.5% men) using opioids for chronic pain or maintenance treatment for opioid addiction, 63% (95% CI, 55%-70%) had low serum testosterone. Men taking fentanyl, methadone, or oxycodone had increased odds for testosterone deficiency compared with those taking hydrocodone (odds ratios, 25.7, 7.3, and 3.2, respectively), and patients taking higher dosages and longer-acting opioids were more likely to have a low serum testosterone level than those taking lower dosages and shorter-acting opioids. In addition to opioid dosage, duration of opioid action, and duration of opioid use, other potential factors postulated to increase susceptibility of suppression the hypothalamic-pituitary-gonadal axis by opioids include older age, use of opioids for cancer pain, and increased adiposity. With respect to symptoms, in the aforementioned meta-analysis, reduced libido and erectile dysfunction were reported in 89% of opioid-using male patients. However, the severity of this man's hypogonadism was unusual, as most opioid users present with nonspecific androgen deficiency-like symptoms and more modest reductions in serum testosterone.

Management options for opioid-induced hypogonadism include opioid cessation, which, if successful, leads to recovery of the hypothalamic-pituitary-gonadal axis. If opioid cessation is not feasible, testosterone treatment should be considered. However, the evidence supporting testosterone treatment in patients who take opioids is limited, with the aforementioned meta-analysis identifying 6 studies with a total of 280 men taking opioids and receiving testosterone treatment. Five were observational studies, and while patients generally reported improvements in sexual function and mental quality of life, the studies did not include control groups. Evidence from randomized controlled trials is scant. In 1 randomized controlled trial, 65 men (aged 18-64 years) with opioid-induced androgen deficiency and chronic noncancer pain were treated with transdermal testosterone for 14 weeks, which resulted in greater improvements in pain perception, sexual desire, body composition, and some domains of quality of life compared with placebo. However, in a 24-week randomized controlled trial of 41 men (aged 44-59 years), testosterone treatment did not change pain perception or quality of life. Given the severity of his hypogonadism, this man was started on topical testosterone treatment while opioids were weaned. Topical testosterone is preferable in this situation, given that injectable testosterone (especially long-acting testosterone undecanoate) may delay endogenous hypothalamic-pituitary-gonadal axis recovery.

As seen in this case, opioids can also suppress the hypothalamic-pituitary-adrenal axis. Opioids mainly act at the hypothalamic-pituitary level, where they inhibit corticotropin-releasing hormone and antidiuretic hormone secretion, resulting in decreased ACTH release. The aforementioned meta-analysis reported that the prevalence of hypocortisolism as assessed by dynamic and nondynamic testing was 15% (95% CI: 6%-28% [5 studies, 205 patients, 57.5% males]) and 24% in studies using insulin tolerance tests (95% CI: 16%-33% [2 studies, 97 patients]). However, the clinical significance of hypoadrenalism in men taking opioids (especially in those with mild/suboptimal responses to dynamic tests) is not clear, and routine glucocorticoid replacement is not indicated. There are, however, published reports of patients receiving opioids developing adrenal crises or clinical manifestations resembling those of adrenal insufficiency, which improved after glucocorticoid replacement, suggesting that suppression of the hypothalamic-pituitary-adrenal axis requires attention in some patients. The degree of hypothalamic-pituitary-adrenal suppression seen in this patient was unusually severe, and glucocorticoid treatment was warranted. While this current patient had unusually profound suppression of the hypothalamic-pituitary-gonadal and hypothalamic-pituitary-adrenal axes, in the absence of other pathology, opioid-induced suppression was the most likely diagnosis. Of note, he gradually weaned off opioid medications over the next 10 months, and his pituitary axis recovered fully. Hydrocortisone and testosterone treatment was ceased. Twelve months later, he remains off opioids, and his hypothalamic-pituitary-gonadal and hypothalamic-pituitary-adrenal axes are normal.

Educational Objective

Identify opioids as a cause of hypogonadotropic hypogonadism, which can be associated with suppression of other pituitary axes (eg, hypothalamic-pituitary-adrenal axis).

Reference(s)

de Vries F, Bruin M, Lobatto DJ, et al. Opioids and their endocrine effects: a systematic review and meta-analysis. *J Clin Endocrinol Metab.* 2019;105(3):1020-1029. PMID: 31511863

Fountas A, Van Uum S, Karavitaki N. Opioid-induced endocrinopathies. *Lancet Diabetes Endocrinol.* 2020 8(1):68-80. PMID: 31624023

Basaria S, Travison TG, Alford D, et al. Effects of testosterone replacement in men with opioid-induced androgen deficiency: a randomized controlled trial. *Pain.* 2015;156(2):280-288. PMID: 25599449

Glintborg D, Vaegter HB, Lehmann Christensen L, et al. Testosterone replacement therapy of opioid-induced male hypogonadism improved body composition but not pain perception: a double-blind, randomized, and placebo-controlled trial. *Eur J Endocrinol.* 2020;182(6):539-548. PMID: 32213659

24 ANSWER: E) Increase in vitamin D catabolism due to phenytoin

While this patient may, in fact, have primary hyperparathyroidism (Answer C), hypercalciuria (Answer B), or frequent falls (Answer D), there is nothing in the history that suggests these issues. Regarding the direct effects of phenytoin on bone, it remains unclear whether this medication has effects on osteoblasts to reduce bone formation (Answer A).

Phenytoin, along with carbamazepine, activates the cytochrome P450 system, including enzymes involved in vitamin D catabolism (Answer E). While the mechanism that increases vitamin D metabolism is not completely understood, it is thought to be related to induction of the steroid and xenobiotic receptor SXR, which can then activate CYP24, the enzyme that deactivates 25-hydroxyvitamin D and 1,25-dihydroxyvitamin D. Ultimately, these medications can lead to chronic vitamin D deficiency, higher bone turnover, and lower bone mineral density.

Educational Objective

Determine the cause of vitamin D deficiency in a patient on antiseizure medication.

Reference(s)

Pack AM, Morrell MJ, Marcus R, et al. Bone mass and turnover in women with epilepsy on antiepileptic drug monotherapy. *Ann Neurol.* 2005;57(2):252-257. PMID: 15668966

Zhou C, Assem M, Tay JC, et al. Steroid and xenobiotic receptor and vitamin D receptor crosstalk mediates CYP24 expression and drug-induced osteomalacia. *J Clin Invest.* 2006;116(6):1703-1712. PMID: 16691293

25 **ANSWER: D) Stop insulin glargine and administer NPH insulin at the start of peritoneal dialysis**
When prescribing basal insulin, one must consider the time of onset, peak, and duration of action for the various formulations (*see figure*). As in this case, hyperglycemia often occurs shortly after the start of peritoneal dialysis and lasts for the duration of dialysis and a few hours after completion. During peritoneal dialysis, the dialysate (which contains glucose) flows into the peritoneal cavity and stays there for a prescribed period (ie, the dwell time), which is usually 4 to 6 hours. Given the onset of NPH insulin (1 to 2 hours), a peak effect of 4 to 6 hours, and duration of action of about 12 hours, it is an ideal insulin to mitigate hyperglycemia that is induced by the dialysate. Thus, the best next step in this patient's management is to stop insulin glargine and administer NPH insulin at the start of peritoneal dialysis (Answer D). NPH may have a longer duration of action in the setting of kidney failure, but the duration would be shorter than that of insulin glargine and the cumulative effect during the day would be less.

Basal (Long-Acting) Insulin Formulations

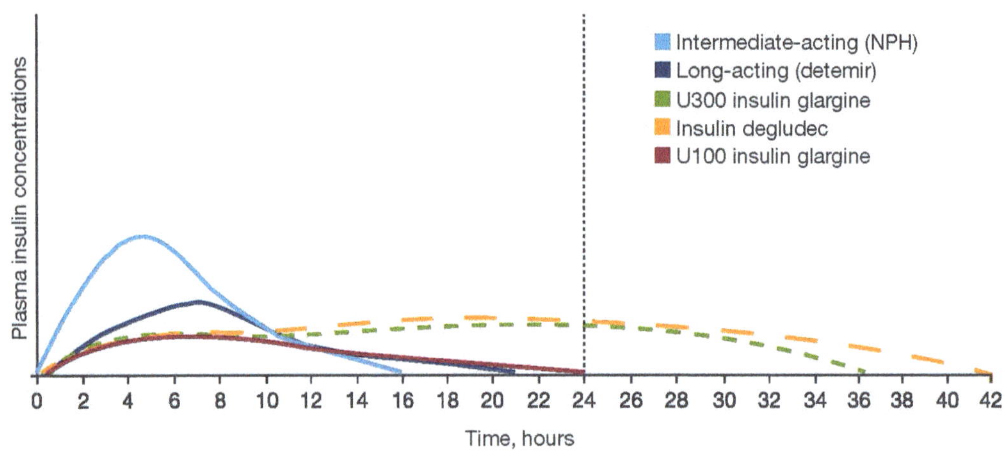

Adapted from Hirsch IB. Insulin analogues. N Engl J Med. 2005;352(2):174-183; Flood TM. Appropriate use of insulin analogs in an increasingly complex type 2 diabetes mellitus (T2DM) landscape. *J Fam Pract.* 2007;56(Suppl 1):S1-S2; Lamos EM, Younk LM, Davis SN. Concentrated insulins: the new basal insulins. *Ther Clin Risk Manag.* 2016;12:389-400.

Insulin glargine is not a good option to manage the hyperglycemia associated with peritoneal dialysis because its duration of action exceeds the length of the peritoneal dialysis session and it lacks a peak to address the hyperglycemia that will occur during dialysis. Thus, neither switching insulin glargine administration to the evening (Answer E) nor changing the insulin glargine dosage to 25 units twice daily (Answer A) will have the desired effect, especially because the total daily dose is not being changed. This patient would continue to have the current glucose profile that reflects suboptimal glycemic control.

Reducing the dosage of insulin glargine and adding glimepiride (Answer B) would not address the current glycemic excursions, and the patient would most likely continue to have episodes of hypoglycemia after completion of the peritoneal dialysis sessions. Likewise, reducing the insulin glargine dosage and adding prandial insulin lispro (Answer C) would also not address this patient's pattern of hyperglycemia and hypoglycemia.

His problems are nocturnal hyperglycemia associated with peritoneal dialysis and episodes of hypoglycemia long after completion of peritoneal dialysis sessions because of the action of the once-daily insulin glargine. The only intervention of the choices listed that will address both of these issues is stopping the insulin glargine and initiating NPH insulin.

Educational Objective

Adjust diabetes therapy for patients with type 2 diabetes mellitus who receive peritoneal dialysis and determine when alternative measures to assess glycemic control may be warranted.

Reference(s)

Gianchandani RY, Neupane S, Iyengar JJ, Heung M. Pathophysiology and management of hypoglycemia in end-stage renal disease patients: a review. *Endocr Pract.* 2017;23(3):353-362. PMID: 27967230

Hirsch IB. Insulin analogues. *N Engl J Med.* 2005;352(2):174-183. PMID: 15647580

Flood TM. Appropriate use of insulin analogs in an increasingly complex type 2 diabetes mellitus (T2DM) landscape. *J Fam Pract.* 2007;56(Suppl 1):S1-S2. PMID: 17217893

Lamos EM, Younk LM, Davis SN. Concentrated insulins: the new basal insulins. *Ther Clin Risk Manag.* 2016;12:389-400. PMID: 27022271

26 ANSWER: E) Start NPH insulin, 6 units daily, with tube feeding, in addition to 15 units regular insulin in parenteral nutrition and 5 units insulin glargine

Patients who undergo total pancreatectomy require insulin for long-term glycemic management. In the immediate postoperative setting, factors that can affect glycemic excursions include the type of nutrition the patient is receiving, use of medications that can increase blood glucose, and the development of postoperative complications that can cause stress hyperglycemia. The goal blood glucose concentration in hospitalized patients is 140 to 180 mg/dL (7.8 to 10.0 mmol/L).

This patient has 2 sources of nutrition: central parenteral nutrition that is infused over 24 hours into a central vein and enteral nutrition with a semi-elemental formula that is infused over 12 hours into the small intestine. Each source of carbohydrate should be covered with an insulin profile that most closely matches delivery of that specific carbohydrate.

The carbohydrate source in parenteral nutrition is hydrous dextrose, which provides 3.4 kcal per g. Parenteral nutrition–induced hyperglycemia is associated with poor clinical outcomes. The glycemic target in hospitalized patients on parenteral nutrition is the same as that in hospitalized patients not on parenteral nutrition. Because parenteral nutrition involves continuous dextrose administration, continuous insulin administration at a ratio that is adjusted for the carbohydrate content of the formula works best. In this patient, blood glucose readings are mostly at goal when the only source of carbohydrate is parenteral nutrition, suggesting sufficient insulin coverage in parenteral nutrition and adequate basal insulin coverage with glargine.

This patient is persistently hyperglycemic while on tube feeding and has required several correction doses of insulin. Since there is no anticipated change to her nutrition program, it would be reasonable to introduce a small amount of NPH insulin specifically to cover the tube-feeding program. NPH insulin has a duration of action of about 12 hours. As the tube feeds last only 12 hours, administering NPH insulin once daily (Answer E) rather than twice daily (Answer A) is appropriate. Regular insulin, which has a duration of action of approximately 8 hours, could also work well to cover glycemic excursions with tube feeds.

Recommending no changes (Answer D) does not address the fact that she develops hyperglycemia with the initiation of tube feeding.

Increasing the concentration of insulin in parenteral nutrition (Answer C) would not specifically address the hyperglycemia during the tube-feed period and may risk hypoglycemia overnight, after the enteral feeds are discontinued each evening.

Similarly, an increase in basal insulin (Answer B) does not specifically address the tube feeding–induced hyperglycemia, and it may risk hypoglycemia overnight, after tube feeds are discontinued each evening.

This patient who has undergone pancreatectomy requires basal insulin coverage (glargine), in addition to the management of tube feed–induced hyperglycemia, so discontinuing insulin glargine (Answer A) is incorrect.

Educational Objective

Manage hyperglycemia in a hospitalized patient after total pancreatectomy while on tube feeding and parenteral nutrition.

Reference(s)

American Diabetes Association Professional Practice Committee; Draznin B, Aroda VR, Bakris G, et al. 16. Diabetes care in the hospital: standards of medical care in diabetes-2022. *Diabetes Care.* 2021;45(Suppl 1):S244-S253. PMID: 34964884

Pasquel FJ, Spiegelman R, McCauley M, et al. Hyperglycemia during total parenteral nutrition: an important marker of poor outcome and mortality in hospitalized patients. *Diabetes Care.* 2010;33(4):739-741. PMID: 20040658

27 ANSWER: D) Ovarian/adrenal venous sampling

This patient presents with irregular periods and infertility after discontinuing oral contraceptives. Her periods were regular in adolescence, and they have become progressively more irregular, with total testosterone continuing to rise over the last year. The progression of symptoms is concerning, and even though the total testosterone concentration has not reached the general threshold of greater than 200 ng/dL (>6.9 nmol/L), which should trigger further evaluation for a tumoral source, although more recent data suggest that a lower threshold of 147 ng/dL (5.1 nmol/L) is appropriate with more universal use of liquid chromatography–tandem mass spectrometry.

In this case, there is enough evidence to pursue further evaluation for a source of the testosterone increase and to consider surgical intervention given the patient's desire to conceive and her age. Her high concentrations of testosterone would most likely interfere with her ability to conceive spontaneously.

Combined ovarian/adrenal venous sampling (Answer D) (selective venous sampling) is performed to help guide treatment decisions in the evaluation of women with hyperandrogenism when clinical suspicion for an androgen-producing tumor is high, findings on pelvic ultrasonography are normal, and findings on adrenal imaging are either normal or a nodule or mass is identified with benign features. This test is also used in the evaluation of premenopausal women with very high testosterone concentrations who desire fertility to determine whether unilateral or bilateral ovarian treatment is necessary. The procedure includes selective catheterization of the ovarian and adrenal veins to demonstrate a gradient in androgen concentrations and localize the source. This procedure is technically difficult and should only be performed by highly experienced interventional radiologists who have been trained in the sampling technique. The elevated androgen is measured from samples of ovarian and adrenal vein effluent, although many protocols include total testosterone, androstenedione, DHEA-S, and cortisol to help interpret results if there is a concern for confirming catheter placement.

Results of ovarian/adrenal venous sampling:

Measurement	Right ovarian vein	Left ovarian vein	Right adrenal vein	Left adrenal vein	Inferior vena cava
Total testosterone	749 ng/dL (SI: 26.0 nmol/L)	65 ng/dL (SI: 2.3 nmol/L)	49 ng/dL (SI: 1.7 nmol/L)	47 ng/dL (SI: 1.6 nmol/L)	60 ng/dL (SI: 2.1 nmol/L)
Androstenedione	>4000 ng/dL (SI: 139.7 nmol/L)	180 ng/dL (SI: 6.3 nmol/L)	212 ng/dL (SI: 7.4 nmol/L)	184 ng/dL (SI: 6.4 nmol/L)	160 ng/dL (SI: 5.59 nmol/L)

Unstimulated testosterone concentrations with a ratio greater than 3 from the ovarian or adrenal vein to the peripheral (inferior vena cava) measurement and a ratio greater than 1.4 from 1 side indicate a unilateral source. In this case, the ratio of the right ovarian vein-to-inferior vena cava is 12.4; the ratio of the left ovarian vein-to-interior vena cava is 1.1; and the ratio of the right ovarian vein-to-left ovarian vein is 11.5. Some protocols might include ACTH or hCG stimulation, but the doses reported vary and low numbers make it difficult to determine utility or prognostic ability.

Regarding pregnancy and live birth rates in clinical trials for women with polycystic ovary syndrome, clomiphene citrate has been shown to be significantly better than metformin (Answer C), and letrozole (Answer B) has been shown to be significantly better than clomiphene citrate. Although ovulation induction with either letrozole or clomiphene citrate would be first-line treatment of infertility for women with polycystic ovary syndrome, the pace of this patient's symptom development and her high testosterone level should prompt additional testing to exclude an androgen-producing tumor.

Laparoscopic ovarian drilling (Answer E) (laparoscopic ovarian diathermy or electrocoagulation) is offered as second-line treatment if pharmacologic ovulation induction is unsuccessful in women with polycystic ovary syndrome. Ovarian drilling replaced widely used wedge resection of the ovaries because of a lower risk of adhesions. Although used for years, ovarian drilling has not been standardized regarding the technique, dose of energy per puncture, number of punctures, or whether both ovaries should be treated.

A 48-hour dexamethasone-suppression test (Answer A) can be helpful to increase or decrease suspicion of an androgen-producing tumor or ovarian hyperthecosis. Dexamethasone is prescribed, 0.5 mg every 6 hours for 2 days, and androgen concentrations are measured before and after dexamethasone. A total testosterone decrease of more than 40% is seen in patients with benign causes of androgen excess that respond to medical therapy such as oral contraceptives or spironolactone. In this case, if the patient wanted to be reassured before medical therapy, a 48-hour dexamethasone-suppression test could be the best next step. However, medical therapy, such as combined oral contraceptives or spironolactone, would not be recommended to help her conceive in the short term, which is her primary goal.

This patient should undergo combined ovarian/adrenal venous sampling to confirm an ovarian source and whether unilateral oophorectomy vs bilateral laparoscopic ovarian drilling should be recommended to improve fertility and her chances of conceiving spontaneously.

Educational Objective

Guide the evaluation of significantly elevated total testosterone levels in a woman with infertility.

Reference(s)

Levens ED, Whitcomb BW, Csokmay JM, Nieman LK. Selective venous sampling for androgen-producing ovarian pathology. *Clin Endocrinol (Oxf).* 2009;70(4):606-614. PMID: 18721192

Sharma A, Kapoor E, Singh RJ, Chang AY, Erickson D. Diagnostic thresholds for androgen-producing tumors or pathologic hyperandrogenism in women by using total testosterone concentrations measured by liquid-chromatography-tandem mass spectrometry. *Clin Chem.* 2018;64(11):1636-1645. PMID: 30068692

Teede JH, Misso ML, Costello MF, et al; International PCOS Network. Recommendations from the International evidence-based guideline for assessment and management of polycystic ovary syndrome. *Fertil Steril.* 2018;110(3):364-379. PMID: 30033227

Martin KA, Anderson RR, Chang RJ, et al. Evaluation and treatment of hirsutism in premenopausal women: an Endocrine Society clinical practice guideline. *J Clin Endocrinol Metab.* 2018;103(4):1233-1257. PMID: 29522147

Farquhar C, Brown J, Marjoribanks J. Laparoscopic drilling by diathermy or laser for ovulation induction in anovulatory polycystic ovary syndrome. *Cochrane Database Syst Rev.* 2012;(6):CD001122. PMID: 22696324

28 **ANSWER: E) Insulin autoantibody measurement**

The patient in this vignette presented with postprandial neuroglycopenic symptoms that improved following intake of carbohydrates. He has autoimmune thyroid dysfunction and may be at risk for other autoimmune conditions such as Addison disease. However, he has no symptoms suggestive of adrenal insufficiency such as fatigue, dizziness, or low blood pressure. Measuring cortisol (Answer A) would not be the first step in this patient's workup.

The pattern of initial postmeal hyperglycemia followed by hypoglycemia can be seen in patients with diabetes who also have gastroparesis. This is thought to happen when mealtime insulin and nutrient absorption occur at discordant times. This patient does not have a history of diabetes or insulin use, so gastroparesis is unlikely and a gastric-emptying study (Answer C) is incorrect.

This glucose pattern can also be seen in patients who develop insulin antibodies. Insulin autoimmune syndrome, known as Hirata disease, has mostly been described in persons of East Asian descent. Affected individuals develop insulin autoantibodies. This can occur in persons who do not have diabetes or previous exposure to insulin, but it is more likely in those with diabetes who are treated with insulin. Several medications have been implicated in causing a rise in insulin autoantibodies. Methimazole (which this patient has been taking) and α-lipoic acid have the strongest association with presence of insulin autoantibodies. The antibodies bind to insulin-forming complexes, reducing insulin attachment to the insulin receptor. This results in higher postmeal blood glucose concentrations. Over time, insulin is released from the complexes, which leads to hypoglycemia. Insulin autoimmune syndrome is diagnosed when insulin autoantibodies are noted in the blood. It is self-remitting, and treatment of insulin autoimmune syndrome is supportive. Given this patient's blood glucose pattern, absence of insulin use, and use of methimazole, insulin autoimmune syndrome is the most likely diagnosis and measurement of insulin antibodies (Answer E) is the correct answer.

Although a 72-hour fast (Answer B) and hypoglycemia panel (Answer D) are standard tests to determine the cause of hypoglycemia when the etiology is unknown, in this patient whose presentation is suggestive of insulin autoimmune syndrome, neither test would be as likely to determine etiology. (Note: at some institutions, both sulfonylurea and meglitinide screens are included in one panel, while at other institutions each has to be ordered separately.)

Educational Objective

Diagnose hypoglycemia related to insulin autoantibodies.

Reference(s)

Cappellani D, Macchia E, Falcorni A, Marchetti P. Insulin autoimmune syndrome (Hirata disease): a comprehensive review fifty years after its first description. *Diabetes Metab Syndr Obes.* 2020;13:963-978. PMID: 32308449

29 ANSWER: A) Change calcium citrate to calcium carbonate

Hypoparathyroidism is often challenging to manage, especially in patients with undetectable intact PTH. The risk of hypoparathyroidism after neck surgery has been reported to be 0.12% to 4.6%, with lower rates when performed by surgeons with extensive experience in neck exploration. If hypoparathyroidism is present for 6 months after neck surgery, it is considered chronic, as the chances of recovery are very low. Other etiologies of hypoparathyroidism include pathogenic variants in the *CASR, GNA11, GATA3, AIRE,* and *GCM2* genes; contiguous gene deletion syndromes of chromosome 22 causing DiGeorge syndrome; and rare mitochondrial pathogenic variants. Infiltrative disorders such as sarcoidosis, Wilson disease, and iron deposition have been described. Severe hypomagnesemia can also mimic hypoparathyroidism.

Serum calcium and phosphate levels and urinary calcium excretion are controlled using a combination of calcium supplements, calcitriol, thiazide diuretics, and occasionally more potent phosphate binders. This patient's serum calcium concentration of 8.4 mg/dL (2.0 mmol/L) is at goal (8.0-8.5 mg/dL [2.0-2.1 mmol/L]). Attempts to further increase calcium usually lead to worsening hypercalciuria due to insufficient renal reclamation of filtered calcium, even with a thiazide diuretic.

The only laboratory value of concern in this patient is the phosphate. An elevated calcium:phosphate product, especially when greater than 55, can result in ectopic calcification, so phosphate is an important laboratory analyte to monitor. One strategy would be to decrease the calcitriol dosage (Answer B) to reduce gut phosphate absorption, leading to a reduction in serum phosphate. However, this would simultaneously reduce serum calcium.

The addition of sevelamer (Answer E), by sequestering dietary phosphate, would also reduce serum phosphate, but this medication is expensive and not a first choice. With this strategy, however, the current calcium regimen could remain.

Increasing the chlorthalidone dosage (Answer C) or prescribing magnesium oxide (Answer D) would have minimal effects on serum phosphate.

The patient is currently taking calcium citrate, which has a marginal ability to bind dietary phosphorus. Compared with calcium citrate, calcium carbonate binds dietary phosphorus better. Given its lower cost, changing this patient's regimen to calcium carbonate (Answer A) is a reasonable choice.

Educational Objective

Manage hyperphosphatemia in a patient with hypoparathyroidism.

Reference(s)

Asari R, Passler C, Kaczirek K, Scheuba C, Niederle B. Hypoparathyroidism after total thyroidectomy: a prospective study. *Arch Surg.* 2008;143(2):132-137. PMID: 18283137

Brandi ML, Bilezikian JP, Shoback D, et al. Management of hypoparathyroidism: summary statement and guidelines. *J Clinical Endocrinol Metab.* 2016;101(6):2273-2283. PMID: 26943719

Sheikh MS, Maguire JA, Emmett M, et al. Reduction of dietary phosphorus absorption by phosphorus binders. A theoretical, in vitro, and in vivo study. *J Clin Invest.* 1989;83(1):66-73. PMID: 2910921

30 ANSWER: A) Autobrewery syndrome secondary to Roux-en-Y gastric bypass

Autobrewery syndrome (Answer A), or gut fermentation syndrome, is a rare complication of gastric bypass surgery. In this condition, an excessive amount of ethanol is produced by fermentation of carbohydrates by certain bacteria or fungi in the gut. Although endogenous alcohol production occurs naturally in very small amounts during digestion, overgrowth of these pathogens can cause high levels of blood ethanol with clinical consequences. Bariatric surgery is known to induce changes to the structure and composition of gut microbes, which predispose to the development of bacterial overgrowth. The true incidence of autobrewery syndrome after gastric bypass is unknown because it is most likely underdiagnosed. Autobrewery syndrome has also been reported in patients with gastrointestinal tract diseases such as short-bowel syndrome, gastroparesis, and Crohn disease, as well as in patients with no history of gastrointestinal surgery.

Patients with this condition present with symptoms suggestive of alcohol intoxication, and symptoms can occur randomly. Sometimes carbohydrate consumption triggers symptoms, but this is not always the case. Affected patients are diagnosed when blood alcohol levels are found to be elevated after confirmation of abstinence from alcohol, typically in the presence of a known risk factor such as prior gastrointestinal surgery. This condition is treated with a low-carbohydrate, high-protein diet and with antibiotics. This particular patient had significant symptom improvement after being placed on long-term rifaximin therapy. Long-term resolution of symptoms has also been reported after fecal transplant.

Dumping syndrome (Answer C) is characterized by postprandial symptoms that occur about an hour after eating and typically consist of gastrointestinal and vasomotor symptoms such as abdominal cramping, tachycardia, and sweating. Dumping symptoms are almost always precipitated by the consumption of food and drink, particularly those containing simple carbohydrates. When severe, dumping syndrome can result in postprandial hypoglycemia. An elevated ethanol concentration is not an expected consequence of dumping.

Although nutritional deficiencies (Answer D) are relatively common after gastric bypass surgery, they are not expected to cause the symptoms described in this vignette and would not explain the elevated ethanol level.

Autonomic neuropathy (Answer B) is a recognized complication of gastric bypass surgery and is related to rapid weight loss. However, the presentation in this vignette is not consistent with this diagnosis, and it would not explain the elevated ethanol level.

Although rare, providers should be aware that gastric bypass can predispose to the development of autobrewery syndrome and should not assume patients are lying about alcohol ingestion (Answer E) when they present with intoxication. Conversely, it is also important to recognize that patients who undergo gastric bypass surgery are at high risk for developing alcohol use disorders postoperatively, thought in part to be secondary to anatomic changes that alter the metabolism of alcohol. A sensitive and empathetic approach to these patients can help make the correct diagnosis.

Educational Objective

Diagnose autobrewery syndrome as a rare complication of gastric bypass surgery.

Reference(s)

Steinert RE, Rehman A, Souto Lima EJ, et al. Roux-en-Y gastric bypass surgery changes fungal and bacterial microbiota in morbidly obese patients-a pilot study. *PLoS One*. 2020;15(7):e0236936. PMID: 32735609

Vandekerckhove E, Janssens F, Tate D, De Looze D. Treatment of gut fermentation syndrome with fecal microbiota transplantation. *Ann Intern Med*. 2020;173(10):855. PMID: 32805128

Dinis-Oliveira RJ. The auto-brewery syndrome: a perfect metabolic "storm" with clinical and forensic implications. *J Clin Med*. 2021;10(20):4637. PMID: 34682761

31 ANSWER: D) Increase in HDL cholesterol

Androgen-deprivation therapy (ADT) has established roles in the neoadjuvant treatment of high-risk localized prostate cancer together with radiotherapy and in biochemically recurrent nonmetastatic and metastatic disease. Use of GnRH analogues as a means of blocking testosterone production is currently the most commonly used ADT modality. As long-term survival in men with localized prostate cancer receiving ADT has become the norm, identifying and mitigating adverse effects of this therapy are important parts of prostate cancer survivorship.

ADT causes profound hypogonadism, leading to constitutional (eg, fatigue, low mood), sexual, and vasomotor symptoms, as well as accelerated bone loss that increases fracture risk. Of note, cardiovascular disease is a common cause of death in men with prostate cancer, so assessment of cardiometabolic health in men commencing ADT should be a routine part of clinical care.

Given that ADT causes profound hypogonadism (reducing both serum testosterone and estradiol to castrate concentrations), it promotes sarcopenic obesity with reductions in muscle mass (thus, Answer E is incorrect) and increases in fat mass (thus, Answer A is incorrect). Therefore, reliance on body weight may underestimate the deleterious changes in body composition that occur during ADT. In a meta-analysis of 16 observational studies of ADT on body composition, the mean increase in body weight was 2.1% (95% CI, 1.4%-2.9%). Fat mass increased by 7.7% (95% CI, 4.3%-11.2%) and lean mass decreased by 2.8% (95% CI, –3.6% to –2.0%). Of note, obesity at diagnosis is consistently associated with prostate cancer progression and an increased risk of prostate cancer–specific mortality. It is unclear whether this reflects differences in the biology of prostate cancer arising in men with obesity, or an effect of obesity-induced adipokines, insulin resistance, IGF-1 pathway alterations, or other factors on transforming prostate cancer once it develops. The possibility of the latter provides an impetus to prevent ADT-associated weight gain.

Sarcopenic obesity is associated with adverse metabolic outcomes. In prospective controlled studies, ADT is associated with increases in insulin resistance within 12 months of ADT commencement (thus, Answer B is incorrect). In a meta-analysis of observational studies of men with prostate cancer receiving ADT compared with men with prostate cancer not receiving ADT, the relative risk was 1.75 (95% CI, 1.27-1.41) for incident metabolic syndrome and 1.36 (95% CI, 1.17-1.58) for diabetes. However, whether ADT increases the risk of cardiovascular events remains uncertain. While observational studies report a consistent association between ADT and cardiovascular disease (including coronary heart disease, myocardial infarction, and sudden cardiac death), secondary analyses from randomized controlled trials have failed to demonstrate such a link. One potential explanation may be that ADT-associated metabolic changes differ from those seen in conventional metabolic syndrome. In contrast to conventional metabolic syndrome, ADT is associated with preferential accumulation of subcutaneous rather than visceral fat, and with increases rather than decreases in circulating adiponectin, a lipokine with potentially favorable cardiometabolic effects. Moreover, the effects of ADT on lipids are thought to be cardiovascularly neutral. While ADT has been associated with increases in total cholesterol, LDL cholesterol (thus, Answer C is incorrect), and triglycerides, it also increases HDL cholesterol (thus, Answer D is correct).

Men initiating ADT should undergo a holistic assessment of their cardiovascular risk. Absolute cardiovascular risk should be calculated using a validated risk prediction model for the particular patient population. Management of modifiable risk factors should be personalized based on absolute cardiometabolic risk and individual comorbidities, with attention to lifestyle factors and appropriate medical therapy following recommendations for the general population.

Educational Objective

Counsel a patient with prostate cancer regarding the adverse cardiometabolic effects of androgen-deprivation therapy.

Reference(s)

Haseen F, Murray LJ, Cardwell CR, O'Sullivan JM, Cantwell MM. The effect of androgen deprivation therapy on body composition in men with prostate cancer: systematic review and meta-analysis. *J Cancer Surviv.* 2010;4(2):128-139. PMID: 20091248

Grossmann M, Zajac JD. Management of side effects of androgen deprivation therapy. *Endocrinol Metab Clin North Am.* 2011;40(3):655-671. PMID: 21889727

32 **ANSWER: E) Start metformin**

The gold standard of diabetes therapy during pregnancy (either gestational or preexisting diabetes complicating pregnancy) is insulin therapy. Insulin is required to achieve the recommended targets:

- Fasting blood glucose less than 95 mg/dL (<5.3 mmol/L)
- 1-Hour postprandial blood glucose less than 140 mg/dL (<7.8 mmol/L) or 2-hour postprandial glucose less than 120 mg/dL (<6.7 mmol/L)
- Due to alterations in red blood cell turnover that lower the normal hemoglobin A_{1c} level in pregnancy, the target in pregnancy is less than 6.0% (42 mmol/mol) if this can be achieved without significant hypoglycemia

Strict monitoring of carbohydrate intake is also required. However, in some instances, the intensity of managing glycemia during pregnancy can be overwhelming, which may lead to patients being nonadherent to blood glucose checks, insulin dosing, or carbohydrate intake.

Given that this patient is already 32 weeks pregnant, starting carbohydrate counting (Answer C) or referring her for nutritional counseling again (Answer A) is unlikely to have a meaningful impact in such a short period before delivery. Learning to count carbohydrates, assess serving sizes, and dose insulin depending on grams of carbohydrate usually requires many months (if not years) of practice and education. Ideally, this education would have been undertaken with her prior pregnancies or much earlier during the current pregnancy.

In instances when intensive insulin therapy during pregnancy is too burdensome for patients, leading to nonadherence, use of metformin (Answer E) or glyburide (Answer D) is an option. In this case, given that the patient has been struggling with hypoglycemia and this has been contributing to the nonadherence, initiating an agent that could improve glycemia while avoiding hypoglycemia would be best. Both glyburide and metformin cross the placenta and have positives and negatives associated with their use in pregnancy. Usually, neither of these agents can achieve the strict glycemic targets recommended during pregnancy, but at this point, given the current situation with this patient's nonadherence, some improvement would still benefit maternal and fetal outcomes. Tolerating metformin is sometimes an issue because of gastrointestinal adverse effects, and there is uncertainty whether metformin is associated with an increased risk of premature birth. Glyburide can increase the risk of hypoglycemia and has been associated with multiple adverse neonatal outcomes (neonatal intensive care unit admissions, large-for-gestational-age infants, hypoglycemia, respiratory distress, and birth injury) vs insulin therapy. Prescribing metformin is the best next step.

No data are available to conclude whether DPP-4 inhibitors (Answer B) are safe in pregnancy. While DPP-4 inhibitors are listed as pregnancy category B because of studies in rats and rabbits, the limited data available in pregnant women are not sufficient to inform a drug-associated risk for major birth defects and miscarriage.

Educational Objective

Determine when noninsulin therapy may be indicated to control glycemia and reduce the risk of adverse maternal and fetal outcomes in women with gestational diabetes mellitus (or preexisting diabetes complicating pregnancy).

Reference(s)

American Diabetes Association. 14. Management of diabetes in pregnancy: standards of medical care in diabetes-2020. *Diabetes Care.* 2020;43(Suppl 1):S183-S192. PMID: 31862757

Rowan JA, Hague WM, Gao W, Battin MR, Moore MP; MiG Trial Investigators. Metformin versus insulin for the treatment of gestational diabetes. *N Engl J Med.* 2008;358(19):2003-2015. PMID: 18463376

Camelo Castillo W, Boggess K, Stürmer T, Brookhart MA, Benjamin DK Jr, Jonsson Funk M. Association of adverse pregnancy outcomes with glyburide vs insulin in women with gestational diabetes. *JAMA Pediatr.* 2015;169(5):452-458. PMID: 25822253

Ryu RJ, Hays KE, Hebert MF. Gestational diabetes mellitus management with oral hypoglycemic agents. *Semin Perinatol.* 2014;38(8):508-515. PMID: 25315294

33

ANSWER: C) Left adrenalectomy

This patient has primary aldosteronism and mild autonomous cortisol excess. The source(s) of aldosterone excess correlate poorly with cross-sectional imaging findings because: (1) clinically overt primary aldosteronism can originate in 1 or more subcentimeter aldosterone-producing nodule, and (2) nonfunctional adrenal adenomas are highly prevalent in the age group commonly affected by primary aldosteronism (older than 50 years). Consequently, adrenal venous sampling is the test of choice whenever surgery is being considered. Conversely, autonomous cortisol excess is typically associated with cortical nodules that are at least 1 cm in size. This patient has primary aldosteronism and very mild ACTH-independent hypercortisolism (incomplete suppression of cortisol after 1-mg dexamethasone suppression and normal 24-hour urinary cortisol excretion). For adrenal venous sampling data interpretation, cortisol is used for 2 reasons: (1) to ensure that the catheters were correctly placed in the adrenal veins (suggested by a ratio of $cortisol_{adrenal\ vein}/cortisol_{peripheral}$ ≥2 before cosyntropin and ≥5 after cosyntropin); and (2) to "normalize" the aldosterone concentrations measured in each location to account for variability in dilution with mixed venous blood. A ratio of aldosterone-to-cortisol of 4 or greater between the 2 adrenal veins (also known as the lateralization index) is commonly used to recommend unilateral adrenalectomy.

Coexistence of an adrenal cortical adenoma that produces cortisol autonomously in a patient with primary aldosteronism can lead to ACTH suppression and consequent suppression of cortisol production from the contralateral adrenal gland. In such cases, the suppressed contralateral cortisol artificially enhances the aldosterone-to-cortisol ratio in the gland without a nodule and favors lateralization to this side.

A mild degree of hypercortisolism, particularly without baseline ACTH suppression (ACTH >10 pg/mL), is unlikely to skew adrenal venous sampling results. Nevertheless, even if it did, and adrenal venous sampling still lateralizes to the adrenal gland harboring a nodule (as it did in this patient), that would reinforce correct primary aldosteronism lateralization, despite suppressed contralateral cortisol. Surgical removal of the nodular gland is expected to cure both primary aldosteronism and mild hypercortisolism (in this case, the left adrenal gland [Answer C]). Further evaluation for cortisol excess (Answer D) is not needed in this patient with subtly abnormal results from 1-mg dexamethasone-suppression testing and normal 24-hour urinary cortisol excretion before surgery.

If adrenal venous sampling lateralizes robustly to the adrenal without a nodule, the clinical decision is more complex, and it must consider the severity of primary aldosteronism and hypercortisolism in each individual patient. If primary aldosteronism is profound and hypercortisolism is minor, removing the gland without a nodule can be offered. Conversely, in patients with large nodules and clinically meaningful hypercortisolism, surgery should prioritize hypercortisolism, primarily because effective medical options are available for primary aldosteronism but are limited for hypercortisolism. Treatment with a mineralocorticoid receptor antagonist (Answer B) would be appropriate in such a case.

Adrenal nodule biopsy (Answer A) is not indicated for lipid-rich cortical adenomas.

Right adrenalectomy (Answer E) is incorrect, as adrenal venous sampling demonstrated aldosterone lateralization to the left adrenal gland. In addition, the right adrenal gland is anatomically normal.

Educational Objective

Interpret adrenal venous sampling results for primary aldosteronism lateralization in the context of an adrenal nodule and mild hypercortisolism.

Reference(s)

Turcu AF, Auchus R. Approach to the patient with primary aldosteronism: utility and limitations of adrenal vein sampling. *J Clin Endocrinol Metab.* 2021;106(4):1195-1208. PMID: 33382421

O'Toole SM, Sze WCC, Chung TT, et al. Low-grade cortisol cosecretion has limited impact on ACTH-stimulated AVS parameters in primary aldosteronism. *J Clin Endocrinol Metab.* 2020;105(10):dgaa519. PMID: 32785656

34 ANSWER: E) Switch to zoledronic acid

The patient in this vignette has developed recurrent kidney stones in the setting of teriparatide (PTH 1-34) therapy for osteoporosis over the past year. His laboratory findings confirm hypercalciuria despite hydrochlorothiazide use. While his bone mineral density has improved with this therapy, continuing teriparatide (Answer A) is not the best option given his active nephrolithiasis. In fact, the prescribing information for teriparatide lists hypercalciuria and urolithiasis as warnings and advises that this agent be used with caution in patients with kidney stones because of risk of exacerbation. A similar warning is listed for abaloparatide (Answer C), a PTHrP analogue used as an osteoanabolic agent in the treatment of osteoporosis. Abaloparatide is not currently approved by the US FDA for the treatment of osteoporosis in men.

Romosozumab (Answer D) is a monoclonal antibody to sclerostin, an endogenous inhibitor of bone formation. In 2019, the US FDA approved romosozumab for the treatment of postmenopausal osteoporosis. Although treatment with romosozumab for 12 months increased spine and hip bone mineral density compared with placebo and was well tolerated in a randomized controlled trial of 245 men with osteoporosis, romosozumab has not yet been approved by the US FDA for the treatment of osteoporosis in men. In addition, romosozumab has a black box warning of the potential risk of myocardial infarction, stroke, and cardiovascular death and should not be initiated in patients who have had a myocardial infarction or stroke within the preceding year. Since this patient had a myocardial infarction 6 months ago, switching to romosozumab would not be appropriate at this time.

While alendronate (Answer B) may be a good treatment option for patients without upper gastrointestinal pathology, it should be avoided in this patient because of his gastroparesis. Switching to zoledronic acid (Answer E), an intravenous bisphosphonate, is the best choice to treat his osteoporosis now. Zoledronic acid is contraindicated in the setting of chronic kidney disease with an estimated glomerular filtration rate less than 35 mL/min per 1.73 m^2.

Patients with active nephrolithiasis should be counseled to decrease their dietary oxalate intake. Other dietary risk factors for recurrent nephrolithiasis include higher sodium intake (which increases urinary calcium excretion) and lower fluid intake. If urine volume is less than 2 L in 24 hours, patients should increase their fluid intake with the goal of consistently producing at least 2 L of urine per day. The effect of dietary calcium intake on kidney stones is paradoxical, as increased dietary calcium intake is associated with a decreased risk of kidney stones.

Educational Objective

Recommend the most appropriate intervention for a patient who has osteoporosis and recurrent kidney stones and is treated with teriparatide.

Reference(s)

Lewiecki EM, Blicharski T, Goemaere S, et al. A phase III randomized placebo-controlled trial to evaluate efficacy and safety of romosozumab in men with osteoporosis. *J Clin Endocrinol Metab.* 2018;103(9):3183-3193. PMID: 29931216

Gennari L, Bilezikian JP. New and developing pharmacotherapy for osteoporosis in men. *Expert Opin Pharmacother.* 2018;19(3):253-264. PMID: 29350069

Heilberg IP, Goldfarb DS. Optimum nutrition for kidney stone disease. *Adv Chronic Kidney Dis.* 2013;20(2):165-174. PMID: 23439376

35 ANSWER: A) Craniopharyngioma

The patient has undergone thelarche (onset of secondary breast development) and pubarche (appearance of pubic hair) within a normal timeframe but has not experienced menarche. Delayed puberty is typically diagnosed if breast development does not start before age 13 years or if menstruation has not occurred within 3 years of thelarche or by age 15 years, although thresholds may vary with ethnic background. In contrast, pubertal arrest signifies that puberty has started normally, but has not progressed, which in young female patients includes when menses start and then stop. However, it is important to bear in mind that an insult arising in the window between onset of puberty and menarche may result in primary (as opposed to secondary) amenorrhea, as occurred in this case.

In this clinical context, with hyperprolactinemia and hypogonadotropic hypogonadism, imaging of the hypothalamus and pituitary must be performed to allow timely detection of a structural abnormality. Here, MRI shows a complex, mixed solid and cystic lesion (*yellow arrows*), which appears discrete and superior to the normal pituitary gland (*white arrows*).

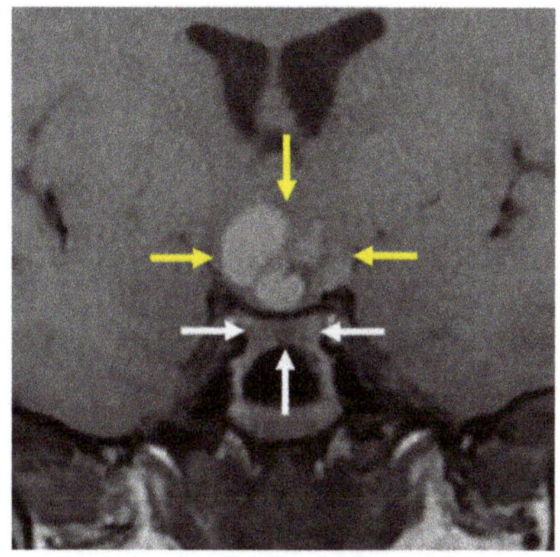

The appearance is consistent with a craniopharyngioma (Answer A). These tumors are often large, with a lobulated appearance, and display a predilection for extending superiorly into the third ventricle, encasing vessels, and adhering to adjacent structures. On T1-weighted MR sequences, craniopharyngiomas are typically isointense to hyperintense (the latter due to high protein content, corresponding to the "engine oil" appearance of cystic components drained at surgery). Following intravenous contrast, there is often marked enhancement of solid components, and peripheral enhancement may also be seen (as in this case). T2-weighted MRI confirms hyperintense cystic components. Areas of calcification may also be seen, but they are often better appreciated on CT.

Macroprolactinomas (Answer B) can have significant suprasellar and parasellar extension and undergo cystic degeneration. However, they usually have an intrasellar epicenter, with pituitary fossa expansion. In addition, the serum prolactin level in this patient is only mildly elevated (<2.5 × upper limit of normal), although exclusion of an artifactual low reading due to the "hook effect" should be undertaken if a primary pituitary adenoma is suspected on radiologic grounds.

Intracranial germ-cell tumors (germinomas) (Answer C) typically arise in the midline and are most commonly seen in the pineal gland followed by the suprasellar region (hypothalamus and third ventricle). Dual lesions involving both sites are virtually pathognomonic of this condition. Presentation of a suprasellar germ-cell tumor may include symptoms and signs of a local mass effect (eg, visual disturbance) and/or endocrine dysfunction (in particular diabetes insipidus). Although appearances vary, MRI most commonly demonstrates a soft-tissue mass that is isointense or slightly hyperintense to adjacent brain, with vivid and homogeneous enhancement. However, cyst formation may be seen, and some lesions exhibit calcification. Given the different management pathways of craniopharyngioma vs germ-cell tumor, if there is any doubt, further investigation should include measurement of serum (± cerebrospinal fluid) tumor markers, consideration of alternative MRI sequences (eg, diffusion-weighted imaging), and even biopsy.

Rathke cleft cysts (Answer D) may enlarge into the suprasellar region, but most are completely or mostly intrasellar and unilocular. Typically, there is no solid or enhancing component following contrast injection, and calcification is rare.

Although suprasellar meningiomas (Answer E) may be seen as discrete from the normal pituitary gland, their morphology and signal characteristics on MRI are quite distinct from those seen in this case. On close inspection, evidence of a dural origin can be seen in up to two-thirds of cases (eg, arising from the planum sphenoidale), and T1-weighted MRI reveals a homogeneous, isointense mass, with moderate to avid uniform postcontrast enhancement. On T2-weighted sequences, meningiomas may be hypointense, isointense, or hyperintense. Endocrine function is often surprisingly well preserved even with sizeable lesions. In addition, outside the context of an inherited tumor syndrome (eg, neurofibromatosis type 2 where multiple tumors may be seen), suprasellar meningiomas rarely present in patients of this age.

Educational Objective

Construct a differential diagnosis for pubertal arrest in a young woman and identify typical radiologic features of craniopharyngioma.

Reference(s)

Otte A, Muller HL. Mini-review: childhood-onset craniopharyngioma. *J Clin Endocrinol Metab.* 2021;106(10):e3820-e3836. PMID: 34086900

Jipa A, Jain V. Imaging of the sellar and parasellar regions. *Clin Imaging.* 2021;77(1):254-275. PMID: 34153590

36 ANSWER: A) Alirocumab

Familial hypercholesterolemia is an autosomal dominant disorder characterized by high levels of LDL cholesterol. Its most frequent presentation is the heterozygous form in which affected individuals inherit a pathogenic variant. Such individuals are at risk for atherosclerotic cardiovascular events early in life, so treatment should be started as soon as the condition is diagnosed. Most affected patients require combination therapy with 2 or more agents. Statins, cholesterol-absorption inhibitors, and bile acid sequestrants are typically used as initial therapy. This patient has been unable to tolerate these medications and has been undergoing LDL apheresis, but she would like to find an alternative treatment option.

Alirocumab (Answer A) is a monoclonal antibody against PCSK9. By binding to circulating PCSK9, it prevents its interaction with surface LDL-cholesterol receptors and leads to less destruction of these receptors. Alirocumab has been approved in the United States to be used by patients with clinical atherosclerotic cardiovascular events or by patients with heterozygous familial hypercholesterolemia whose LDL cholesterol is not at goal despite taking the maximally tolerated statin dosage. It comes in 2 doses: 75 mg and 150 mg. Patients administer alirocumab every 14 days subcutaneously. They also have the option to administer 450 mg monthly. The ODYSSEY FH I and FH II studies included patients with heterozygous familial hypercholesterolemia whose LDL cholesterol was not at goal on maximally tolerated lipid-lowering therapy. Patients were randomly assigned to alirocumab, 75 mg every 14 days, or placebo and the dosage was increased by week 12 if LDL cholesterol was not at goal (>70 mg/dL [>1.81 mmol/L]). By week 24, the treatment groups had a mean LDL-cholesterol decrease of 49% in both the FH I and FH II studies. The most commonly reported adverse effects were injection site reactions, flulike symptoms, and back pain. The patient described in this vignette is a candidate for this medication; she stopped LDL apheresis and started alirocumab, 75 mg every 14 days. Evolocumab, another monoclonal antibody against PCSK9, would have been a possible treatment option.

Bempedoic acid (Answer B) is an ATP citrate lyase inhibitor that decreases cholesterol synthesis. In the United States, it is approved for use in patients with atherosclerotic cardiovascular disease or in patients with heterozygous familial hypercholesterolemia whose LDL-cholesterol concentration is not at goal. It comes as a tablet (180 mg daily). The Clear Harmony Trial was a phase 3, randomized, placebo-controlled trial that included patients with atherosclerotic cardiovascular disease, heterozygous familial hypercholesterolemia, or both who were already on maximally tolerated statin therapy. A 12.6% reduction in LDL cholesterol was observed in the bempedoic acid treatment group compared with a 1% increase in the placebo group. The most frequent adverse effects are hyperuricemia, gout, thrombocytopenia, leukopenia, and upper respiratory tract infections. This patient has gout, so bempedoic acid would not be the best first choice because it could raise her uric acid level. Also, compared with alirocumab, bempedoic acid provides less LDL-cholesterol lowering.

Lomitapide (Answer D) is a microsomal triglyceride transfer protein inhibitor. Microsomal triglyceride transfer protein is involved in the transfer of triglycerides and phospholipids to apolipoprotein B. Blocking this protein results in lower levels of apolipoprotein B–containing lipoproteins such as VLDL and accumulation of triglycerides in the liver, leading to steatosis. Lomitapide comes as a capsule and the starting dosage is 5 mg daily. The dosage can be increased to 60 mg daily. A single-arm, open-label, phase 3 study of patients with homozygous hypercholesterolemia showed an LDL-cholesterol decrease of 50% at week 26. The most frequent adverse effects are gastrointestinal disturbances, liver enzyme elevation, and increased liver fat. Long-term risks of this medication include steatohepatitis and liver fibrosis. This medication provides similar LDL-cholesterol lowering to that of alirocumab; however, its long-term adverse effects make it a less desirable choice when other options are available.

Mipomersen (Answer E) is an antisense oligonucleotide that binds to the messenger RNA of apolipoprotein B and leads to its degradation. Preventing the formation of apolipoprotein B reduces apolipoprotein B–containing lipoproteins. Mipomersen comes in one dose (200 mg), and it is administered weekly via a subcutaneous injection. A phase 3, randomized, double-blind, placebo-controlled study in patients with homozygous familial hypercholesterolemia showed a 25% reduction in LDL cholesterol after 26 weeks of mipomersen treatment. The most common adverse effects are injection site reactions and liver enzyme elevation. The risk of hepatotoxicity makes this medication less appealing when there are other treatment options. Also, mipomersen is no longer available in the United States.

Evinacumab (Answer C) is a monoclonal antibody to angiopoietin-like 3 (ANGPTL3). ANGPTL3 is a hepatic protein that inhibits lipoprotein lipase and endothelial lipase activity leading to increased triglycerides and LDL cholesterol. Individuals with loss-of-function variants in the *ANGPTL3* gene have lower levels of triglycerides and LDL cholesterol. The recommended dosage of evinacumab is 15 mg/kg administered intravenously every 4 weeks. The ELIPSE HoFH study is a phase 3, double-blind, placebo-controlled trial that included patients with homozygous familial hypercholesterolemia. It showed a 47% LDL-cholesterol reduction at week 24 in the treatment arm. The most frequent adverse events included nasopharyngitis, flulike symptoms, dizziness, and nausea.

Lomitapide, mipomersen, and evinacumab are approved only for patients with homozygous familial hypercholesterolemia. This patient has heterozygous familial hypercholesterolemia.

Educational Objective

Describe treatment options for patients with heterozygous familial hypercholesterolemia and coronary artery disease.

Reference(s)

Kastelein JJ, Ginsberg HN, Langslet G, et al. ODYSSEY FH I and FH II: 78 week results with alirocumab treatment in 735 patients with heterozygous familial hypercholesterolemia. *Eur Heart J*. 2015;36(43):2996-3003. PMID: 26330422

Cuchel M, Meagher EA, du Toit Theron H, et al; Phase 3 HoFH Lomitapide Study Investigators. Efficacy and safety of microsomal triglyceride transfer protein inhibitor in patients with homozygous familial hypercholesterolemia: a single-arm, open-label, phase 3 study. *Lancet*. 2013;381(9860):40-46. PMID: 23122768

Raal FJ, Santos RD, Blom DJ, et al. Mipomersen, an apolipoprotein B synthesis inhibitor, for lowering of LDL cholesterol concentrations in patients with homozygous familial hypercholesterolaemia: a randomised, double-blind, placebo-controlled trial. *Lancet*. 2010;375(9719):998-1006. PMID: 20227758

Ray KK, Bays HE, Catapano AL, et al. Safety and efficacy of bempedoic acid to reduce LDL cholesterol. *N Engl J Med*. 2019;380(11):1022-1032. PMID: 30865796

Raal FJ, Rosenson RS, Reeskamp LF, et al; ELIPSE HoFH Investigators. Evinacumab for homozygous familial hypercholesterolemia. *N Engl J Med*. 2020;383(8):711-720. PMID: 32813947

37 ANSWER: C) Percutaneous ethanol ablation

This patient has a cystic thyroid nodule that has been aspirated several times, but it recurs after each aspiration. The patient is experiencing compressive symptoms due to the size of this cystic nodule and she does not want thyroid surgery. Therefore, percutaneous ethanol ablation (Answer C) should be considered. Within a thyroid cyst, the ethanol results in permanent tissue damage with subsequent fibrosis, necrosis, and thrombosis of cyst wall blood vessels, which reduces the cyst volume and lessens compressive symptoms. This procedure is performed in the outpatient setting, and it is well tolerated. Depending on practices across the United States or the world, this procedure may be performed by radiologists, endocrinologists, or endocrine surgeons. Furthermore, percutaneous ethanol ablation may not be widely available in the United States or in other countries.

Per the 2015 American Thyroid Association guidelines on thyroid nodules, pure cystic thyroid nodules have a minimal risk of malignancy (<1%), and partially cystic thyroid nodules without suspicious features are also considered to have a very low risk of malignancy (<3%). Therefore, FNA biopsy is not required to check for malignancy in a purely cystic thyroid nodule. Once thyroid cancer is excluded, treatment of a thyroid nodule is recommended according to the presence or absence of compressive symptoms. Treatment options for symptomatic benign cystic or predominately cystic thyroid nodules include needle aspiration, minimally invasive techniques such as percutaneous ethanol injection under ultrasound guidance, or surgery. Recurrence rates are high with needle aspiration (60%-90%). Although surgical management is considered to be definitive treatment, it can be associated with complications, and some patients may decline this treatment modality. In addition, surgery may be contraindicated in some patients because of medical comorbidities.

In a recent publication, 20 patients with cystic thyroid nodules were treated with percutaneous ethanol ablation. Of these 20 patients, 12 had complex cystic thyroid nodules (>50% cystic component) and 8 had purely cystic nodules. Before ethanol ablation, the largest median diameter of the thyroid cyst was 4.5 cm (range, 2.3-8.0 cm), and the median volume was 19.6 mL (range, 2.8-118.1 mL). The median amount of ethanol administered was 3 mL (range, 0.5-20 mL). At a median follow-up of 2 years, 89% of patients were asymptomatic, and 70% had a 50% or greater reduction in thyroid nodule volume. The median decrease in volume was 75.6%. Temporary adverse effects such as vagal reaction, slight pain, and bleeding into the cyst were observed in 4 patients (20%). Overall, the procedure was well tolerated and deemed to be safe. Percutaneous ethanol ablation is the best management strategy for this patient's thyroid nodule.

Levothyroxine suppressive therapy (Answer A) has not been shown to decrease thyroid nodule size, and this patient's TSH concentration is within the reference range.

Because her TSH concentration is normal, thyroid scan (Answer D) is not indicated.

The patient opted out of thyroid surgery, so total thyroidectomy (Answer E) should not be considered. If surgery were chosen, right hemithyroidectomy rather than total thyroidectomy would be the surgical choice.

Her compressive symptoms are explained by her large cystic thyroid nodule, and neck CT (Answer B) is not necessary to evaluate her symptoms.

Educational Objective

List indications for ethanol ablation in the management of thyroid nodules.

Reference(s)

Haugen BR, Alexander EK, Bible KC, et al. 2015 American Thyroid Association management guidelines for adult patients with thyroid nodules and differentiated thyroid cancer: the American Thyroid Association Guidelines Task Force on Thyroid Nodules and Differentiated Thyroid Cancer. *Thyroid.* 2016;26(1):1-133. PMID: 26462967

Iñiguez-Ariza NM, Lee RA, Singh-Ospina NM, Stan MN, Castro MR. Ethanol ablation for the treatment of cystic and predominantly cystic thyroid nodules. *Mayo Clin Proc.* 2018;93(8):1009-1017. PMID: 30078409

38 ANSWER: D) Normal pituitary gland

Therapy with immune checkpoint inhibitor monoclonal antibodies has emerged during the recent years as an effective therapeutic option for several malignant tumors. The 3 main classes of immune checkpoint inhibitors currently available are anti-CTLA-4 antibodies, anti-PD-1 antibodies, and anti-PD-L1 antibodies. Immune checkpoint inhibitor therapy may cause adverse effects related to activation of the immune system. The endocrine system seems to be particularly susceptible to immune-related adverse events. Thyroiditis (often with a thyrotoxic phase followed by hypothyroidism) is particularly frequent with anti-PD-1 and anti-PD-L1 antibodies. Hypophysitis is more likely to be caused by anti-CTLA-4 antibodies or by combination therapy. This form of hypophysitis differs from the classic form of lymphocytic hypophysitis, as it does not have a high prevalence in females, it is rarely associated with diabetes insipidus, and the pituitary enlargement is not marked and sometimes absent. Typically, the highest risk of anti-CTLA-4–induced hypophysitis occurs 8 to 10 weeks after therapy is started. While ACTH deficiency is almost invariably seen, affected patients often have secondary hypothyroidism and hypogonadism. Recently, adrenal insufficiency due to isolated ACTH deficiency has been reported to be associated with immune checkpoint inhibitors. This syndrome is most frequently caused by monotherapy with the anti-PD-1 antibodies nivolumab and pembrolizumab. The median time to develop this syndrome is 6 months, but it may occur after longer periods. Symptoms are often nonspecific but are consistent with what would be expected with adrenal insufficiency such as fatigue and anorexia. In addition to low serum cortisol and ACTH, hyponatremia and eosinophilia can be seen. Interestingly, in most cases of anti-PD-1–induced isolated ACTH deficiency (>90%), the pituitary gland appears normal on MRI (Answer D).

Diffuse pituitary enlargement (Answer A) is more likely to be observed in anti-CTLA-4–induced hypophysitis in which pituitary enlargement occurs in approximately 60% of cases.

Empty sella (Answer B) would not be expected in this clinical scenario (isolated ACTH deficiency). Additionally, most patients with empty sella have normal pituitary function.

A large pituitary mass suggestive of metastasis (Answer C) would obviously be considered in the differential diagnosis of a patient with cancer who presents with ACTH deficiency. However, metastasis would be unlikely to cause isolated ACTH deficiency. Additionally, pituitary metastases typically cause diabetes insipidus, and this patient does not have polyuria or polydipsia (even after glucocorticoid therapy was started, which may unmask latent diabetes insipidus).

Finally, thickening of the pituitary stalk (Answer E) is a radiologic sign that can result from inflammatory causes (sarcoidosis, infundibulitis), infectious causes (tuberculosis), or neoplastic causes (Langerhans-cell histiocytosis, Erdheim-Chester disease, lymphoma, germinoma), and it is usually associated with diabetes insipidus, which this patient does not have.

Educational Objective

Construct a differential diagnosis of secondary adrenal insufficiency in a patient with cancer being treated with immunotherapy.

Reference(s)

Iglesias P, Sánchez JC, Díez JJ. Isolated ACTH deficiency induced by cancer immunotherapy: a systematic review. *Pituitary.* 2021;24(4):630-643. PMID: 33761049

Di Dalmazi G, Ippolito S, Lupi I, Caturegli P. Hypophysitis induced by immune checkpoint inhibitors: a 10-year assessment. *Expert Rev Endocrinol Metab.* 2019;14(6):381-398. PMID: 31842671

Wehbeh L, Alreddawi S, Salvatori R. Hypophysitis in the era of immune checkpoint inhibitors and immunoglobulin G4-related disease. *Expert Rev Endocrinol Metab.* 2019;14(3):167-178. PMID: 30939947

39

ANSWER: E) Switch insulin lispro to regular insulin

Unfortunately, diabetic gastroparesis can cause great difficulty in controlling postprandial glucose excursions because food absorption is often unpredictable in these patients. Thus, many different management approaches may be needed. Patients with gastroparesis who take prandial insulin may need to delay their insulin doses until after they eat to ensure that nausea and vomiting does not occur after insulin administration. In addition, shorter-acting insulin formulations (insulin lispro and insulin aspart) have a quicker onset of action and peak effect that may occur prior to stomach emptying and digestion, resulting in frequent postprandial hypoglycemia (*see figure*).

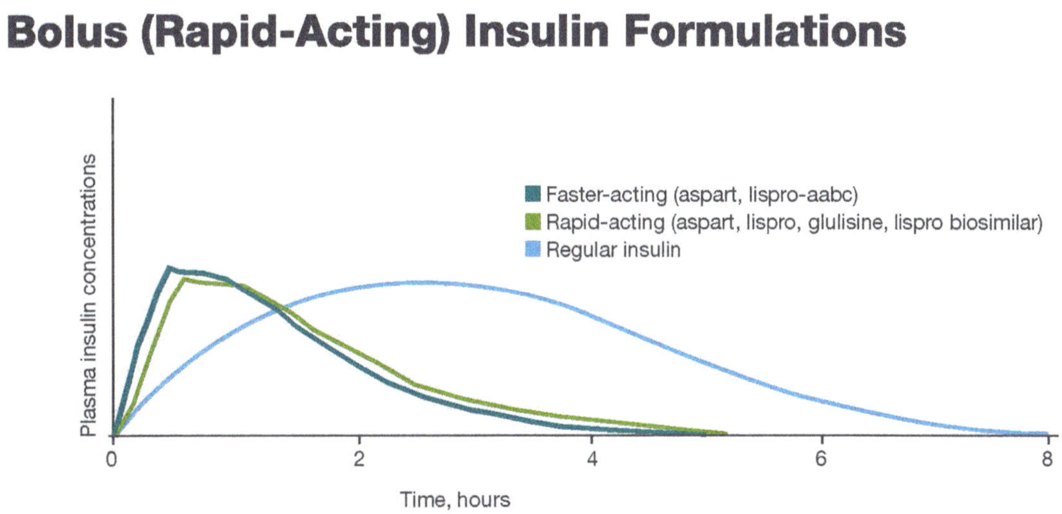

Adapted from Hirsch IB. Insulin analogues. *N Engl J Med.* 2005;352(2):174-183 and Flood TM. Appropriate use of insulin analogs in an increasingly complex type 2 diabetes mellitus (T2DM) landscape. *J Fam Pract* 2007;56(Suppl 1):S11-S12.

In some cases, patients may need to inject prandial insulin hours after a meal in an attempt to make the insulin bolus match the late absorption of the food consumed. Alternative strategies include switching the prandial insulin to one that has a delayed onset and peak action (ie, regular insulin).

Reducing the dose of basal insulin (Answer A) or switching from one basal insulin to another (Answer C) is incorrect, as neither strategy would address the postprandial hypoglycemia that is being driven by the underlying gastroparesis, and decreased insulin doses will further worsen her glycemic control.

Reducing the insulin lispro dose (Answer B) may initially seem like a reasonable approach, but not in a patient with a hemoglobin A_{1c} level of 7.8% (62 mmol/mol), which is above her individualized goal of less than

7.0% (<53 mmol/mol). The issue here is not really the insulin dose, but rather the delayed gastric emptying resulting in a mismatch between the peak effect of insulin lispro and the peak glucose absorption. The best approach is to try to match up these peaks, rather than to reduce the insulin dose. Thus, switching prandial insulin to regular insulin (Answer E), which has a delayed onset of action and peak effect vs that of insulin lispro, is the best step. This change would more consistently match up the peak action of the prandial insulin with the peak (delayed) absorption of glucose, thereby helping to reduce the frequency of postprandial hypoglycemia.

Switching insulin lispro to insulin lispro-aabc (Answer D), an insulin formulation with an even faster onset of action and peak effect than that of insulin lispro, would only exacerbate the current problem. Insulin lispro-aabc is faster acting than insulin lispro because the insulin lispro-aabc formulation contains insulin lispro with 2 additional ingredients. Tiny amounts of treprostinil, an analogue of prostacyclin, and sodium citrate, were added to relax blood vessels near the injection or infusion site, speeding up insulin's absorption/action.

Moving the administration of insulin lispro to after meals would have been reasonable to try before switching to regular insulin, but that was not provided as an answer choice.

Educational Objective

Determine when older insulin formulations that provide a delayed peak effect may be more appropriate in patients with gastroparesis experiencing postprandial hypoglycemia.

Reference(s)

Hirsch IB. Insulin analogues. *N Engl J Med.* 2005;352(2):174-183. PMID: 15647580

Flood TM. Appropriate use of insulin analogs in an increasingly complex type 2 diabetes mellitus (T2DM) landscape. *J Fam Pract* 2007;56(Suppl 1):S11-S12. PMID: 17217893

Young CF, Moussa M, Shubrook JH. Diabetic gastroparesis: a review [published correction appears in *Diabetes Spectr.* 2020;33(4):358]. *Diabetes Spectr.* 2020;33(3):290-297. PMID: 32848351

40 ANSWER: B) DICER1 syndrome

The co-occurrence of ovarian Sertoli-Leydig–cell tumors and thyroid cancer or familial multinodular goiter is highly suggestive of DICER1 syndrome (Answer B). DICER1 is an endoribonuclease that promotes normal processing of RNA into small RNAs, including miRNA. Germline pathogenic variants in the *DICER1* gene are associated with an autosomal dominant syndrome characterized by pleuropulmonary blastomas, lung cysts, cystic nephroma, Sertoli-Leydig–cell tumors, embryonal rhabdomyosarcoma, benign and malignant thyroid lesions, and other rare tumors. Clinical manifestations of DICER1 syndrome most frequently occur in infancy, childhood, and adolescence. Multinodular goiter is the most common associated condition, and the lifetime risk of thyroid cancer is estimated to be 16 times higher in patients with DICER1 syndrome than in the general population. Follicular variant of papillary thyroid carcinoma and minimally invasive follicular thyroid carcinoma are common. Most thyroid cancers are diagnosed before age 40 years with peak incidence between age 10 and 20 years. Initiation of neck ultrasonography as a screening test is recommended at age 8 years. This patient underwent ultrasound-guided FNA biopsy of her largest thyroid nodule in the context of a known history of DICER1 syndrome. In patients with a higher pretest probability of thyroid cancer, such as those familial syndromes, the 2015 American Thyroid Association Guidelines for Adult Patients with Thyroid Nodules and Differentiated Thyroid Cancer suggest that lower size cutoffs for FNA can be used.

Early-onset medullary thyroid carcinoma is the hallmark of multiple endocrine neoplasia type 2B (Answer C). While pheochromocytoma and nonendocrine manifestations (intestinal ganglioneuromatosis, mucosal neuromas/neurofibromas, and marfanoid body habitus) may occur, ovarian Sertoli-Leydig–cell tumors are not characteristic of multiple endocrine neoplasia type 2B.

PTEN hamartoma tumor syndrome (Cowden syndrome) (Answer D) results from pathogenic variants in the *PTEN* gene and is associated with an increased risk of benign thyroid nodules, as well as papillary and follicular thyroid carcinoma. Colonic polyps are characteristic and there is an elevated risk of breast, endometrial, and renal cell carcinoma. Macrocephaly can be observed in individuals with Cowden syndrome or DICER1 syndrome. The absence of colonic polyps and any of the malignancies commonly associated with Cowden syndrome makes this diagnosis unlikely.

Carney complex (Answer A) is an autosomal dominant multiple endocrine neoplasia syndrome that is associated with pathogenic variants in the protein kinase A type I alpha regulatory subunit gene (*PRKAR1A*). Cushing syndrome due to primary pigmented nodular adrenocortical disease and acromegaly are common endocrine manifestations. Benign large-cell calcifying Sertoli-cell tumors are also often seen in males, while Leydig-cell tumors are less common. Thyroid nodules are observed in 75% of patients with Carney complex, but papillary and follicular thyroid carcinoma affect less than 10%. Nonendocrine manifestations of Carney complex include characteristic pigmented lesions of the skin (lentigines), blue nevi, and cutaneous and cardiac myxomas. The absence of any of the classic clinical findings of Carney complex in this patient makes the diagnosis extremely unlikely.

Werner syndrome (Answer E) is an autosomal recessive disorder that is most common in Japan and is associated with pathogenic variants in the *WRN* gene. Clinical manifestations include premature aging, short stature, nonmedullary thyroid cancer (papillary thyroid cancer, follicular thyroid cancer, and anaplastic thyroid cancer), soft-tissue sarcoma, and meningioma. There is no description of premature aging or short stature in this vignette to suggest a diagnosis of Werner syndrome.

Educational Objective

Describe the association between differentiated thyroid cancer and DICER1 syndrome.

Reference(s)

Bakhuizen JJ, Hanson H, van der Tuin K, et al; SIOPE Host Genome Working Group; CanGene-CanVar Clinical Guideline Working Group; Expert Network Members. Surveillance recommendations for DICER1 pathogenic variant carriers: a report from the SIOPE Host Genome Working Group and CanGene-CanVar Clinical Guideline Working Group. *Fam Cancer.* 2021;20(4):337-348. PMID: 34170462

Cameselle-Teijeiro JM, Mete O, Asa SL, LiVolsi V. Inherited follicular epithelial-derived thyroid carcinomas: from molecular biology to histological correlates. *Endocr Pathol.* 2021;32(1):77-101. PMID: 33495912

Durieux E, Descotes F, Mauduit C, Decaussin M, Guyetant S, Devouassoux-Shisheboran M. The co-occurrence of an ovarian Sertoli-Leydig cell tumor with a thyroid carcinoma is highly suggestive of a DICER1 syndrome. *Virchows Arch.* 2016;468(5):631-636. PMID: 26983701

41 ANSWER: B) Ethinyl estradiol

Evaluation of patients who present with new-onset hypertriglyceridemia should start by ruling out secondary etiologies that cause this condition. Secondary etiologies of hypertriglyceridemia are uncontrolled type 2 diabetes mellitus, nephrotic syndrome, medications, pregnancy, excess alcohol intake, and excess carbohydrate intake.

Medications known to raise triglycerides include thiazides, β-adrenergic blockers, oral estrogen, isotretinoin, corticosteroids, bile acid sequestrants, antiretroviral protease inhibitors, immunosuppressants, and antipsychotic agents. Oral estrogen (Answer B) increases triglyceride levels by 10% to 50%. The degree of hypertriglyceridemia depends on the type and the dosage of the estrogen preparation. Estrogen raises triglycerides by increasing hepatic VLDL production. The mechanism by which it affects lipoprotein lipase activity is uncertain; however, some investigators propose that it reduces triglyceride catabolism by lowering lipoprotein lipase activity. One theory as to why oral estrogen, but not transdermal estrogen, affects triglycerides is that oral estrogens are delivered to hepatocytes by the portal circulation in high concentrations after intestinal absorption. These high intrahepatic estrogen levels lead to increases in VLDL production.

Norgestimate (Answer D) is a progestin with weak androgenic properties. A study showed that progesterone alone did not alter VLDL, so it does not influence triglyceride concentrations.

There is no evidence that ranitidine (Answer E), amlodipine (Answer A), or metformin (Answer C) is associated with hypertriglyceridemia.

Educational Objective

Identify medications that cause secondary hypertriglyceridemia.

Reference(s)

Berglund L, Brunzell J, Goldberg A, et al; Endocrine Society. Evaluation and treatment of hypertriglyceridemia: an Endocrine Society clinical practice guideline. *J Clin Endocrinol Metab.* 2012;97(9):2969-2989. PMID: 22962670

Walsh B, Schiff I, rosner B. Effects of postmenopausal estrogen replacement on the concentrations and metabolism of plasma lipoproteins. *N Engl J Med.* 1991;325(17):1196-1204. PMID: 1922206

Goldberg RB, Chait A. A comprehensive update on the chylomicronemia syndrome. *Front Endocrinol.* 2020;11:593931. PMID: 33193106

Jiang Y, Tian W. The effects of progesterone on blood lipids in hormone replacement therapy. *Lipids Health Dis.* 2017;16(1):219. PMID: 29157280

42 **ANSWER: D) Klinefelter syndrome**

This man presented to his primary care physician with established osteoporosis. Potential contributing factors are found in up to 60% in men with osteoporosis, with major causes of secondary osteoporosis including hypogonadism, glucocorticoid exposure, and excess alcohol consumption. Recommended initial laboratory testing for men with osteoporosis includes serum testosterone measurement. In this patient, serum testosterone was low, prompting measurement of gonadotropins, which were elevated, findings indicative of primary hypogonadism. On examination, he had features consistent with hypogonadism (ie, gynecomastia and loss of muscle bulk) and testes were small and firm to palpation, consistent with a clinical diagnosis of Klinefelter syndrome (Answer D) that was subsequently confirmed by karyotype testing. On specific questioning, the patient reported a history of a left wrist facture after a fall from standing height 2 years prior to presentation, although this was not investigated at the time. He also reported a history of infertility. Testosterone replacement was initiated, with noticeable improvements in energy levels, libido, and muscle strength. Given his established osteoporosis and the lack of fracture data with testosterone treatment, antiresorptive treatment with a bisphosphonate was commenced, consistent with Endocrine Society recommendations.

Klinefelter syndrome is the most common cause of organic hypogonadism in men, with an estimated prevalence of 1 in 600 of liveborn males. Affected men present with uniformly elevated gonadotropins, while testosterone concentrations are either frankly low or, especially in younger men, normal to low-normal. Therefore, pubertal androgenization can occur, and men may not appear to be frankly hypogonadal. However, more than 95% of affected men have very small (prepubertal-sized) 3- to 4-mL testes that are firm to palpation. Infertility is typical, although some men have sperm that can be retrieved by testicular sperm extraction. Given that genital examination is not routine in men, the Klinefelter diagnosis can be missed, and registry data suggest that only one-third of men with Klinefelter syndrome are diagnosed in their lifetime, with a median age at diagnosis of 27 years, around the time affected men present with infertility. Missed or delayed diagnosis and ensuing untreated hypogonadism is associated with reduced quality of life and increased morbidity, including osteoporosis and increased risk of obesity, diabetes, sarcopenia, and cardiovascular disease.

While this man's glucocorticoid exposure was clinically evident and most likely contributed to his osteoporosis, glucocorticoid excess (Answer C)—whether exogenous or endogenous—is associated with central suppression of the hypothalamic-pituitary-testicular axis and therefore causes hypogonadotropic (secondary) rather than primary hypogonadism.

Likewise, obesity (Answer E), especially class III or higher (BMI >40 kg/m^2) is associated with central hypothalamic-pituitary-testicular axis suppression and presents with hypogonadotropic hypogonadism.

Whether depression (Answer B) is associated with low serum testosterone remains controversial, and multiple large, population-based epidemiologic studies have failed to find a consistent association between circulating endogenous testosterone concentrations and depression. Certainly, depression would not be expected to cause severe primary hypogonadism as seen in this case. Of note, untreated organic hypogonadism can cause low mood in some patients, and testosterone replacement is expected to improve low mood if present.

Finally, while advanced age (Answer A) has been associated with somewhat diminished Leydig-cell reserve in some men, age-related primary hypogonadism manifests predominantly with modest elevations in LH (<2 times the upper normal limit) and modest reductions in serum testosterone (mean ~220 ng/dL [7.5 nmol/L]). In age-related primary hypogonadism, testicular size is typically normal or low-normal, and testes are soft, rather than firm. Severe hypogonadism with clinical features as described in the case vignette would not be consistent with hypogonadism due to advanced age alone.

Educational Objective

Diagnose Klinefelter syndrome as a cause of secondary osteoporosis in men.

Reference(s)

Diab DL, Watts NB. Updates on osteoporosis in men. *Endocrinol Metab Clin North Am.* 2021;50(2):239-249. PMID: 34023041

Gravholt CH, Chang S, Wallentin M, Fedder J, Moore P, Skakkebaek A. Klinefelter syndrome: integrating genetics, neuropsychology, and endocrinology. *Endocr Rev.* 2018;39(4):389-423. PMID: 29438472

Watts NB, Adler RA, Bilezikian JP, et al; Endocrine Society. Osteoporosis in men: an Endocrine Society Clinical Practice Guideline. *J Clin Endocrinol Metab.* 2012;97(6):1802-1822. PMID: 22675062

Bhasin S, Seidman S. Testosterone treatment of depressive disorders in men: too much smoke, not enough high-quality evidence. *JAMA Psychiatry.* 2019;76(1):9-10. PMID: 30428087

Tajar A, Forti G, O'Neill TW, et al; EMAS Group. Characteristics of secondary, primary, and compensated hypogonadism in aging men: evidence from the European Male Ageing Study. *J Clin Endocrinol Metab.* 2010;95(4):1810-1818. PMID: 20173018

43 ANSWER: B) Order x-ray of the left femur

Paget disease of bone is an osteoclast disorder that has been hypothesized to be due to viral infection. Rarely, the disease is due to pathogenic variants in genes that encode sequestosome 1, RANK, and others. In most cases, Paget disease can be easily controlled with bisphosphonates such as a dose of zoledronic acid, 5 mg, infused as infrequently as every 6 years.

Osteosarcoma is a rare complication of Paget disease of bone, occurring in 0.2% to 1% of patients. Increasing pain and swelling are concerning in patients whose pain had previously been controlled with a bisphosphonate. Osteosarcoma is usually identified by x-ray (Answer B), and this is the best next step in this patient's evaluation. X-ray imaging would also detect fractures that can occur within pagetic lesions. If findings on bone x-ray are normal, MRI should be considered due to higher sensitivity in detecting osteosarcoma.

Repeating the nuclear medicine bone scan (Answer E) would be reasonable to identify new pagetic lesions if the patient had reported new bone pain in an area without previous increased scintographic uptake. However, the sensitivity of this test would be lower because of previous bisphosphonate administration.

Administration of a third zoledronic acid infusion soon after the second infusion (Answer A) or prescribing calcitonin (Answer C) is unlikely to alleviate bone pain.

Acetaminophen (Answer D) may reduce pain, but this strategy could delay diagnosis of a more serious complication.

Educational Objective

Evaluate for osteosarcoma as a complication of Paget disease.

Reference(s)

Singer FR, Bone HG 3rd, Hosking DJ, et al. Paget's disease of bone: an Endocrine Society clinical Practice Guideline. *J Clin Endocrinol Metab.* 2014;99(12):4408-4422. PMID: 25406796

Singer FR. Paget's disease of bone-genetic and environmental factors. *Nat Rev Endocrinol.* 2015;11(11):662-671. PMID: 26284446

44 ANSWER: D) *HNF4A* (maturity-onset diabetes of the young type 1)

This patient was diagnosed with type 1 diabetes, but she has detectable C-peptide 5 years after diagnosis and an absence of antibodies commonly associated with the autoimmune basis of this disease. Moreover, she has no history of diabetic ketoacidosis, and her family history suggests an autosomal dominant pattern of inheritance. For these reasons, either type 2 diabetes mellitus or a monogenic cause of diabetes should be considered. Her age, normal BMI, and lack of response to metformin makes type 2 diabetes (Answer E) a less likely diagnosis. Indeed, use of the maturity-onset diabetes of the young (MODY) probability calculator (https://www.diabetesgenes.org/exeter-diabetes-app/) yielded an approximately 1 in 4 chance that this patient has MODY. Since she is on insulin therapy, the C-peptide concentration has important utility in modulating the risk assessment: a C-peptide concentration greater than 0.6 ng/mL (>0.2 nmol/L) further increases the likelihood of MODY, and a C-peptide concentration less than 0.6 ng/mL (<0.2 nmol/L) decreases the probability to less than 1%. The use of such calculators may help practitioners identify patients at risk. Standard clinical criteria (age at diagnosis <25 years, use of oral agents, and an affected parent) identify only 48% of patients with MODY.

The different forms of MODY have unique characteristics that make it possible to predict which genetic abnormality may be responsible for disease. The most common causes of MODY are pathogenic variants in the *HNF1A* gene (Answer B), *GCK* gene (Answer A), and *HNF4A* gene (Answer D), accounting for approximately 50% to 60%, 20% to 30%, and 10% to 20% of cases, respectively. *HNF1B*-associated MODY (Answer C) is less common.

GCK-associated MODY (Answer A) has a stable disease course without a risk for complications, and affected individuals do not require pharmacologic treatment. Her increasing need for medication makes this diagnosis unlikely.

HNF1B-associated MODY (Answer C) is caused by a β-cell developmental defect. Also, it is associated with exocrine pancreas insufficiency and extrapancreatic findings, typically kidney, in approximately 40% of affected individuals. None of these findings are present in this patient.

The apparent progression to insulin therapy is consistent with the clinical course of both *HNF1A*-associated MODY and *HNF4A*-associated MODY. *HNF1A*-associated MODY (Answer B) is often characterized by glycosuria, which is absent in this patient.

Patients with *HNF4A*-MODY (Answer D) often have a history of being large-for-gestational-age; this patient's birth weight was 3500 g at 34 weeks. Neonatal hypoglycemia is also reported in patients with this condition, presumably due to hyperinsulinism; she also had neonatal hypoglycemia. Interestingly, carriers of *HNF4A* pathogenic variants who have not yet been identified as having diabetes have been studied and found to have a mean duration of hypoglycemia of 10.4% on 72-hour continuous glucose monitoring, with most episodes found to be nocturnal or in the 2- to 3-hour postprandial period. Notably, her brother has a history of so-called reactive hypoglycemia. Therefore, *HNF4A*-associated MODY (Answer D) is the most likely diagnosis.

Educational Objective

Identify clinical features and relevant family history that distinguish *HNF4A*-associated maturity-onset diabetes of the young from other causes of monogenic diabetes.

Reference(s)

Pihoker C, Gilliam LK, Ellard S, et al; SEARCH for Diabetes in Youth Study Group. Prevalence, characteristics and clinical diagnosis of maturity onset diabetes of the young due to mutations in HNF1A, HNF4A, and glucokinase: results from the SEARCH for Diabetes in Youth. *J Clin Endocrinol Metab.* 2013;98(10):4055-4062. PMID: 23771925

Hattersley AT, Patel KA. Precision diabetes: learning from monogenic diabetes. *Diabetologia.* 2017;60(5):769-777. PMID: 28314945

Bacon S, Kyithar MP, Condron EM, Vizzard N, Burke M, Byrne MM. Prolonged episodes of hypoglycaemia in HNF4A-MODY mutation carriers with IGT. Evidence of persistent hyperinsulinism into early adulthood. *Acta Diabetol.* 2016;53(6):965-972. PMID: 27552834

45 ANSWER: B) Levothyroxine

In a young woman with symptoms and signs of hyperprolactinemia, no confounding medication use, and a mildly elevated serum prolactin level (2.3 times upper normal limit), the most likely diagnosis is a microprolactinoma. Consistent with this, formal visual field assessment is reassuring with no evidence of a compressive optic neuropathy. Unexpectedly, pituitary MRI shows a sella-based mass with homogeneous contrast enhancement, which is not typical of a pituitary adenoma, and suprasellar extension abutting the optic chiasm.

The degree of serum prolactin elevation is not consistent with a prolactinoma of this size (especially in the absence of cystic degeneration or apoplexy), and therefore a trial of dopamine agonist therapy (Answer A) is unlikely to induce shrinkage of the mass, and alternative diagnoses should be considered. In this case, both pituitary stalk compression and primary hypothyroidism (with raised TRH) may be contributory to hyperprolactinemia.

A nonfunctioning pituitary adenoma (with pituitary stalk compression) is possible but less likely in a patient of this age. As her IGF-1 level is low-normal, a somatotroph tumor is also unlikely. Although formal screening for Cushing disease has not been undertaken, most corticotroph tumors are microadenomas. The finding of a markedly elevated serum TSH level and a raised free T_4 level might suggest a thyrotroph adenoma. However, a number of features make this less likely, not least the rarity of this pituitary tumor subtype. In addition, TSH levels are typically inappropriately normal or only mildly elevated in most patients with thyrotropinomas. Somatostatin receptor ligand therapy (Answer D) is therefore not indicated, as there is no evidence of pathologic GH and/or TSH secretion.

Importantly, the patient has a history of primary thyroid disease and, assuming the original clinical presentation was consistent with Graves disease (ie, fully suppressed serum TSH, positive thyroid antibodies, and typical histologic features at thyroidectomy), then a possible link should be explored. Here, the patient reports a number of symptoms that are more typical of hypothyroidism than hyperthyroidism, despite a prescribed daily levothyroxine dosage greater than 3 mcg/kg and overtly raised serum free T_4. In this context, the possibility of intermittent or poor adherence to levothyroxine therapy should be considered. Failure to take levothyroxine reliably may result in the development of significant hypothyroidism, with a markedly elevated TSH level. If continued over several months, expansion of pituitary thyrotrophs with hyperplasia is well recognized and may be misinterpreted as a pituitary tumor, as in this case. In contrast to TSH normalization, which requires sustained adequate T_4 replacement, taking several doses of levothyroxine in the days prior to blood testing, or even a single large dose on the morning of the test, can be sufficient to temporarily restore blood levels of free T_4 to the reference range or above. In this patient, supervised levothyroxine administration (Answer B) permitted the exclusion of malabsorption and normalized serum TSH and serum free T_4 over several weeks and was accompanied by subsequent resolution of the pituitary mass and correction of hyperprolactinemia.

Transsphenoidal surgery (Answer E) and radiotherapy (Answer C) were therefore not indicated and indeed would likely have predisposed the patient to additional pituitary deficits.

Educational Objective

Explain how thyrotroph hyperplasia can complicate inadequately treated primary hypothyroidism and may be mistaken for a pituitary adenoma, leading to unnecessary medical therapy, pituitary surgery, or radiotherapy.

Reference(s)

Johnston PC, Ellis PK, Hunter SJ. Thyrotroph hyperplasia. *Postgrad Med J.* 2014;90(1059):56-57. PMID: 24096682

Joshi AS, Woolf PD. Pituitary hyperplasia secondary to primary hypothyroidism: a case report and review of the literature. *Pituitary.* 2005;8(2):99-103. PMID: 16195776

Koulouri O, Gurnell M. TSH-secreting pituitary adenomas. In: Huhtaniemi I, Martini L, eds. *Encyclopedia of Endocrine Diseases.* 2nd ed. Academic Press; 2018:261-266.

46 ANSWER: A) Convert insulin to a simple continuous subcutaneous insulin infusion (CSII) "patch-like therapy," which delivers a fixed dose of hourly insulin and adjustable dose of meal-time insulin

When partnering with patients for insulin management and titration, one of the most important steps is to assess, in a nonjudgmental way, whether there are any barriers to taking insulin and the actual dose of insulin they are currently taking. Barriers to taking insulin can be fear of needles and hypoglycemia, embarrassment about injecting while in public places, busy schedules, etc. Asking open-ended questions such as, "Many people have difficultly taking their insulin. In a typical week, how often do you find taking insulin challenging?" or, "If your blood glucose is 100 or less when you check, what do you do with your meal-time insulin or bedtime insulin?" Both questions are examples of ways to elicit information and start the conversation about the total insulin dose.

The patient in this vignette acknowledges finding it difficult to take insulin at lunch, which is often his largest meal, and he has high glucose values (200-300 mg/dL [11.1-16.7 mmol/L]) before dinner because he is not taking prandial insulin at lunchtime. However, he also reports hypoglycemia after dinner. Thus, increasing the prandial insulin dose (Answer D) is incorrect, as his issue is not being able to take prandial insulin at lunch and he is already taking an insulin dose at dinnertime that may be too high, especially when he exercises.

Mixed insulin (typically a combination of short/regular-acting insulin at ratio of 25% to 50% with 50% to 75% NPH insulin) (Answer B) is also not the best choice for this patient. Mixed insulin along with insulin-sparing agents may be a good option for some patients to simplify the insulin regimen and minimize injection burden, especially for patients who commonly eat 2 meals daily. However, as compared with analogue basal insulins, NPH insulin has a more significant peak 4 to 6 hours after administration and may put patients at greater risk for nocturnal hypoglycemia. In this patient's case, he has stated that lunch is his largest meal. He is at risk for low glucose later in the day and overnight given his preferred pattern of evening exercise, and the higher cumulative dose of insulin makes mixed insulin a less ideal choice.

Discouraging exercise in a patient living with diabetes (Answer E) is not the best choice when insulin dosing is the primary issue.

Increasing the basal insulin dosage to 38 units (Answer C) is incorrect because the patient's fasting glucose levels are already optimized. Increasing his basal insulin dosage would put him at increased risk for hypoglycemia.

This patient's main issue is missing his lunchtime insulin dose. Thus, finding a means to facilitate lunchtime dosing, especially given that it is his largest meal, is the best approach. Being familiar with all available technology for patients with diabetes is important. Converting insulin to a simple continuous subcutaneous insulin infusion "patch-like therapy," system, which delivers fixed hourly insulin and adjustable meal-time insulin (Answer A) may be the best choice for this patient. Patch insulin therapy delivers a basal insulin dose hourly for a total of 20 to 40 units daily and allows patients to select a dose of prandial insulin with a click of the patch device. Each click delivers 2 units of prandial insulin with a maximum total daily dose of 48 units. Thus, as long as there is no barrier to wearing a small device, this patient would have enhanced access to prandial insulin at lunch with easy instructions (eg, "Take 4 clicks [8 units] at dinner on nights you will be exercising instead of your typical 5 mealtime clicks [10 units]"). The tool that increases access to delivery of prandial insulin and the ability to make simple dose adjustments is the best choice when one considers this patient's individual characteristics.

Educational Objective

Explain how diabetes technology can be used to help patients optimize their diabetes management.

Reference(s)

Rosenstock J, Dailey G, Massi-Benedetti M, Fritsche A, Lin Z, Salzman A. Reduced hypoglycemia risk with insulin glargine: a meta-analysis comparing insulin glargine with human NPH insulin in type 2 diabetes. *Diabetes Care.* 2005;28(4):950-955. PMID: 15793205

Grunberger G, Rosenfeld CR, Bode BW, et al. Effectiveness of V-Go® for patients with type 2 diabetes in a real-world setting: a prospective observational study. *Drugs Real World Outcomes.* 2020;7(1):31-40. PMID: 31833010

47 ANSWER: D) Menopause

Although hCG is not routinely measured in perimenopausal or postmenopausal women, it might be measured as part of a preoperative or preprocedural protocol or before imaging or treatments that could affect a fetus. This hormone is also measured as a tumor marker or marker of disease activity for trophoblastic disease, germ-cell tumors, and other malignancies. Up to 10% of hCG measurements are elevated in perimenopausal or postmenopausal women without disease or a tumor, and this finding can lead to additional laboratory evaluation, delayed treatment, unnecessary worry, and invasive testing and/or surgery.

The heterodimeric glycoprotein hCG has a β-subunit, as well as an α-subunit identical to that of LH, FSH, and TSH. The β-subunit is different and specific to each hormone's function. Pituitary hCG was first identified by hCG staining of pituitary gland extracts. Pituitary hCG production was confirmed when GnRH administration resulted in a 2- to 3-fold increase in hCG in healthy nonpregnant women and hCG suppression was observed in postmenopausal women given combined estrogen and progesterone. As women get older, hCG levels, like those of FSH and LH, rise due to loss of negative feedback inhibition from estrogen and progesterone.

A 2-site noncompetitive sandwich immunoassay is usually used to measure hCG, where hCG is first bound to capture antibodies and then exposed to detection antibodies, allowing quantitative measurement of an enzymatic reaction tagged to the detection antibodies. False-positive results can occur from antibody interference (Answer A), cross-reactivity with other serum glycoproteins, or heterophilic antibodies that bind to the antibodies in the hCG assay. In this case, the repeated hCG measurement with a different commercial assay showed persistent elevation in hCG, making antibody interference a less likely explanation.

Fibroelastoma (Answer E) is not a tumor type known to produce hCG. With a tumoral source, hCG concentrations can be very high (in the several hundred to thousands range), and α-fetoprotein can be elevated as well, which differs from the undetectable α-fetoprotein in this case. These findings argue against the presence of a malignancy, such as a germ-cell tumor (Answer C).

Ectopic pregnancy (Answer B) would also be associated with much higher hCG concentrations, and this patient's elevated FSH value makes this diagnosis far less likely.

An FSH concentration greater than 40.0 or 45.0 mIU/mL with an hCG concentration less than 14.0 mIU/mL is consistent with pituitary/physiologic hCG elevations and no further evaluation is necessary. If hCG is 14 mIU/mL or greater with an FSH value less than 40.0 mIU/mL, the next step would be to evaluate for assay interference using multiple commercial quantitative assays by sending the sample to different laboratories or asking the laboratory director for assistance in acquiring different test kits/immunoassays. Greater than 10% variance (or percent difference between test results) indicates a likely false-positive result. When less than 10% variance occurs, the next step is to confirm whether a pituitary source is likely by suppressing pituitary hCG with either high-dosage estrogen birth control pills for 3 weeks or a GnRH analogue injection 10 days before repeat hCG testing. If hCG is suppressed, there is no need for further evaluation. If hCG is not suppressed, further evaluation for underlying malignancy is indicated.

In this patient, an FSH concentration greater than 45.0 mIU/mL was reassuring, along with relatively low (and stable) hCG levels. The most likely etiology of her elevated hCG is menopause (Answer D), and she elected not to be treated with hormone therapy to suppress hCG. Follow-up measurement 3 months later was 8.0 mIU/mL.

Educational Objective

Evaluate elevated hCG in a postmenopausal woman.

Reference(s)

Cole LA, Khanlian SA, Muller CY. Normal production of human chorionic gonadotropin in perimenopausal and menopausal women and after oophorectomy. *Int J Gynecol Cancer.* 2009;19(9):1556-1559. PMID: 19994471

Gronowski AM, Frantz CR, Parvin CA, et al. Use of serum FSH to identify perimenopausal women with pituitary hCG. *Clin Chem.* 2008;54(4):652-656. PMID: 18258666

Cole LA, Laidler LL, Muller CY. USA hCG reference service, 10-year report. *Clin Biochem.* 2010;43(12):1013-1022. PMID: 20493830

48 ANSWER: A) Initiate oral cinacalcet

The elderly woman in this vignette has severe hypercalcemia (albumin-corrected calcium >14 mg/dL [>3.5 mmol/L]) in the setting of advanced chronic kidney disease and a significantly elevated PTH concentration. Primary hyperparathyroidism is typically characterized by hypercalcemia in the setting of inappropriately normal or elevated PTH levels. When hypercalcemia develops because of autonomous parathyroid function and excess PTH secretion after longstanding secondary hyperparathyroidism (such as in patients with end-stage kidney disease and after kidney transplant), this is referred to as tertiary hyperparathyroidism. This patient most likely has tertiary hyperparathyroidism that needs to be treated given the severity of her hypercalcemia. Elevations in the calcium concentration, particularly greater than 14 mg/dL (>3.5 mmol/L), may lead to severe volume depletion and acute kidney injury. Most patients with significant degrees of hypercalcemia exhibit clinical evidence of intravascular volume depletion. Patients with an acute rise in serum calcium to more moderate levels (total albumin-corrected calcium between 12 and 14 mg/dL [3.0 and 3.5 mmol/L]) who have changes in altered mental status also require aggressive therapy. Initial treatment with intravenous isotonic saline to reverse volume depletion often lowers the serum calcium concentration 1 to 2 mg/dL (0.25 to 0.5 mmol/L) due to expanding the intravascular space. Saline therapy beyond what is necessary to restore euvolemia is not recommended, and loop diuretics such as oral furosemide (Answer B) should not be used unless needed to reverse overly aggressive fluid replacement.

Oral cinacalcet (Answer A) is the medical treatment of choice for patients with severe hypercalcemia secondary to hyperparathyroidism. Cinacalcet is a calcimimetic agent that activates the calcium-sensing receptor in the parathyroid gland, thereby inhibiting PTH secretion. Cinacalcet is effective at quickly lowering, and often normalizing, serum calcium and increasing serum phosphate in patients with primary hyperparathyroidism. Cinacalcet is indicated for the treatment of hypercalcemia due to hyperparathyroidism in adult patients for whom parathyroidectomy would be indicated on the basis of serum calcium levels, but who are unable to undergo parathyroidectomy, as well as in patients with hypercalcemia due to parathyroid carcinoma. Common adverse effects include nausea, diarrhea, myalgias, dizziness and paresthesias, unfortunately requiring discontinuation of the medication on occasion.

Immediate treatment with subcutaneous calcitonin therapy (not provided as an option) or an intravenous bisphosphonate infusion would be appropriate in a patient with severe hypercalcemia due to excessive bone resorption, although intravenous bisphosphonates are not approved for the treatment of hypercalcemia due to hyperparathyroidism and have potential nephrotoxicity. Zoledronic acid (Answer E) is contraindicated in the setting of chronic kidney disease in patients with an estimated glomerular filtration rate less than 35 mL/min per 1.73 m^2. Off-label treatment with intravenous pamidronate (not provided as an option in this vignette) could be considered at a reduced dosage with a slower infusion rate, with close monitoring of kidney function, although limited data exist for pamidronate use in patients with creatinine clearance less than 30 mL/min.

While subcutaneous denosumab therapy (Answer C) is an approved treatment for osteoporosis and hypercalcemia of malignancy, it is not approved for the treatment of hypercalcemia secondary to hyperparathyroidism. It may be considered as an off-label option if needed, especially in patients with severe kidney impairment, but it would not be the most appropriate next step in this case.

Hemodialysis with little or no calcium in the dialysis fluid effectively lowers calcium concentrations but is considered to be a treatment of last resort. Referral for dialysis (Answer D) may be indicated for patients with kidney insufficiency or heart failure in whom hydration cannot be safely administered and in whom medical therapy is either inadequate or contraindicated.

Educational Objective

Recommend appropriate therapy in a hospitalized patient with severe hypercalcemia due to hyperparathyroidism.

Reference(s)

Maier JD, Levine SN. Hypercalcemia in the intensive care unit: a review of pathophysiology, diagnosis, and modern therapy. *J Intensive Care Med.* 2015;30(5):235-252. PMID: 24130250

Silverberg SJ, Rubin MR, Faiman C, et al. Cinacalcet hydrochloride reduces the serum calcium concentration in inoperable parathyroid carcinoma. *J Clin Endocrinol Metab.* 2007;92(10):3803-3808. PMID: 17666472

49 ANSWER: C) Initiate therapy with pegvisomant

Mild to moderate hyperprolactinemia is a common finding that brings patients to the attention of endocrinologists. Prolactin is often measured during workup of symptoms that are common and not necessarily related, such as menstrual irregularity in women or erectile dysfunction in men. Simply repeating prolactin measurement (either with a regular blood test or after placing an indwelling venous catheter 2 hours prior) results in a normal prolactin level in about one-fourth of the cases of mild-to-moderate hyperprolactinemia.

Sometimes, however, transiently elevated prolactin brings a patient to the attention of an endocrinologist, as in this case. This patient endorsed some symptoms consistent with excessive GH (ie, enlargement of digits and feet, loud snoring), and she had elevated serum IGF-1. While about 15% of GH-secreting adenomas cosecrete prolactin, this patient's repeated prolactin measurement was normal. Results of her glucose-suppression test are abnormal. While the 2014 acromegaly Endocrine Society clinical practice guidelines set a normal postglucose GH nadir level at less than 1.0 ng/mL (1.0 μg/L), most experts consider a GH nadir below 0.4 ng/mL (<0.4 μg/L) to be normal. Independently, the diagnosis of acromegaly has been established in this patient with the abnormal results of the glucose-suppression test (thus, Answer D is incorrect). While in most cases, acromegaly is caused by GH-secreting pituitary adenomas, acromegaly can be occasionally caused by a GHRH-secreting neuroendocrine tumor. In these cases, a discrete pituitary adenoma is not visible. The patient's normal GHRH plasma concentration excludes this possibility, making the presence of a small GH-secreting pituitary adenoma the most likely diagnosis despite the normal MRI. This is a rare occurrence, as adenomas are most often visible at the time of diagnosis.

First-line therapy for acromegaly is generally surgery (Answer E). However, in this case, because MRI failed to show a discrete adenoma, surgery would not be advisable, as it is unlikely to be curative in the absence of an obvious surgical target.

Cabergoline (Answer B) is a reasonable first-line medical therapy for mild-to-moderate acromegaly, although only a small percentage of patients (20%-30%) respond with IGF-1 normalization. Conversely, serum IGF-1 normalizes in about 50% of patients treated with a somatostatin receptor agonists (eg, octreotide or lanreotide) (Answer A). Both cabergoline and somatostatin receptor agonists, when they are effective, also likely prevent adenoma growth. As such, if they were to work in this case, the patient would probably be committed to lifelong medical therapy, as additional MRIs would most likely continue to not show a surgical target.

The GH-receptor antagonist pegvisomant (Answer C), while successful in normalizing IGF-1 in about two-thirds of patients with acromegaly, would not prevent adenoma growth. Controlling acromegaly with pegvisomant in the hope that the presumed adenoma will grow and become a possible visible surgical target is the most logical strategy in this patient. Importantly, there is currently no evidence that treatment with pegvisomant accelerates the growth of GH-secreting adenomas. In this case, after 18 months of pegvisomant therapy (with good control of serum IGF-1 levels and improvement of acromegaly symptoms), an adenoma was identified on MRI and the patient underwent transsphenoidal surgery.

Educational Objective

Interpret results of a GH-suppression test and recommend the best therapeutic approach in a patient with elevated IGF-1 and no obvious pituitary lesion.

Reference(s)

Whyte MB, Pramodh S, Srikugan L, et al. Importance of cannulated prolactin test in the definition of hyperprolactinaemia. *Pituitary.* 2015;18(3):319-325. PMID: 24879500

Giustina A, Barkan A, Beckers A, et al. A consensus on the diagnosis and treatment of acromegaly comorbidities: an update. *J Clin Endocrinol Metab.* 2020;105(4):dgz096. PMID: 31606735

Fleseriu M, Führer-Sakel D, van der Lely AJ, et al. More than a decade of real-world experience of pegvisomant for acromegaly: ACROSTUDY. *Eur J Endocrinol.* 2021;185(4):525-538. PMID: 34342594

50 **ANSWER: C) Perform a low-intensity cool-down routine for 10 to 15 minutes after each run**

This patient's initial problem was the occurrence of hypoglycemia during aerobic exercise. Reasons for this include: (1) an inability to match the normal physiologic decrease in insulin, (2) increased insulin absorption due to increased subcutaneous blood flow, (3) increased muscle uptake of glucose due to insulin-independent GLUT4 trafficking to the cell membranes during muscle contraction, and (4) impaired counterregulatory hormone responses that may depend on the duration of exercise.

To correct this problem, he suspended his basal insulin, but he now has postexercise hyperglycemia. Hyperglycemia during exercise can occur with anerobic activity such as heavy weightlifting or sprinting, and blood glucose elevations can be substantial. Hyperglycemia after exercise can occur after any type of exercise and often happens during early recovery. Mechanisms for this early postexercise hyperglycemia include excessive reduction of insulin before exercise (as was done in this case), higher levels of glucose counterregulatory hormones, and lactate build-up. Education is important, as patients often feel discouraged by exercise-related glucose fluctuation, believing it to be an error on their part when such changes are, in fact, related to physiologic responses to exercise. Making the reduction of basal insulin less aggressive by asking the patient to not suspend the pump but leave the basal rates running with 80% reduction is a reasonable first step. But if hyperglycemia persists after his runs, additional action is needed.

Consumption of small quantities of high glycemic–index carbohydrates during prolonged aerobic exercise (Answer B) is important for both hypoglycemia prevention and performance. Although 15 to 20 g per hour may be sufficient to prevent hypoglycemia if insulin is appropriately reduced, 75 g per h may be required for optimal performance or for activities lasting 2.5 hours or longer. Regardless, consumption of carbohydrates during exercise will not help the postexercise hyperglycemia problem.

Administering a correction bolus (Answer A) has the disadvantage of requiring 30 minutes to take effect and then having a duration of action of 3 to 5 hours, which may cause hypoglycemia at a later point.

Interestingly, weightlifting (Answer D) is associated with a slight increase in blood glucose through unclear mechanisms. It is a recommended strategy to help prevent hypoglycemia occurring early in exercise, but it would not reduce the hyperglycemia this patient experiences after he runs.

A low-intensity cool-down routine for 10 to 15 minutes (Answer C) is the recommended activity to address this problem, as it helps reduce the build-up of lactate and increases muscle contraction-related uptake of glucose via GLUT4, thus overcoming potential elevations of counterregulatory hormones.

Consumption of high glycemic–index snacks before a workout (Answer E) would not be anticipated to reduce postexercise hyperglycemia. Many patients consume snacks in this way to prevent low glucose levels during aerobic workouts, but low glycemic–index snacks are preferred before workouts, with consumption of simple carbohydrates during exercise to prevent midexercise hypoglycemia.

Educational Objective

Advise appropriate measures to mitigate hyperglycemia after exercise in patients with type 1 diabetes mellitus and recommend appropriate next steps.

Reference(s)

Riddell MC, Gallen IW, Smart CE, Taplin CE, et al. Exercise management in type 1 diabetes: a consensus statement. *Lancet Diabetes Endocrinol.* 2017;5(5):377-390. PMID: 28126459

51 ANSWER: B) Hypocortisolism

Safe management of hyponatremia is critically dependent on accurate assessment of the patient's clinical status and careful review of laboratory results. It is important to exclude "spurious" causes of hyponatremia including:

- Factitious hyponatremia: when a venous blood sample is collected from a site proximal to a hypoosmolar intravenous infusion.
- Pseudohyponatremia: artifactually low sodium resulting from the way a blood sample is processed. This may be seen when using flame emission spectrophotometry or indirect ion-selective electrode potentiometry—both require sample dilution and assume a fixed proportion of water (93%) and solutes (7%) in plasma. However, if the fraction of solid-phase particles is increased, the same amount of diluent results in greater dilution, leading to underestimation of serum sodium. Importantly, however, measured serum osmolality is normal. Hypertriglyceridemia and abnormally high levels of protein (both native [eg, multiple myeloma] or exogenous [eg, intravenous immunoglobulin therapy]) may result in pseudohyponatremia when sodium is measured using susceptible laboratory methods. Direct ion-selective electrode potentiometry, which does not require sample dilution, is not affected, and many laboratory and blood gas analyzers now use this methodology. In this patient, the measured serum osmolality is low, thus effectively excluding a spurious reading due to increased serum immunoglobulins (Answer C).

The presence of osmotically active solutes, such as mannitol or glucose, can result in significant fluid shifts that are associated with true low serum sodium (dilutional hyponatremia). However, measured serum osmolality is typically not low because of the osmotically active solute. This patient is therefore unlikely to have hyperglycemia (Answer A).

Estimation of volume status is a key step in the evaluation of true hyponatremia and provides an important clue to the underlying etiology:

- Hypervolemia:
  - States of secondary hyperaldosteronism (eg, congestive cardiac failure, cirrhosis, nephrotic syndrome)
  - Chronic kidney failure
  - Iatrogenic (eg, excessive glucose infusion)
  - Water intoxication

- Hypovolemia:
  - Excessive renal loss (eg, diuretic usage, salt-wasting nephropathy, mineralocorticoid deficiency)
  - Extra-renal loss (eg, vomiting/diarrhea, small-bowel obstruction, pancreatitis, excessive sweating, burns)

- Euvolemia:
  - Syndrome of inappropriate antidiuretic hormone secretion (SIADH)/antidiuresis
  - Physiologically increased antidiuretic hormone release (eg, anesthesia, nausea, pain)
  - Endocrine (eg, glucocorticoid deficiency, hypothyroidism)
  - Water intoxication

This patient has no reported clinical or laboratory features to indicate a hypervolemic state. Similarly, although she is tachycardic with borderline-low blood pressure, these findings are consistent with systemic infection and there is no evidence of kidney impairment.

Primary (psychogenic/dipsogenic) polydipsia (Answer D) is typically associated with polyuria and dilute urine. However, in this case the urine is relatively concentrated and is not suggestive of excessive fluid ingestion.

The laboratory and clinical findings (euvolemia with hypoosmolar hyponatremia, urine osmolality >100 mOsm/kg, and inappropriate urinary sodium excretion) are potentially consistent with SIADH (Answer E). However, the latter is a diagnosis of exclusion, and the demonstration of normal kidney, thyroid, and adrenal status is required before SIADH can be confirmed. Accordingly, screening for both hypocortisolism and hypothyroidism is indicated. The former is of particular importance in this case given the history of significant asthma requiring maximal therapy, which almost certainly would have included oral corticosteroids in addition to high-dosage inhaled corticosteroids. The recent introduction of biological therapies (eg, antiinterleukin-5 receptor monoclonal antibody) has transformed the management of many patients with severe eosinophilic asthma, often allowing a steroid-sparing approach to be pursued with discontinuation of oral corticosteroid therapy. However, in this setting, a recent study has highlighted that many patients (60%) are at risk of secondary hypoadrenalism (sometimes referred to as tertiary hypoadrenalism in the context of exogenous glucocorticoid therapy), at least in the initial months after oral corticosteroid withdrawal. Accordingly, active screening is recommended to ensure appropriate physiological replacement, as well as ensuring that additional coverage for intercurrent illness is instituted in a timely manner. Therefore, while it is appropriate to exclude hypothyroidism in this patient, hypocortisolism (Answer B) should be assumed until proven otherwise.

Educational Objective

Explain that patients who have recently weaned off higher dosages of exogenous corticosteroids may have unrecognized hypothalamic-pituitary-adrenal axis suppression and require glucocorticoid coverage during intercurrent illness.

Reference(s)

Spasovski G, Vanholder R, Allolio B, et al; Hyponatremia Guideline Development Group. Clinical practice guideline on diagnosis and treatment of hyponatraemia. *Eur J Endocrinol.* 2014;170(3):G1-G47. PMID: 24569125

Menzies-Gow A, Gurnell M, Heaney LG, et al. Oral corticosteroid elimination via a personalised reduction algorithm in adults with severe, eosinophilic asthma treated with benralizumab (PONENTE): a multicentre, open-label, single-arm study. *Lancet Respir Med.* 2022;10(1):47-58. PMID: 34619104

52 ANSWER: A) Intravenous bisphosphonate therapy

This patient has differentiated thyroid cancer with several bone metastases. The prognosis of patients who have thyroid cancer with localized/regional disease is excellent, with a 5-year survival rate of 99%. Survival is reduced in the presence of distant metastases. Bone metastases occur in 2% to 13% of all patients with differentiated thyroid cancer and result in high morbidity due to the occurrence of skeletal-related events, including pathologic fractures leading to pain and spinal cord compression and the need for bone irradiation or surgery. Hypercalcemia is also among the skeletal-related events. Bone metastases can be treated via multiple modalities such as:

- Radioiodine treatment
- Surgery
- External radiotherapy
- Radiofrequency ablation
- Palliative embolization
- Systemic chemotherapy (eg, tyrosine kinase inhibitors)

However, systemic therapy with bone-directed agents such as bisphosphonates or RANKL inhibitors should be considered for patients with thyroid cancer and diffuse bone metastases, and intravenous bisphosphonate therapy (Answer A) is the best next step in this patient's management. Bisphosphonates, including zoledronic acid, inhibit osteoclast-mediated bone resorption. Denosumab is a fully human monoclonal antibody that binds and inactivates receptor activator of nuclear factor kappaB ligand (RANKL), an important ligand that regulates bone remodeling. By binding to RANKL, denosumab affects the important pathway involved in bone remodeling and disrupts the cycle of bone destruction stimulated by tumor cells. Most of the published studies have used intravenous bisphosphonates in the treatment of bone metastases in patients with thyroid cancer. In a study of patients with bone metastases from differentiated thyroid cancer, treatment with intravenous zoledronic acid reduced skeletal-related events or delayed their appearance in that cohort. This benefit has not been seen in some other studies, probably due to small numbers of patients with thyroid cancer and bone metastases in those studies. Before prescribing these medications, a basic metabolic panel should be obtained to assess kidney function and measure serum calcium. In addition, all adverse effects should be reviewed with the patient, and a dental evaluation should be undertaken given the related adverse effects (ie, osteonecrosis of the jaw). Bone-directed agents prescribed for patients with solid tumors delay time to occurrence of subsequent skeletal-related adverse events. A few studies of patients with differentiated thyroid cancer receiving bisphosphonate therapy suggest some benefit. In this patient with several bone metastases and bone pain, bisphosphonate therapy should be initiated. For patients with thyroid cancer and bone metastases, zoledronic acid is typically administered every 3 to 6 months instead of monthly as in solid tumors with bone metastases. Data from randomized controlled trials are not available to definitively determine the frequency and duration of bone-directed agents in patients with bone metastases from thyroid cancer.

In a study based on SEER Medicare data involving 30,063 patients with thyroid cancer (medullary, follicular, papillary, and anaplastic), 9.4% had either bone metastasis or a skeletal-related event. The presence of bone metastases was an indicator of poor prognosis. The likelihood of developing bone metastases or a skeletal-related event was higher in patients with follicular or medullary thyroid cancer than in patients with papillary thyroid cancer.

Radioiodine treatment of iodine-avid bone metastases has been associated with improved survival. However, patients with bone metastases may require other aforementioned treatments. External radiotherapy (Answer B) may be indicated for painful bone lesions or prevention of impending fractures, particularly for patients with persistent back pain despite radioiodine and intravenous bisphosphonate therapy.

Tyrosine kinase inhibitors (Answer D) are prescribed to patients with distant metastases that are iodine refractory. This is not the case in this patient.

As the radioiodine scan demonstrated iodine-avid vertebral bone metastases, PET/CT scan (Answer C) or bone scan (Answer E) is not indicated.

Educational Objective

Manage bone metastases in a patient with differentiated thyroid cancer.

Reference(s)

Haugen BR, Alexander EK, Bible KC, et al. 2015 American Thyroid Association management guidelines for adult patients with thyroid nodules and differentiated thyroid cancer: the American Thyroid Association Guidelines Task Force on Thyroid Nodules and Differentiated Thyroid Cancer. *Thyroid.* 2016;26(1):1-133. PMID: 26462967

Choksi P, Papaleontiou M, Guo C, Worden F, Banerjee M, Haymart M. Skeletal complications and mortality in thyroid cancer: a population-based study. *J Clin Endocrinol Metab.* 2017;102(4):1254-1260. PMID: 28324052

Iñiguez-Ariza NM, Bible KC, Clarke BL. Bone metastases in thyroid cancer. *J Bone Oncol.* 2020;21:100282. PMID: 32154098

Matta-Coelho C, Simoes-Pereira J, Vilar H, Leite V. Bone metastases from thyroid carcinoma of follicular origin: a single institutional experience. *Eur Thyroid J.* 2019;8(2):96-101. PMID: 31192149

Farooki A, Leung V, Tala H, Tuttle RM. Skeletal-related events due to bone metastases from differentiated thyroid cancer. *J Clin Endocrinol Metab.* 2012;97(7):2433-2439. PMID: 22564664

Orita Y, Sugitani I, Toda K, Manabe J, Fujimoto Y. Zoledronic acid in the treatment of bone metastases from differentiated thyroid carcinoma. *Thyroid.* 2011;21(1):31-35. PMID: 21058881

53 ANSWER: D) Type 1 diabetes mellitus

In the United States, Canada, and Europe, about 90% of diabetes cases can be attributed to type 2 diabetes. Type 1 diabetes accounts for 5% to 10%, and maturity-onset diabetes of the young (MODY) and other specific syndromes account for the rest of the cases. The classification of diabetes by the American Diabetes Association and the World Health Organization does not reflect the heterogeneity present in the population.

Two recent consensus statements from the American Diabetes Association and the European Association for the Study of Diabetes help clarify diagnostic and treatment strategies for patients with diabetes. Two major factors in determining the etiology of diabetes are age and BMI, with younger age (<35 years) and lower BMI (<25 kg/m^2) increasing the likelihood of type 1 diabetes and MODY. In this 21-year-old woman who has a BMI of 23 kg/m^2, the likelihood of type 2 diabetes (Answer E) is quite low.

The relationship between alcohol consumption and glucose levels is complex, and there is evidence of improved insulin sensitivity with alcohol use in persons without diabetes. Other studies demonstrate increased insulin resistance in patients with chronic alcohol use. In this patient without significant alcohol consumption, alcohol-induced hyperglycemia (Answer A) is unlikely to be the reason for diabetes.

Single gene pathogenic variants can also result in hyperglycemia, collectively termed MODY. The most common pathogenic variants are seen in *HNF1A*, *GCK* (glucokinase), and *HNF4A*. This patient has no features suggestive of MODY such as (1) hemoglobin A_{1c} at diagnosis less than 7.5% (<58 mmol/mol), (2) a parent with a diagnosis of diabetes, or (3) presence of specific clinical features seen in MODY (eg, kidney cysts, partial lipodystrophy, maternally inherited deafness, or severe insulin resistance in the absence of obesity). A calculator is available to determine risk of MODY (https://www.diabetesgenes.org/exeter-diabetes-app/ModyCalculator). Calculated risk greater than 5% is considered to be significant and should prompt genetic testing. This patient's risk is 1.7%, so screening for MODY type 3 (Answer C) is therefore incorrect.

Latent autoimmune diabetes in adults (Answer B) has the following features: (1) older age (>30 years), (2) lack of insulin requirement for initial management (in first 6 months), and (3) presence of autoantibodies. This patient is younger than 30 years, needed insulin at the time of diagnosis, and had negative insulin autoantibodies, so her condition would not be designated as latent autoimmune diabetes in adults.

The consensus statement recommendation when evaluating for type 1 diabetes is to start by testing glutamic acid decarboxylase (GAD) 65 antibodies, followed by insulinoma-associated protein antibody 2, and/or zinc transporter antibodies if GAD 65 antibodies are not detected and clinical suspicion is high. About 5% to 10% of patients with type 1 diabetes of European ancestry have negative antibodies. A low random C-peptide concentration (<0.6 ng/mL [<0.2 nmol/L]) is also suggestive of type 1 diabetes. This patient's level C-peptide level was low (0.4 ng/mL [0.13 nmol/L]). Considering all available information, this patient most likely has type 1 diabetes (specifically type 1b) (Answer D) despite having negative antibody levels.

Educational Objective

Guide the classification of diabetes mellitus.

Reference(s)

Holt RIG, DeVries JH, Hess-Fischl A, et al. The management of type 1 diabetes in adults. A consensus report by the American Diabetes Association (ADA) and the European Association for the Study of Diabetes (EASD). *Diabetes Care.* 2021;44(11):2589-2625. PMID: 34593612

Buzzetti R, Tuomi T, Mauricio D, et al. Management of latent autoimmune diabetes in adults: a consensus statement from an International Expert Panel. *Diabetes.* 2020;69(10):2037-2047. PMID: 32847960

54 ANSWER: D) Prescribe a physical activity regimen focused on resistance exercises

Perturbations in energy balance result in changes in body weight. Energy intake is most often assessed through dietary recall, while energy expenditure can be assessed in several different ways. Both components are important to understand when evaluating a patient with obesity.

Dietary recall alone notoriously underestimates true energy intake by up to 30% when validated against total energy expenditure measured by doubly labeled water. Some food journals allow uploading of photographs of food, which are sent to a dietician for review. While this can overcome some of the general underreporting of energy intake, problems of incomplete record-keeping or undereating during the study period often persist, creating a challenge to accurately determine a person's true energy intake.

An individual's total energy expenditure is composed of the following: basal energy expenditure and adaptive thermogenesis (60%-80%), activity-related expenditure (20%-30%), and the thermic effect of food (5%-10%). Basal energy expenditure can be predicted using validated equations (eg, Harris-Benedict or Mifflin-St. Jeor), with the doubly labeled water method, or by measuring via indirect calorimetry. In patients with obesity, there is variable concordance of these predictive equations when compared with indirect calorimetry measurement.

Patients who do not lose weight despite good adherence to an appropriately calculated calorie deficit are potential candidates for measured energy expenditure. Indirect calorimetry uses the principles of gas exchange (VO_2 and VCO_2) to determine metabolic activity. To exclude the thermic effect of food, patients are asked to fast and to avoid strenuous activity and consumption of stimulants such as caffeine for at least 6 hours. Indirect calorimetry measures the differences in concentrations of O_2 and CO_2 between the inspired and expired gases and the flow of gas. Energy expenditure is then calculated using the Weir equation. The measured resting (or basal) energy expenditure is compared with predicted resting energy expenditure derived from the above-mentioned equations. In this vignette, low measured basal energy expenditure is the most likely explanation for why the patient has not experienced adequate weight loss with his current degree of calorie restriction.

Fat-free mass is the best predictor of basal energy expenditure. Resistance exercises can increase fat-free mass and therefore basal energy expenditure. However, outcomes of exercise intervention studies with respect to alterations in body composition are influenced by the type of exercise, with intensity, frequency, and duration of exercise as limiting factors. In this particular patient, prescribing a physical activity program focusing on resistance exercises (Answer D) with the goal of increasing lean body mass, is the best option to help him lose weight. Another option (although not offered in this vignette) would be to further restrict calories to approximately 2100 calories per day (as measured by indirect calorimetry).

Dietary macronutrient composition may have some effect on the thermic effect of food and therefore total energy expenditure. However, higher dietary protein intake alone (Answer A) has not been shown to influence basal energy expenditure in the absence of physical activity.

Although biochemical hypothyroidism decreases basal energy expenditure, a mild increase in TSH does not. Thus, even though supplementing with levothyroxine (Answer E) may increase his basal energy expenditure, this is not a reason to treat mild subclinical hypothyroidism in this patient.

There is no indication in the vignette that hypercortisolism should be suspected and obtaining 24-hour urine collection to measure free cortisol (Answer C) is not necessary.

Untreated sleep apnea may contribute to difficulty losing weight, and patients should be screened for sleep apnea (Answer B) if there is clinical suspicion for the condition. However, starting treatment for sleep apnea alone would not influence this patient's primary driver of difficulty achieving weight loss (reduced basal energy expenditure).

Educational Objective

Interpret results of a resting energy expenditure study in a patient who has difficulty losing weight.

Reference(s)

Frankenfield D, Roth-Yousey L, Compher C. Comparison of predictive equations for resting metabolic rate in healthy nonobese and obese adults: a systematic review. *J Am Diet Assoc.* 2005;105(5):775-789. PMID: 15883556

Stiegler P, Cunliffe A. The role of diet and exercise for the maintenance of fat-free mass and resting metabolic rate during weight loss. *Sports Med.* 2006;36(3):239-262. PMID: 16526835

55

ANSWER: E) Refer to behavioral health/social work services

Although this patient has symptoms of polycystic ovary syndrome, androgen excess based on the Ferriman-Gallwey score, and irregular menses, these concerns are less immediately relevant than treatment of his gender dysphoria and type 2 diabetes. Therefore, evaluation for and treatment of polycystic ovary syndrome (Answer A) is not the best next step.

The first step in treating his type 2 diabetes would be initiation of metformin, not a GLP-1 receptor agonist (Answer C). However, addition of a GLP-1 receptor agonist might be helpful in the future if his type 2 diabetes is not controlled with metformin, and particularly with the treatment goal of losing weight before any surgical intervention given his BMI of 41 kg/m^2.

Several aspects of this patient's history indicate that referral to behavioral health/social work services (Answer E) should be the next step. The patient has experienced numerous challenges accessing health care that illustrate the importance of addressing the social determinants of health to optimize patient outcomes. A comprehensive evaluation includes several spheres in a patient's environment and social needs assessment, including family support, work/school environment, faith/cultural perspective, home, financial, peer social support, and legal aspects—all of which contribute to health care access. Lack of family support and financial dependence on family have had a significant role in preventing this patient from seeking gender-affirming therapy. Treating type 2 diabetes is important to improve outcomes if surgery is eventually pursued, but the patient has been avoiding follow-up for diabetes care because he fears being misgendered. This highlights the degree to which medical mistrust might develop from patient experiences at the pharmacy, laboratory, and clinic, as well as the degree to which minority stress interferes with health care delivery and outcomes. The minority stress model of sexual-minority health describes how exposure to environmental stressors of discrimination and verbal or physical abuse leads to chronic stress levels that negatively affect both mental and physical health and outcomes.

Although initiating testosterone therapy to treat dysphoria (Answer D) would be expected to eventually assist in decreasing misgendered experiences, the patient needs immediate help to overcome his demonstrated resistance to engaging and following up with medical providers. Thus, referral to behavioral health/social work services is the best strategy now. He needs help to follow through with picking up prescriptions and attending appointments for follow-up laboratory testing and monitoring hormone therapy. Assisting the patient in seeking employment and achieving financial independence and independent living arrangements would be important. He could also benefit from vocal therapy to limit misgendering and triggering of dysphoria. This comprehensive approach to his care is not meant to be obstructive to his goals of gender-affirming therapy but rather supportive of his transition.

Identifying local resources for support groups and gender therapists (Answer B) would also be an important part of optimizing this patient's gender transition to avoid isolation and improve support systems, but it is not the best next step to improve his overall health outcomes.

Educational Objective

Describe the importance of social determinants of health for transgender/gender-diverse individuals.

Reference(s)

Deutsch MB, ed. *Guidelines for the Primary and Gender-Affirming Care of Transgender and Gender Nonbinary People.* 2nd ed. 2016. Available at: www.transhealth.ucsf.edu/guidelines. Accessed April 2022.

Hembree WC, Cohen-Kettenis PT, Gooren L, et al. Endocrine treatment of gender-dysphoric/gender-incongruent persons: an Endocrine Society clinical practice guideline. *J Clin Endocrinol Metab.* 2017;102(11):3869-3903. PMID: 28945902

Office of Disease Prevention and Health Promotion. Determinants of Health. Available at: https://www.healthypeople.gov/2020/about/foundation-health-measures/Determinants-of-Health. Accessed April 2022.

56 ANSWER: E) Serum 17-hydroxyprogesterone measurement

This patient's symptoms are suggestive of compensated primary adrenal insufficiency, and his "tan" skin and hormone concentrations (low-normal cortisol, elevated ACTH, elevated renin) support the diagnosis. Abdominal CT shows severe bilateral adrenal enlargement and left myelolipomas. In addition, the patient has firm, enlarged testes due to testicular adrenal rest tumors (TARTs). TARTs are testicular masses composed of adrenal-like tissue, typically located within the rete testis, which enlarge during sustained ACTH elevation. Taken together, these clinical features are highly suggestive of congenital adrenal hyperplasia due to 21-hydroxyalse deficiency. Uncontrolled 21-hydroxylase deficiency is associated with excessive production of adrenal androgens (testosterone and adrenal-specific androgens, such as 11β-hydroxyandrostenedione and 11-ketotestosterone), which suppress gonadotropins. Additionally, TARTs might obstruct seminiferous tubules. Both processes can contribute to infertility, as observed in this patient.

Screening for congenital adrenal hyperplasia is performed with a baseline serum 17-hydroxyprogesterone measurement (Answer E). For indeterminate values, a high-dose (250-mcg) cosyntropin-stimulation test (Answer B) typically clarifies the diagnosis. Genetic testing is only necessary when biochemical results are borderline or when genetic counseling is desired before conception.

FDG-PET scan (Answer C) can be useful in patients with suspected malignancy. Myelolipomas are benign, lipid-rich adrenal masses. Pituitary-directed MRI (Answer D) is not indicated in cases of primary adrenal insufficiency.

Adrenal biopsy (Answer A) is rarely useful for adrenal masses, and it cannot distinguish between benign and malignant cortical tumors. Adrenal biopsy might be useful when adrenal metastases of unclear origin are suspected based on imaging.

Educational Objective

Diagnose classic congenital adrenal hyperplasia in a patient who presents with bilateral adrenal enlargement.

Reference(s)

Speiser PW, Arlt W, Auchus RJ, et al. Congenital adrenal hyperplasia due to steroid 21-hydroxylase deficiency: an Endocrine Society clinical practice guideline [*J Clin Endocrinol Metab.* 2019;104(1):39-40]. *J Clin Endocrinol Metab.* 2018;103(11):4043-4088. PMID: 30272171

57 ANSWER: A) Continue methimazole at the current dosage

Methimazole is the preferred antithyroid drug (thionamide) for the treatment of Graves hyperthyroidism except during the first trimester of pregnancy. Liver toxicity (typically cholestasis) and agranulocytosis can occur with treatment. Agranulocytosis affects between 1 in 300 and 1 in 500 persons on antithyroid drug therapy overall and occurs within the first 90 days of treatment in 85% of patients. The risk of agranulocytosis with methimazole is dosage-dependent.

Methimazole is often discontinued in patients with Graves disease after 12 to 18 months of therapy; however, relapse rates are high after treatment cessation. Using this approach, durable remission is achieved in only 20% to 40% of patients. Half of relapses occur within 1 year of stopping treatment. Reported predictors of relapse include the presence of moderate to severe Graves ophthalmopathy, higher serum T_3 levels at diagnosis, lower serum TSH values at the time of treatment discontinuation, and persistently elevated TRAb. Conversely, undetectable TRAb at diagnosis or the disappearance of measurable TRAb at the completion of therapy predicts lower likelihood of recurrent hyperthyroidism.

In a recent prospective, unblinded trial of 302 consecutive patients with an untreated first episode of Graves hyperthyroidism, participants were randomly assigned to 18 to 24 months of low-dosage methimazole (conventional group) or 60 to 120 months of therapy (long-term group). At study entry, the patient characteristics of the conventional and long-term groups were not significantly different regarding age, sex, smoking status, presence of Graves orbitopathy (26% and 29%), baseline thyroid function test values (all TSH <0.1 mIU/L; free T_4, 37.8 pmol/L and 37.9 pmol/L; T_3, 407 ng/dL and 393 ng/dL), and TRAb (16 IU/L and 16.1 IU/L). Following discontinuation of methimazole, hyperthyroidism recurred within 48 months in 15% of patients on long-term therapy vs in 53% of patients in the conventional group. Longer treatment courses with low-dosage methimazole should thus be considered for patients with a lower likelihood of durable remission after completing conventional treatment unless definitive therapy (radioactive iodine or surgery) is preferred by the patient.

The patient described in this vignette has been treated with methimazole for a total of 16 months and has been on low-dosage methimazole for 1 year. Although her thyroid function tests have normalized, TRAb remains positive. The patient's risk of recurrent hyperthyroidism would be close to 85% if methimazole were stopped now, making discontinuation of therapy (Answer B) an incorrect choice, while continuing methimazole at the current dosage (Answer A) would be appropriate. Using a "block and replace" approach, which involves increasing the methimazole dosage and starting levothyroxine (Answer C), has been shown to result in a higher rate of adverse effects related to antithyroid drug therapy and is not generally recommended.

Although referral for radioactive iodine therapy (Answer D) or surgery (Answer E) could be considered, the patient is satisfied with her current management approach and is tolerating low-dosage methimazole without adverse effects. She may achieve durable remission following a longer course of methimazole treatment.

Educational Objective

Identify predictors of Graves disease remission with thionamide therapy.

Reference(s)

Azizi F, Amouzegar A, Tohidi M, et al. Increased remission rates after long-term methimazole therapy in patients with Graves' disease: results of a randomized clinical trial. *Thyroid.* 2019;29(9):1192-1200. PMID: 31310160

Ross DS, Burch HB, Cooper DS, et al. 2016 American Thyroid Association guidelines for diagnosis and management of hyperthyroidism and other causes of thyrotoxicosis. *Thyroid.* 2016;26(10):1343-1421. PMID: 27521067

Thewjitcharoen Y, Karndumri K, Chatchomchuan W, et al. Serum T3 level and duration of minimum maintenance dose therapy predict relapse in methimazole-treated Graves disease [published correction in *J Endocr Soc.* 2021;5(4):bvab015]. *J Endocr Soc.* 2020;5(1):bvaa170. PMID: 33305160

Tun NNZ, Beckett G, Zammitt NN, Strachan MWJ, Seckl JR, Gibb FW. Thyrotropin receptor antibody levels at diagnosis and after thionamide course predict Graves' disease relapse. *Thyroid.* 2016;26(8):1004-1009. PMID: 27266892

58 ANSWER: E) Apolipoprotein E

Apolipoproteins are the principal proteins carried by lipoproteins. Together with different amounts of lipids, they make lipoproteins of varying size and density. Functionally, apolipoproteins can be structural proteins, enzyme activators, ligands for different receptors, or cofactors for different enzymes (*see table*).

Table. Summary of Apolipoproteins

Apolipoprotein	Location	Function
A-1	HDL	• Activate lecithin cholesterol acyl transferase • Ligand for ATP-binding cassette transporters
B_{100}	VLDL, IDL, LDL	• Ligand for the LDL receptor • Ligand for hepatic chylomicron and VLDL remnant receptor
CII	VLDL, HDL	• Cofactor for lipoprotein lipase
E	VLDL, HDL	• Ligand for the LDL receptor • Ligand for hepatic chylomicron and VLDL remnant receptor
(a)	Lipoprotein (a)	• Inhibits fibrinolysis

Apolipoprotein E (Answer E) is present in VLDL and HDL and it is a ligand for the LDL receptor. The apolipoprotein E gene has 3 different alleles: *E2, E3,* and *E4,* which generate 6 apolipoprotein E phenotypes: *APO*E2/E2, APO*E3/E3, APO*E4/E4, APO*E2/E3, APO*E2/E4,* and *APO*E3/E4.* APO E3 and APO E4 bind to the LDL receptor with high affinity, but the binding of APO E2 is 50 to 100 times weaker. This explains the lipid abnormalities seen in affected patients. APO E3 is the most common isoform. Familial dysbetalipoproteinemia is associated with *APO*E2/E2.* Patients with this condition have elevated triglycerides and cholesterol due to the accumulation of chylomicron remnant and intermediate-density lipoprotein. The presence of *APO*E2/E2* alone is not sufficient to cause dysbetalipoproteinemia. The onset of this condition requires a second metabolic stressor such as insulin resistance, type 2 diabetes mellitus, obesity, etc. Palmar crease xanthomas are specific for this disease. Affected individuals are predisposed to premature coronary artery disease and peripheral artery disease. This patient has obesity and prediabetes, which combined with his likely genotype of *APO*E2/E2* explains his lipid panel and presentation.

Apolipoprotein A-1 (Answer A) is the main apolipoprotein in HDL particles. Apolipoprotein A-1 activates lecithin cholesterol acyl transferase and is the ligand for ATP-binding cassette transporters. Pathogenic variants in the gene encoding apolipoprotein A-1 lead to very low HDL cholesterol (<10th percentile), premature coronary artery disease, and corneal opacification. Patients with a pathogenic variant in the gene encoding apolipoprotein A-1 do not have elevated triglycerides or total cholesterol. Also, they do not present with palmar crease xanthomas.

Apolipoprotein (a) (Answer B) binds to apolipoprotein B from an LDL-cholesterol particle and forms lipoprotein (a). The size of apolipoprotein (a) varies depending on the number of kringle IV type 2 repeats. There is an inverse relationship between the size of apolipoprotein (a) and lipoprotein (a) plasma concentrations. Apolipoprotein (a) is similar to plasminogen and may inhibit fibrinolysis by inhibiting the generation of plasmin. High concentrations of lipoprotein (a) are associated with atherosclerotic cardiovascular disease and the development of aortic stenosis. Patients with elevated lipoprotein (a) do not have any distinct physical examination findings or elevated total cholesterol or triglycerides.

Apolipoprotein B_{100} (Answer C) is made by the liver. It is the major apolipoprotein in VLDL, intermediate-density lipoprotein, and lipoprotein (a), and it is the only apolipoprotein in LDL. Apolipoprotein B_{100} is a ligand for the LDL receptor. Pathogenic variants in the gene encoding apolipoprotein B_{100} can cause either low or high levels of LDL cholesterol. Patients who have familial hypercholesterolemia due to a pathogenic variant in the apolipoprotein B_{100} gene present with personal or family history of premature atherosclerotic disease, have elevated LDL cholesterol, and have corneal arcus and/or Achilles tendon xanthomas on physical examination. This patient does not have familial hypercholesterolemia, as his physical examination findings are not characteristic of this condition and his lipid problem is mainly high triglycerides and high cholesterol.

Apolipoprotein C-II (Answer D) is found in chylomicrons, VLDL, and HDL. It is a cofactor of lipoprotein lipase. Individuals with pathogenic variants in the apolipoprotein C-II gene have hypertriglyceridemia, chronic pancreatitis, and eruptive xanthomas on physical examination. Due to the size of the chylomicron particle, affected patients are not at risk of premature cardiovascular disease. This patient does not have a pathogenic variant in the gene encoding apolipoprotein C because his triglycerides are not high enough (usually >1000 mg/dL [>11.30 mmol/L]) and he has no history of pancreatitis.

The laboratory where the patient had his lipid panel done used the Friedewald equation to provide a calculated LDL-cholesterol value. When using this equation, calculated LDL-cholesterol is not given when triglycerides are greater than 400 mg/dL (>4.52 mmol/L). If the laboratory used the National Institutes of Health equation, a calculated LDL-cholesterol value would have been provided, as this formula gives valid LDL-cholesterol results in patients with a triglyceride concentration up to 800 mg/dL (9.04 mmol/L).

Educational Objective

Identify the apolipoprotein responsible for familial dysbetalipoproteinemia.

Reference(s)

Reyes-Soffer G, Ginsberg HN, Ramakrishnan R. The metabolism of lipoprotein (a): an ever-evolving story. *J Lipid Res.* 2017;58(9):1756-1764. PMID: 28720561

Patsch W, Gorro AM Jr. Apolipoproteins: pathophysiology and clinical implications. *Methods Enzymol.* 1996;263:3-32. PMID: 8748998

Ramasamy I. Update on the molecular biology of dyslipidemias. *Clin Chim Acta.* 2016;454:143-185. PMID: 26546829

59 ANSWER: D) Nephrotic syndrome

An increased levothyroxine requirement in a patient treated with this medication can be due to various etiologies. The most common reasons for needing a higher dosage are weight gain, pregnancy, malabsorption syndrome due to celiac disease or Roux-en-Y gastric bypass, and medications and supplements. Some medications worsen underlying hypothyroidism (tyrosine kinase inhibitors), interfere with absorption (iron, calcium, proton-pump inhibitors), enhance clearance (phenytoin, phenobarbital), or increase thyroxine-binding globulin (estrogen and selective estrogen receptor modulators). In addition, nonadherence to levothyroxine should be considered if the etiology remains undetermined after ruling out common causes.

This patient has lower-extremity edema with elevated TSH, low albumin, elevated LDL cholesterol, elevated total cholesterol, and microalbuminuria. Her urinary protein excretion was 3.8 g/24 h (not shown in the laboratory data). The clinical and biochemical findings are consistent with nephrotic syndrome (Answer D). Nephrotic syndrome is one of the most common glomerular disorders. It is defined by edema, proteinuria greater than 3.5 g/24 h, hypoalbuminemia (<30 g/L [<3.0 g/dL]), and hyperlipidemia. Thromboembolism, infection, vitamin D deficiency, and iron deficiency have been associated with nephrotic syndrome. Endocrine abnormalities have been reported in affected patients. The thyroid gland has a major role in kidney development and function, and the kidneys also have a crucial role in the metabolism and elimination of thyroid hormone. Hypothyroidism and subclinical hypothyroidism have been reported in patients with nephrotic syndrome and chronic kidney disease with no known hypothyroidism. In nephrotic syndrome, there is a loss of thyroid-binding proteins in the urine, leading to loss of thyroid hormones and subsequently an increase in TSH. Therefore, a patient with nephrotic syndrome and known hypothyroidism who is taking levothyroxine needs a higher dosage of levothyroxine to maintain normal thyroid function. However, once proteinuria is resolved, the levothyroxine dosage requirement returns to baseline. Many disorders can cause glomerular damage and lead to nephrotic syndrome, including systemic lupus erythematosus, amyloidosis, diabetic kidney disease, focal segmental glomerulosclerosis, membranous nephropathy, and minimal change disease (mostly seen in children).

This patient takes her levothyroxine tablets as prescribed and has had a gradual dosage increase, but her serum TSH concentration remains elevated. Her levothyroxine dosage should be further adjusted to maintain her TSH concentration within the normal range. Nonadherence to levothyroxine (Answer E) is unlikely because she has nephrotic syndrome and reports taking her levothyroxine.

Biotin interference (Answer A) causes low TSH values when a noncompetitive sandwich method is used and causes elevated thyroid hormone values when a competitive method is used. This patient's serum TSH is elevated, and biotin interference is not the most likely explanation. In addition, she does not take any over-the-counter supplements.

Metformin (Answer C) is known to cause slightly low TSH levels, not elevated TSH as in this vignette.

Malabsorption could be a reason for requiring several adjustments in the levothyroxine dosage. However, celiac disease (Answer B) is mostly seen in patients with type 1 diabetes or other autoimmune diseases. This patient has type 2 diabetes. In addition, this patient's clinical findings are not consistent with celiac disease.

Educational Objective

Diagnose nephrotic syndrome as a cause of abnormal thyroid blood test results in patients with known hypothyroidism.

Reference(s)

Di Mario F, Pofi R, Gigante A, et al. Hypothyroidism and nephrotic syndrome: why, when and how to treat. *Curr Vasc Pharmacol.* 2017;15(5):398-403. PMID: 28176633

Benido Silva VB, Pereira MT, Moreira CL, Monteiro SS, Inacio I, Cardoso MH. Nephrotic syndrome as a cause of transient clinical hypothyroidism. *Case Rep Endocrinol.* 2021;5523929. PMID: 34513097

Karethimmaiah H, Sarathi V. Nephrotic syndrome increases the need for levothyroxine replacement in patients with hypothyroidism. *J Clin Diagn Res.* 2016;10(12):OC10-OC12. PMID: 28208903

60 ANSWER: A) Dementia

Psychosocial factors influence control of both type 1 and type 2 diabetes. These factors can be behavioral, emotional, environmental, social, and cultural. This patient had good glycemic control until 2 years prior to this visit, and there is no evidence that she had difficulty adjusting to her diabetes diagnosis early on. She appears to have acquired self-management skills, and there is no suggestion of low health literacy or lack of comprehension of diabetes management (Answer E).

She has had no change in weight and has no gastrointestinal symptoms that might suggest a secondary cause for suboptimal glycemic control such as adenocarcinoma of the pancreas (Answer D).

Hypothyroidism (Answer C) may be associated with hypoglycemia; one would not expect unexpected rise in blood glucose in this setting.

Depression (Answer B) can certainly affect glycemic control, although this diagnosis appears unlikely in this patient, as she has no difficulty with sleep and reports usual interest in activities.

Her late arrival to the appointment due to confusion about the appointment time, flustered and frustrated demeanor, and elevated blood pressure (suggestive of missed dose[s] of antihypertension medication) raise the real possibility of cognitive dysfunction. Given her age and confusion, a diagnosis of dementia (Answer A) must be considered and a Mini-Mental test should be administered.

The American Diabetes Association recommends personalized, patient-centered psychosocial care. This includes problem identification, screening, therapeutic intervention, and communication. Various behavioral health disorders, including depression, anxiety, adjustment disorders, and cognitive disorders, may affect a patient's ability to engage in self-care. Individual needs should be ascertained before interventions can be initiated. All patients should first be assessed with formal diagnostic tests used as needed at the time of diagnosis and at the time of major clinical changes. The box lists of some of the screening tools available for specific conditions.

Box. Screening Tools for Assessing Psychosocial Conditions Affecting Diabetes Management

Self-management	Diabetes Self Management Questionnaire (DSMQ)
Diabetes distress	Diabetes Distress Scale (DDS-17) or Problem Areas in Diabetes Questionnaires (PAID)
Diabetes numeracy	DNT-15 DNT-15 Latino
Depression	PHQ-9
Anxiety	Beck Anxiety Index (BAI)
Cognitive dysfunction	Mini-Mental State Examination (MMSE)

Educational Objective

Identify psychosocial causes of suboptimal glycemic control.

Reference(s)

Young-Hyman D, de Groot M, Hill-Briggs F, Gonzalez JS, Hood K, Peyrot M. Psychosocial care for people with diabetes: a position statement of the American Diabetes Association. *Diabetes Care.* 2016;39(12):2126-2140. PMID: 27879358

61 **ANSWER: E) Very low-energy diet and referral for bariatric surgery**

Obesity is one of the clinical conditions most strongly associated with decreased serum testosterone in men. Clinical studies in otherwise healthy young to middle-aged men (18-55 years) with obesity have reported 2 main patterns of hypothalamic-pituitary-gonadal (HPG) axis abnormalities. Men with class 1 obesity (BMI 30 to <35 kg/m^2) or class 2 obesity (BMI 35 to <40 kg/m^2) predominantly exhibit low total testosterone concentrations due to obesity-associated reductions in SHBG, while free testosterone (if measured by gold standard equilibrium dialysis) has typically been reported to be normal. Studies in men with class 3 obesity (BMI ≥40 kg/m^2), however, demonstrate not only reductions in total but also in free testosterone concentrations, as evident in this vignette. Of note, if requested, free testosterone is usually calculated (and equations may differ depending on the commercial laboratory used), and calculated free testosterone is a reasonable approximate of gold standard equilibrium dialysis. In the setting of obesity, gonadotropins are typically low to low-normal, indicating that obesity suppresses the HPG axis at the hypothalamic-pituitary level. Exact mechanisms remain unknown, but proinflammatory adipocytokines, impaired insulin signaling in the central nervous system, and dysregulated leptin signaling may contribute to hypothalamic-pituitary suppression. While negative central feedback due to elevation in circulating estradiol has been implicated previously, more recent studies using accurate mass spectrometry–based assays have reported that men with obesity have low rather than high circulating estradiol concentrations.

The association between obesity and decreased testosterone is bi-directional. Obesity reduces testosterone, and reductions in serum testosterone can lead to increased accumulation of adipose tissue. However, a recent bi-directional Mendelian randomization analysis concluded that while BMI had a causal effect on reducing serum testosterone, conversely, serum testosterone did not affect BMI. Overall, therefore, the evidence suggests that adiposity has more dominant effects on the HPG axis than vice versa. Interestingly, the above-mentioned clinical studies in otherwise healthy men with obesity found limited evidence of clinical androgen deficiency or of reduced semen quality, even in men with class 3 obesity. Therefore, the degree to which nonspecific androgen deficiency-like symptoms such as low libido, fatigue, anxiety, and mild depression as seen in this vignette are causally related to reduced serum testosterone rather than driven by obesity and associated complications such as sleep apnea remains unknown.

The best treatment for this man's hypogonadism is weight loss (Answer E). Multiple studies have shown that successful weight loss is not only very effective in reactivating the HPG axis, but it is also associated with many other health benefits. In a recent meta-analysis, diet-associated weight loss (~10% loss of body weight) led to an increase in total testosterone of 83 ng/dL (95% CI, 48-117 ng/dL) (SI: 2.87 nmol/L [95% CI, 1.68-4.07 nmol/L]). Bariatric surgery (~30% loss of body weight) was associated with an even more marked increase in total testosterone of 251 ng/dL (95% CI, 187-315 ng/dL) (SI: 8.73 nmol/L [95% CI, 6.51-10.95 nmol/L]). With sufficient weight loss (≥10% of body weight), increases in gonadotropins and free testosterone also occur, confirming a genuine reactivation of the HPG axis. In several longitudinal studies among men with obesity who underwent bariatric surgery, the degree of weight loss was closely associated with improvements in sexual function and other nonspecific androgen deficiency-like symptoms, but the increase in testosterone was not. This further suggests that clinical features are more closely related to excess adiposity, rather than to the lowered serum testosterone, supporting weight loss as the first-line treatment.

In contrast, testosterone treatment, either topical or intramuscular (Answers B and D), is not the first-line treatment. Whether testosterone treatment should be considered when lifestyle measures fail remains controversial, as there are no clinical trials in men with obesity that provide definitive evidence regarding patient-important long-term benefits and risks of testosterone treatment. Of note, this patient most likely has clinically significant sleep apnea, suggested by his history and the fact that despite his relatively low testosterone, his hematocrit is elevated, which suggests significant hypoxia. Testosterone treatment not only could worsen his sleep apnea, but also worsen his erythrocytosis. Endocrine Society clinical practice guidelines recommend against prescribing testosterone in men with a baseline hematocrit greater than 48%. For all these reasons, testosterone therapy is not the best strategy for treating this man's hypogonadism.

Clomiphene (Answer A), a selective estrogen receptor modulator, acts as an estradiol antagonist at the hypothalamic-pituitary unit. Clomiphene counteracts estradiol-mediated central negative feedback and has been reported to increase gonadotropin concentrations and secondarily testosterone in men with obesity-associated functional suppression of the HPG axis. However, definitive randomized controlled trials demonstrating that this increase in serum testosterone is associated with improvements in clinical symptoms are lacking, and, like testosterone treatment, clomiphene may worsen erythrocytosis.

Finally, the normal iron studies make hemochromatosis, which can be associated with secondary hypogonadism, unlikely and the increased hematocrit is sufficiently explained by his untreated sleep apnea. Although phlebotomy (Answer C) is an appropriate treatment for hemochromatosis, hemochromatosis-associated hypogonadism usually does not revert with this therapy. In men with hemochromatosis-associated hypogonadism, testosterone therapy is usually required, once phlebotomy has decreased the hematocrit to a safe level.

Educational Objective

Manage obesity-associated hypogonadism by encouraging weight loss to reactivate the hypothalamic-pituitary-gonadal axis.

References

Grossmann M. Hypogonadism and male obesity: focus on unresolved questions. *Clin Endocrinol (Oxf)*. 2018;89(1):11-12. PMID: 29683196

Corona G, Rastrelli G, Monami M, et al. Body weight loss reverts obesity-associated hypogonadotropic hypogonadism: a systematic review and meta-analysis. *Eur J Endocrinol.* 2013;168(6):829-843. PMID: 23482592

Bhasin S, Brito JP, Cunningham GR, et al. Testosterone therapy in men with hypogonadism: an Endocrine Society clinical practice guideline. *J Clin Endocrinol Metab.* 2018;103(5):1715-1744. PMID: 29562364

62 ANSWER: A) Hyperthyroidism

The patient described in this vignette has an elevated bone-specific alkaline phosphatase level with no bony pain. There are several etiologies of elevated bone-specific alkaline phosphatase isoenzyme, which is a result of increased osteoblastic activity: Paget disease, metastatic cancer to bone, hyperthyroidism, hyperparathyroidism, and osteomalacia. This patient has an undetectable TSH level, and his whole-body bone scan shows uniform visualization of the axial and appendicular skeleton, without visualization of the kidneys, consistent with a metabolic superscan. The multifocal articular uptake in the left knee, spine, and ankles is most likely degenerative. The combination of these findings should raise suspicion for a diagnosis of hyperthyroidism (Answer A). In fact, he had significantly elevated free T_4 and T_3 levels, along with a thyroid uptake and scan that revealed diffuse abnormal increased radioiodine uptake (24-hour uptake = 73%), consistent with a diagnosis of Graves disease. It is important to remember that hyperthyroidism in older patients may be apathetic, and that older patients with Graves hyperthyroidism are less likely to have a goiter.

An example of a bone scan showing normal kidney and soft-tissue uptake is shown (*see image*).

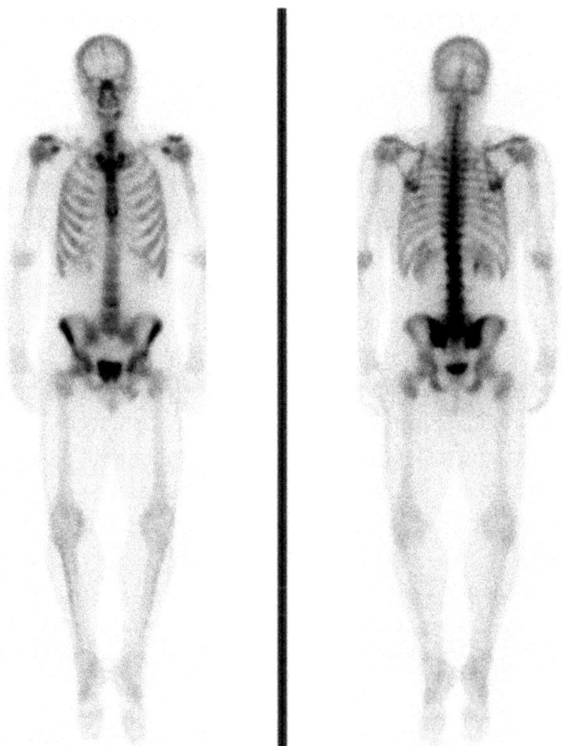

This patient has normal calcium, phosphate, and PTH levels, which essentially rules out primary hyperparathyroidism (Answer D).

His vitamin D level is suboptimal but not low enough to suggest osteomalacia. Individuals with osteomalacia typically present with bone pain, muscle weakness, and difficulty walking. In nutritional osteomalacia, laboratory abnormalities include a very low serum 25-hydroxyvitamin D level (<10 ng/mL [<25 nmol/L]), low to low-normal serum calcium and phosphate levels, high PTH and alkaline phosphatase levels, and low urinary calcium excretion. However, this patient's vitamin D insufficiency (Answer E) does not explain his clinical findings.

Similarly, there is no reason to suspect that he has Paget disease (Answer C) or metastasis (Answer B) given the clinical presentation, lack of history of malignancy, and uptake findings on his bone scan.

Educational Objective

Diagnose hyperthyroidism as a cause of elevated bone-specific alkaline phosphatase and metabolic superscan.

Reference(s)

Love C, Din AS, Tomas MB, Kalapparambath TP, Palestro CJ. Radionuclide bone imaging: an illustrative review. *Radiographics.* 2003;23(2):341-358. PMID: 12640151

Kravets I. Paget's disease of bone: diagnosis and treatment. *Am J Med.* 2018;131(11):1298-1303. PMID: 29752905

Singer FR, Bone HG 3rd, Hosking DJ, et al; Endocrine Society. Paget's disease of bone: an Endocrine Society clinical practice guideline. *J Clin Endocrinol Metab.* 2014;99(12):4408-4422. PMID: 25406796

Sonoda LI, Balan KK. Co-existent Paget's disease of the bone, prostate carcinoma skeletal metastases and fracture on skeletal scintigraphy-lessons to be learned. *Mol Imaging Radionucl Ther.* 2013;22(2):63-65. PMID: 24003400

63

ANSWER: A) Increase the semaglutide dosage to 2.4 mg weekly as tolerated

High-dosage semaglutide therapy was approved by the US FDA in July 2021 for the treatment of obesity. The approval was based on trial data from the STEP studies (Semaglutide Treatment Effect in People with Obesity) that evaluated high-dosage semaglutide regarding its efficacy, tolerability, and role in weight maintenance. STEP was a set of randomized control trials comparing semaglutide with placebo in weight-stable adults with either a BMI of 30 kg/m^2 or higher or a BMI of 27 kg/m^2 with weight-related complications. The dosage of semaglutide was gradually titrated in a step-wise fashion such that participants reached the maximum dosage of 2.4 mg weekly after 16 weeks. All participants were also provided lifestyle intervention advice aiming for 150 minutes of physical activity per week and a 500 kcal deficit per day. After 68 weeks, participants who had been receiving semaglutide lost an average of 15% of their body weight vs 2.4% in the placebo group. When intensive behavioral therapy was added to the intervention, weight loss increased to 16% in the treatment group vs 5.7% in the placebo group. The most commonly reported adverse effects were gastrointestinal symptoms (nausea, constipation, diarrhea) or gallbladder-related symptoms.

Semaglutide, as with other GLP-1 agonists, is relatively contraindicated in patients with a history of pancreatitis or who are at risk for pancreatitis. Adverse effects are related to dosing, and patients who cannot tolerate high-dosage semaglutide should decrease the dosage to the highest tolerated.

In this patient with type 2 diabetes, increasing the semaglutide dosage to 2.4 mg weekly as tolerated (Answer A) may afford additional weight loss and improvement in glycemic control. Her history of nausea with a short-acting GLP-1 receptor agonist does not preclude her from being on a long-acting GLP-1 receptor agonist.

Switching to high-dosage liraglutide (Answer D) is unlikely to offer additional weight-loss benefits. In the SCALE trial, participants lost an average 8% of their body weight on liraglutide, 3 mg daily, when administered as an adjunct to dietary modification and exercise. The STEP 8 placebo-controlled randomized clinical trial showed greater weight loss with high-dosage semaglutide compared with high-dosage liraglutide, when added to counseling for diet and physical activity (15.8% vs 6.4%, respectively). Extended-release phentermine/topiramate (Answer B) is FDA approved for weight loss. However, adding a sympathomimetic agent such as phentermine to the regimen of a patient with uncontrolled hypertension is not recommended. Furthermore, semaglutide has the dual advantage of addressing weight and glycemic control. The combination of naltrexone and bupropion (not offered here as a choice) is also FDA approved for weight loss, but its effectiveness is reportedly lower than semaglutide's.

Meal replacement programs (Answer E) have been proven to help patients lose weight and maintain weight loss. However, they are an impractical long-term strategy and are therefore not the best option for this particular patient.

Finally, recombinant leptin therapy (Answer C) is FDA approved for the treatment of generalized forms of lipodystrophy. Based on this patient's metabolic parameters and clinical phenotype, she does not have generalized lipodystrophy. Her relatively lean extremities in comparison to her increased abdominal girth may raise the suspicion for partial lipodystrophy; however, this does not qualify her for leptin replacement therapy.

Educational Objective

Recommend high-dosage GLP-1 receptor agonists as the most effective drugs for weight loss.

Reference(s)

Wilding JPH, Batterham RL, Calanna S, et al. Once-weekly semaglutide in adults with overweight or obesity. *N Engl J Med.* 2021;384(11):989. PMID: 33567185

Pi-Sunyer X, Astrup A, Fujioka K, et al; SCALE Obesity and Prediabetes NN8022-1839. A randomized, controlled trial of 3.0 mg of liraglutide in weight management. *N Engl J Med.* 2015;373(1):11-22. PMID: 26132939

Rubino DM, Greenway FL, Khalid U, et al; STEP 8 Investigators. Effect of weekly subcutaneous semaglutide vs daily liraglutide on body weight in adults with overweight or obesity without diabetes: the STEP 8 randomized clinical trial. *JAMA.* 2022;327(2):138-150. PMID: 35015037

64 ANSWER: A) Left hemithyroidectomy

Ultrasound-guided FNA biopsy of thyroid nodules for cytopathologic evaluation is the standard procedure to determine whether a thyroid nodule is benign or malignant. The Bethesda System for Reporting Thyroid Cytopathology was first proposed in 2007 as a standard reporting system for thyroid cytopathology, and it was revised in 2017 to include updated studies and the noninvasive follicular thyroid neoplasm with papillary-like nuclear features (NIFTP) category of surgical pathology. However, cytopathology does not provide a definitive diagnosis in a significant minority of cases, with some 20% to 25% of nodules demonstrating indeterminate results (Bethesda categories III, IV, and V). Historically, many patients with indeterminate cytopathology were subjected to diagnostic thyroid lobectomy. As many as 60% were overtreated or undertreated using such an approach.

Molecular testing has become a common approach to help distinguish between indeterminate thyroid nodules that are likely to be benign and can be followed clinically and those that probably represent thyroid cancer or NIFTP. Molecular tests use different approaches to make this determination, which may include assessment for single nucleotide variants (point mutations), insertions/deletions, gene fusions, chromosomal copy number alterations, and/or abnormal gene expression using DNA, mRNA, miRNA, or a combination thereof.

RAS (*HRAS, NRAS, KRAS*) point mutations, which lead to the constitutive activation of downstream *RAS*-mediated signaling pathways, represent the second most common genetic alteration identified in thyroid cancer. However, thyroid nodules with isolated *RAS* variants are equally likely to be benign adenomas, NIFTP, or thyroid cancers. Most *RAS*-related malignancies are follicular variant papillary thyroid cancer, which is associated with a low incidence of cervical lymph node metastases. Reasons to consider total thyroidectomy (Answer D) in the context of an indeterminate thyroid nodule with an identified *RAS* variant include high-risk radiographic findings (eg, evidence of extrathyroidal extension), the co-occurrence of higher risk genetic alterations within the same nodule (eg, *TERT* promoter co-mutation), or a compelling clinical indication (eg, large contralateral nodule). In the absence of such findings, a more conservative operative approach (hemithyroidectomy [Answer A]), should be chosen for thyroid nodules with indeterminate cytology and isolated *RAS* variants to avoid overtreatment. Total thyroidectomy with central neck dissection (Answer E) would also be an overly aggressive surgical approach.

Performing neck CT (Answer B) is not indicated in this case and is generally not required in the preoperative evaluation of most patients with a new thyroid cancer diagnosis except when there is clinical suspicion for advanced disease, such as locally invasive tumors or bulky lymph node involvement.

Lastly, radioactive iodine uptake scanning (Answer C) is not generally performed in patients with an intact thyroid gland except in cases of hyperthyroidism and would thus have no relevance in this case.

Educational Objective

Use molecular testing to help determine the most appropriate management of thyroid nodules with indeterminate (Bethesda III/IV) cytopathology results.

Reference(s)

Haugen BR, Alexander EK, Bible KC, et al. 2015 American Thyroid Association management guidelines for adult patients with thyroid nodules and differentiated thyroid cancer: the American Thyroid Association Guidelines Task Force on Thyroid Nodules and Differentiated Thyroid Cancer. *Thyroid.* 2016;26(1):1-133. PMID: 26462967

Patel SG, Carty SE, McCoy KL, et al. Preoperative detection of RAS mutation may guide extent of thyroidectomy. *Surgery.* 2017;161(1):168-175. PMID: 27863786

Paulson VA, Shivdasani P, Angell TE, Cibas ES, Krane JF, Lindeman NI, Alexander EK, Barletta JA. Noninvasive follicular thyroid neoplasm with papillary-like nuclear features accounts for more than half of "carcinomas" harboring RAS mutations. *Thyroid.* 2017;27(4):506-511. PMID: 28114855

Steward DL, Carty SE, Sippel RS, et al. Performance of a multigene genomic classifier in thyroid nodules with indeterminate cytology: a prospective blinded multicenter study. *JAMA Oncol.* 2019;5(2):204-212. PMID: 30419129

65 ANSWER: A) Administer the Diabetes Numeracy Test (DNT)

This patient, who is a recent immigrant, is on a complicated insulin regimen. She has limited resources and multiple possible reasons for suboptimal glycemic control. Her consistently elevated hemoglobin A_{1c} level of 9.0% (75 mmol/mol) may reflect the high cost of medication, low health literacy, low numeracy skills, and a language barrier that makes diabetes education sessions less fruitful. Each of these possible factors must be assessed and the diabetes regimen simplified if needed.

Gaining self-management skills requires close interaction between patients and health care providers, and this is particularly difficult when patients have limited English proficiency. Latino patients, especially those who have limited English proficiency, have better outcomes if they receive culturally appropriate and relevant information from navigators. Navigators are generally bilingual and help determine social and cultural nuances that might help health care providers deliver personalized patient care. This patient would benefit from working with a navigator rather than seeing a certified diabetes educator (Answer D) in the same setting as she has in the past.

Low health literacy and numeracy skills are associated with less optimal glycemic control, although ascribing causality is difficult. Numeracy is defined as the ability to understand and use numbers in daily life. Addressing numeracy issues with specific educational interventions has resulted in at least short-term improvements in glycemic control. This patient has demonstrated difficulty with insulin dose calculation, so assessing numeracy skills using the Diabetes Numeracy Test (DNT) (Answer A) would be a good next step in her management. Simply reviewing the correction scale (Answer C) if she is unable to understand or implement the plan would be ineffective. The DNT assesses a range of skills, including the ability to read nutrition labels, to sequentially increase the dosage of medications such as metformin, and to take the right dose of insulin. The test can identify specific areas of difficulty, and these findings can be used to tailor future diabetes education sessions, preferably with the help of a navigator.

Use of a smart insulin pen (Answer E) could take some of the calculation issues out of the patient's hands. For some patients, smart pens can be very helpful. However, this patient has financial constraints and may not be able to afford these pens. Carbohydrate counting would still be required. While smart insulin pens are certainly worth considering, their use would not be the best next step in this case.

Finally, although assessing mood and risk of depression is important for all patients with diabetes, this patient gives no history of decreased interest or energy, and administering the Patient Health Questionnaire (PHQ) 9 (Answer B) would not be the best next step in her care.

Educational Objective

Assess health literacy and numeracy skills to improve glycemic control in a patient with suboptimally controlled diabetes.

Reference(s)

Lopez L, Grant RW. Closing the gap: eliminating health care disparities among Latinos with Diabetes using health information technology tools and patient navigators. *J Diabetes Sci Technol.* 2012;6(1):169-176. PMID: 22401336

Cavanaugh K, Huizinga MM, Wallston KA, et al. Association of numeracy and diabetes control. *Ann Intern Med.* 2008;148(10):737-746. PMID: 18490687

White RO 3rd, Osborn CY, Gebretsadik T, Kripalani S, Rothman RL. Development and validation of a Spanish diabetes-specific numeracy measure: DNT-15 Latino. *Diabetes Technol Ther.* 2011;13(9):893-898. PMID: 21714674

Patient Health Questionnaire-9 (PHQ-9). Available at: https://www.apa.org/depression-guideline/patient-health-questionnaire.pdf. Accessed April 2022.

66 ANSWER: C) Follow-up abdominal CT in 3 months

This patient's clinical presentation is consistent with acute primary adrenal insufficiency. Adrenal insufficiency should be suspected in a patient with nonspecific abdominal pain, nausea/vomiting, and hypotension. Electrolyte abnormalities commonly seen in patients with primary adrenal insufficiency (who lack not only cortisol, but also mineralocorticoids) include hyponatremia, hyperkalemia, and mild hyperchloremic acidosis. If not promptly recognized and treated, acute adrenal insufficiency can be fatal.

Causes of acute adrenal insufficiency in a patient without a preestablished diagnosis include bilateral adrenal hemorrhage or infarction. Risk factors for adrenal hemorrhage include anticoagulant/antithrombotic therapy, thromboembolic disease, hypercoagulable disorders, physical trauma, and sepsis, particularly meningococcemia (Waterhouse-Friderichsen syndrome). This patient was treated with warfarin for atrial fibrillation, and he had a supratherapeutic international normalized ratio, which prompted his acute adrenal hemorrhage.

On CT, adrenal hemorrhage appears as nonenhancing, low- or mixed-attenuation, round or oval masses and periadrenal fat stranding. Over time, the size and CT attenuation of adrenal hemorrhage decrease or even completely resolve. Serial imaging (Answer C) is thus indicated. Resolution of the hemorrhage is a good prognostic factor for recovery of adrenal function (this must be evaluated clinically and hormonally).

Adrenal biopsy (Answer A) is rarely indicated. Furthermore, adrenal biopsy cannot generally distinguish between benign and malignant cortical adrenal masses. Adrenal biopsy might be offered for the diagnosis of metastases of uncertain origin in which the adrenal lesion is the most accessible of possible metastatic foci.

FDG-PET/CT (Answer B) can be useful for indeterminate adrenal masses that are suspicious for malignancy.

Screening for congenital adrenal hyperplasia with serum 17-hydroxyprogesterone (Answer D) should be considered in patients with bilateral adrenal enlargement or myelolipomas. Such patients typically have hyperpigmentation due to untreated chronic primary adrenal insufficiency and severe ACTH elevations. Women with untreated congenital adrenal hyperplasia often have clinical and hormonal evidence of androgen excess, and affected men might have testicular adrenal rest tumors.

Elevation of serum ACE (Answer E) can be seen in granulomatous diseases, such as sarcoidosis, but this is not suspected in this patient.

Educational Objective

Identify the imaging characteristics of adrenal hemorrhage and guide management.

Reference(s)

Ali A, Singh G, Balasubramanian SP. Acute non-traumatic adrenal haemorrhage-management, pathology and clinical outcomes. *Gland Surg.* 2018;7(5):428-432. PMID: 30505763

67 ANSWER: A) Functioning gonadotroph adenoma

Gonadotroph adenomas are among the most common pituitary adenoma subtypes. Most are nonsecretory and come to attention only when large enough to cause local mass effect (eg, optic chiasm compression, hypopituitarism). Immunohistochemical studies (LH, FSH, and SF-1) of resected tumors confirm a gonadotroph origin in a significant proportion of clinically nonfunctioning pituitary adenomas.

In contrast, functioning gonadotroph adenomas (Answer A), which express and secrete active hormones (usually FSH), are much rarer. However, in some patients, they can give rise to very distinctive clinical presentations—macroorchidism in men and spontaneous ovarian hyperstimulation in premenopausal women.

A diagnosis of ovarian hyperstimulation is suggested by several clinical, laboratory, and radiologic findings, including the following:

- Abdominal distention and discomfort, pelvic pain, weight gain
- Polymenorrhea
- Raised serum FSH with low/suppressed LH (and elevated FSH-to-LH ratio)
- Hyperestrogenism (with high-normal/high serum estradiol)
- Enlarged ovaries with multiple large cysts

Many of these features are present in this patient, and there is also evidence of pituitary dysfunction with mild/moderate hyperprolactinemia (consistent with stalk interruption) and possible central hypothyroidism with low free T_4, but only mildly raised TSH. Serum cortisol and IGF-1 are also within their lower respective reference ranges, but dynamic testing would be required to exclude or confirm more widespread hypopituitarism. Pituitary MRI in this patient revealed a macroadenoma with suprasellar extension. Following successful transsphenoidal resection of a histologically confirmed gonadotroph adenoma, the patient had complete resolution of her symptoms and normalization of her laboratory results.

Spontaneous ovarian hyperstimulation has also been reported in a small number of patients who harbor pathogenic variants in the FSH receptor (Answer E). The abnormal receptors display increased sensitivity to hCG (±TSH), resulting in spontaneous ovarian hyperstimulation during early pregnancy. The phenotype of a woman with specific constitutive FSH receptor activation, which is not dependent on permissive signaling by hCG, still remains to be discovered.

This patient's clinical presentation and laboratory investigations are not typical of a germ-cell tumor that is secreting hCG (Answer B).

Primary hypothyroidism (Answer C) in females has been linked to the development of multicystic ovaries in both childhood and early adulthood. In addition, if inadequately treated, hypothyroidism can predispose to the development of pituitary thyrotroph hyperplasia, which may be mistaken for a pituitary adenoma. Serum TSH is typically markedly raised, and it has been postulated that cross-signaling through the FSH receptor accounts for the gonadal phenotype. However, in this patient, hypothyroidism is mild and TSH is only marginally above the upper limit of the reference range.

Although this patient's serum FSH concentration is high, the clinical features and laboratory profile are not suggestive of incipient ovarian failure (Answer D).

Educational Objective

Differentiate among the causes of spontaneous (endogenous) ovarian hyperstimulation syndrome and recognize the possibility that some gonadotroph adenomas are clinically functioning.

Reference(s)

Patel S, Pacione D, Fischer I, Maloku E, Agrawal N. Follicle-stimulating hormone-producing pituitary adenoma: a case report and review of the literature. *AACE Clin Case Rep.* 2019;5(3):e175-e180. PMID: 31967028

Caretto A, Lanzi R, Piani C, Molgora M, Mortini P, Losa M. Ovarian hyperstimulation syndrome due to follicle-stimulating hormone-secreting pituitary adenomas. *Pituitary.* 2017;20(5):553-560. PMID: 28676954

De Leener A, Montanelli L, Van Durme J, et al. Presence and absence of follicle stimulating hormone receptor mutations provide some insights into spontaneous ovarian hyperstimulation syndrome pathophysiology. *J Clin Endocrinol Metab.* 2006;91(2):555-562. PMID: 16278261

Rivero-Muller A, Huhtaniemi I. Genetic variants of gonadotrophins and their receptors: impact on the diagnosis and management of the infertile patient. *Best Pract Res Clin Endocr Metab.* 2022;36(1):101596. PMID: 34802912

68 ANSWER: C) Start a carbohydrate- and fat-restricted diet

Starting at the end of the first trimester of pregnancy, both total cholesterol and triglycerides increase. Triglyceride levels rise 2- to 4-fold by the third trimester with higher levels seen in patients with diabetes mellitus. Gestational hypertriglyceridemia is defined as fasting triglycerides above the 95th percentile, and severe gestational hypertriglyceridemia is defined as triglycerides greater than 1000 mg/dL (>11.30 mmol/L). Severe gestational hypertriglyceridemia is seen in patients who have an underlying genetic abnormality due to either a monogenic or polygenic etiology or in patients in whom a secondary factor exacerbates the rise in triglycerides (such as uncontrolled type 2 diabetes). The maternal risks of severe gestational hypertriglyceridemia are acute pancreatitis, hyperviscosity syndrome, and preeclampsia, and the fetal risks are macrosomia, preterm labor, and premature birth.

Evaluation of hypertriglyceridemia during pregnancy is not different from the evaluation in nonpregnant women. This evaluation includes documenting personal or family history of hypertriglyceridemia, reviewing the patient's medications and dietary habits, and ruling out secondary etiologies.

Management of hypertriglyceridemia should always start with dietary intervention (Answer C). Patients should be counseled on adhering to a diet low in simple carbohydrates and low in fat (<20% of calories from fat). Patients should be encouraged to eat mostly complex carbohydrates, 20 to 30 g of fiber daily, and at least 300 mg of omega-3 fatty acids daily. This counseling should be provided by a registered dietitian, when possible, to ensure that the needs of both the mother and the fetus are met.

Gemfibrozil (Answer E) is a fibrate that could be used in the second trimester; however, this should only be started if dietary modifications do not achieve the triglyceride-lowering goal. Multiple case reports of its use during pregnancy have reported no adverse effects. High-dosage omega-3 fatty acids are an alternative treatment option that could also be started after implementing dietary changes.

Atorvastatin (Answer D), like other statins, can be used as third-line therapy to manage hypertriglyceridemia. However, this medication is contraindicated for this patient because of reports of congenital anomalies following its use in pregnancy.

Case reports have detailed the use of therapeutic plasma exchange (Answer B) in the setting of gestational hypertriglyceridemia-induced pancreatitis. This procedure rapidly reduces triglycerides. The role of therapeutic plasma exchange in the absence of pancreatitis is not well established, so it would not be the initial treatment option for this patient.

Hospital admission for observation and parenteral nutrition (Answer A) can be considered when triglycerides remain greater than 1000 mg/dL (>11.30 mmol/L) despite dietary and pharmacologic interventions.

Educational Objective

Guide the management of hypertriglyceridemia during pregnancy.

Reference(s)

Goldberg AS, Hegele RA. Severe hypertriglyceridemia in pregnancy. *J Clin Endocrinol Metab.* 2012;97(8):2589-2596. PMID: 22639290

Wong B, Ooi TC, Keely E. Severe gestational hypertriglyceridemia: a practical approach for clinicians. *Obstet Med.* 2015;8(4):158-167. PMID: 27512474

Simha V. Management of hypertriglyceridemia. *BMJ.* 2020;371:m3109. PMID: 33046451

69 ANSWER: C) Order neck ultrasonography in 6 to 12 months

Noninvasive follicular thyroid neoplasm with papillary-like nuclear features (NIFTP) was previously described as encapsulated follicular variant of papillary carcinoma (EFVPTC). This entity was renamed after an international, multicenter consensus study demonstrated the indolent biological behavior of these tumors (lack of metastasis or recurrence). In a retrospective review of 109 patients (67 patients underwent only lobectomy and none received radioiodine) followed for 10 to 26 years (median follow-up, 13 years), all patients were alive with no evidence of disease.

The NIFTP diagnosis is exclusively based on surgical pathology. Pathologic diagnostic criteria are as follows:

- Encapsulation or clear demarcation
- Follicular growth pattern with less than 1% papillae, no psammoma bodies, and less than 30% of solid/trabecular/insular growth pattern
- Nuclear score of 2 to 3
- No capsular or vascular invasion
- No tumor necrosis
- No high mitotic activity (<3 mitoses per 10 high-power fields)

As this tumor has a very low risk for malignancy, lobectomy is sufficient as the sole treatment. *RAS* pathogenic variants are the most common molecular alterations associated with NIFTP. These tumors have no *BRAF* V600E or *TERT* promoter variants. At this time, length and method of follow-up of patients with NIFTP remain to be established. However, serial neck ultrasonography is appropriate for monitoring these patients.

In a retrospective study of 129 patients with NIFTP (65 patients had lobectomy and none received radioiodine), none developed structural recurrence or had an increase in thyroglobulin or thyroglobulin antibodies in the median follow-up of 72 months after surgery. Another study has also shown that lobectomy appears to be an adequate surgical option for large NIFTP (≥4 cm).

This patient had a right hemithyroidectomy for a thyroid nodule with FNA biopsy–proven Bethesda IV. The surgical pathology revealed noninvasive follicular thyroid neoplasm with papillary-like nuclear features with no capsular or vascular invasion. There were no psammoma bodies. This pathology report is consistent with NIFTP, which considers the tumor to have a low malignancy risk. Therefore, right hemithyroidectomy is acceptable and completion thyroidectomy (Answer D) is unnecessary. The best next step is to repeat neck ultrasonography in 6 to 12 months (Answer C) to check for any abnormal mass or cervical lymph node in her neck.

Her TSH concentration is within the reference range and, therefore, levothyroxine (Answer A) does not need to be initiated.

This patient still has her left thyroid lobe, and this precludes her from having a radioiodine scan (Answer E) or receiving radioiodine treatment. Even if she had total thyroidectomy, the diagnosis of NIFTP refutes the need for a radioiodine scan and radioiodine treatment.

Neck CT (Answer B) is not indicated now.

Educational Objective

Diagnose noninvasive follicular thyroid neoplasm with papillary-like nuclear features and recommend appropriate treatment.

Reference(s)

Nikiforov YE, Seethala RR, Thallini G, et al. Nomenclature revision for encapsulated follicular variant of papillary thyroid carcinoma: a paradigm shift to reduce overtreatment of indolent tumors. *JAMA Oncol.* 2016;2(8):1023-1029. PMID: 27078145

Thompson LD. Ninety-four cases of encapsulated follicular variant of papillary thyroid carcinoma: a name change to noninvasive follicular thyroid neoplasm with papillary-like nuclear features would help prevent overtreatment. *Mod Pathol.* 2016;29(7):698-707. PMID: 27102347

Xu B, Tallini G, Scognamiglio T, Roman BR, Tuttle RM, Ghossein RA. Outcome of large noninvasive follicular thyroid neoplasm with papillary-like nuclear features. *Thyroid.* 2017;27(4):512-517. PMID: 28136139

Rosario PW, Mourão GF, Faria Oliveira LF, Calsolari MR. Long-term follow-up in patients with noninvasive follicular thyroid neoplasm with papillary-like nuclear features (NIFTP) without a suspicion of persistent disease in postoperative assessment. *Horm Metab Res.* 2018;50(3):223-226. PMID: 29121688

70 ANSWER: E) Switch from insulin aspart to fast-acting insulin aspart

To optimize postprandial blood glucose, one must consider the onset, peak, and duration of action of various prandial insulins (*see figure*). Providers can alter the timing of prandial insulin administration or the choice of insulin formulation to address suboptimal postprandial glycemic control.

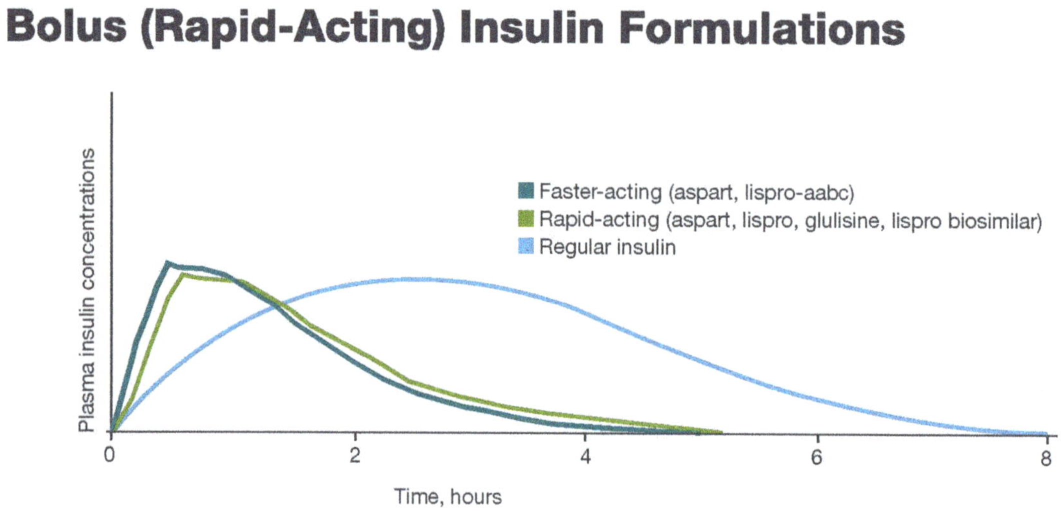

Adapted from Hirsch IB. Insulin analogues. N Engl J Med. 2005;352(2):174-183 and Flood TM. Appropriate use of insulin analogs in an increasingly complex type 2 diabetes mellitus (T2DM) landscape. J Fam Pract 2007;56(Suppl 1):S11-S12.

Of all the interventions listed, only switching from insulin aspart to fast-acting insulin aspart (Answer E) would help to address postprandial hyperglycemia in the 60- to 90-minute timeframe reported by the patient. Another option would be to administer the dose of insulin aspart 15 to 20 minutes before her later meals; however, that is not listed as an option.

Administering insulin aspart after meals (Answer C) or deintensifying the insulin-to-carbohydrate ratio (Answer B) would not fix this patient's postprandial hyperglycemia and would most likely worsen postprandial glucose excursions.

Increasing the basal rate from 11 AM to 4 PM (Answer D) would not be an appropriate method to reduce postprandial glucose excursions.

Lastly, adding a correction bolus of insulin aspart 60 minutes after meals (Answer A) would be reactive to the high glucose readings and would require additional postprandial blood glucose readings that would unnecessarily increase the management burden. Also, frequent administration of insulin doses within a short period can result in stacking and the development of hypoglycemia a few hours later.

The newer ultrafast-acting insulin products (fast-acting insulin aspart, insulin lispro-aabc, and inhaled insulin) address early postprandial hyperglycemia through their quicker onset of action. However, these insulins may result in persistent hyperglycemia or even a rise in glucose 3 to 4 hours after administration because they also have a shorter duration of action.

Educational Objective

Describe the peak action and duration of action of various prandial insulins and explain how the timing of administration in relation to meals may also affect postprandial glucose excursions.

Reference(s)

Hirsch IB. Insulin analogues. *N Engl J Med.* 2005;352(2):174-183. PMID: 15647580

Flood TM. Appropriate use of insulin analogs in an increasingly complex type 2 diabetes mellitus (T2DM) landscape. *J Fam Pract.* 2007;56(Suppl 1):S1-S2. PMID: 17217893

Lyumjev (insulin lispro-aabc). Prescribing information. Lilly USA, LLC; 2020. Accessed: September 2021. https://www.accessdata.fda.gov/drugsatfda_docs/label/2020/761109s000lbl.pdf

Fiasp (insulin aspart). Prescribing information. Novo Nordisk Inc; 2017. Accessed September 2021. https://www.accessdata.fda.gov/drugsatfda_docs/label/2017/208751s000lbl.pdf

Afrezza (insulin inhalation powder). Prescribing information. MannKind Corporation; 2014. Accessed September 2021. https://www.accessdata.fda.gov/drugsatfda_docs/label/2014/022472lbl.pdf

71

ANSWER: C) Perform core biopsy

Thyroid lymphoma is an uncommon diagnosis accounting for only 1% to 5% of thyroid malignancies. The most common subtype of primary thyroid lymphoma is diffuse large B-cell lymphoma, which accounts for approximately half of cases. Extranodal marginal zone lymphoma, also called mucosa-associated lymphoid tissue (MALT) lymphoma, is a clinically indolent B-cell nonHodgkin lymphoma and the second most common subtype of primary thyroid lymphoma. Primary thyroid lymphoma usually presents as a rapidly enlarging neck mass that is often associated with compressive symptoms (the patient described here has both dysphagia and dysphonia). B-type symptoms occur in only 10% of patients. Thyroid lymphoma is associated with Hashimoto thyroiditis in as many as 90% of cases. Characteristic ultrasound findings of thyroid lymphoma include (1) a hypoechoic or markedly hypoechoic solid mass, (2) increased internal vascularity, and (3) the absence of calcifications. Associated cervical lymphadenopathy may be observed. Although FNA biopsy is the recommended diagnostic test in the initial evaluation of most thyroid nodules meeting criteria for biopsy, its diagnostic accuracy in the context of thyroid lymphoma is lower (sensitivity 45%-70%). Core biopsy (Answer A) results in an accurate diagnosis more often (sensitivity 95%) and should be the first diagnostic step when thyroid lymphoma is suspected. Core biopsy provides more tissue for flow cytometry and immunohistochemistry and maintains tissue architecture, which may be needed for accurate subtype determination.

Patients with stage I or II thyroid MALT lymphoma can be treated with localized radiation therapy with a 10-year overall survival of approximately 90%. The patient described in this case was ultimately diagnosed with diffuse large B-cell lymphoma. Large cell transformation denotes a more aggressive phenotype. The patient's B-type symptoms and subsequently detected elevated serum lactate dehydrogenase concentration of 400 U/L (reference range, 85-245 U/L) are consistent with this diagnosis. PET-CT was performed for staging, and it showed a hypermetabolic neck mass (SUV max 30.4) and no hypermetabolic lymphadenopathy. Treatment with R-CHOP (rituximab, cyclophosphamide, doxorubicin, vincristine, and prednisone) was initiated.

Performing another ultrasound-guided FNA biopsy for cytopathology and rapid *BRAF* V600E genetic testing (Answer E) is not the most appropriate next step in this patient's evaluation. Although anaplastic thyroid cancer should be considered in the differential diagnosis of any patient presenting with a rapidly enlarging thyroid mass, the results of the patient's FNA biopsy and her relatively young age at presentation are not consistent with this diagnosis. The cytology results indicating Hashimoto thyroiditis make thyroid lymphoma more likely and thus additional testing to confirm this diagnosis is needed.

Performing total thyroidectomy (Answer D) is not recommended in cases of suspected thyroid lymphoma, as radiation or sometimes chemotherapy would be considered first-line treatment.

Measurement of TPO antibodies (Answer B) could confirm Hashimoto thyroiditis, but their presence would not help determine the etiology of the patient's thyroid mass.

Measurement of calcitonin (Answer A) to screen for medullary thyroid carcinoma is incorrect, as the FNA biopsy results do not point to this diagnosis.

Educational Objective

Diagnose thyroid lymphoma after negative ultrasound-guided FNA biopsy.

Reference(s)

Pavlidis ET, Pavlidis TE. A review of primary thyroid lymphoma: molecular factors, diagnosis and management. *J Invest Surg.* 2019;32(2):137-142. PMID: 29058491

Sharma A, Jasim S, Reading CC, et al. Clinical presentation and diagnostic challenges of thyroid lymphoma: a cohort study. *Thyroid.* 2016;26(8):1061-1067. PMID: 27256107

Watanabe N, Narimatsu H, Noh JY, et al. Long-term outcomes of 107 cases of primary thyroid mucosa-associated lymphoid tissue lymphoma at a single medical institution in Japan. *J Clin Endocrinol Metab.* 2018 Feb 1;103(2):732-739. PMID: 29165612

72 **ANSWER: E) Perform coronary artery calcium scoring with noncontrast CT**

In persons with diabetes mellitus older than 40 years who have no known ASCVD, a moderate-intensity statin in addition to lifestyle therapy is indicated for primary prevention of coronary heart disease. However, it is well recognized that there is risk heterogeneity among individuals. In this vignette, one must consider other factors that may alter the risk assessment because of the patient's concerns. Persons of South Asian descent are at 2-fold increased risk for ASCVD compared with other racial and ethnic groups. The American College of Cardiology/American Heart Association guidelines note that South Asian ancestry is a risk enhancer such that in this patient population, in those without diabetes, a 10-year ASCVD risk of 7.5% or greater should prompt starting statin therapy. However, such information does not help us to refine his individual risk. Therefore, while it is true that the ASCVD Risk Estimator underestimates the risk in persons of south Asian descent (Answer A), communicating this will not help in shared decision-making for this particular patient with diabetes.

Serum biomarkers such as C-reactive protein (Answer B) and lipoprotein (a) (Lp[a]) (Answer C) are associated with an increased risk of ASCVD. Lp(a) is a low-density lipoprotein in which apolipoprotein (a), a large glycoprotein, is bound to apolipoprotein B by a disulfide bridge. High levels of Lp(a) are an independent risk factor for cardiovascular disease and promote atherosclerosis by interfering with fibrinolysis, binding to macrophages to promote foam-cell formation, interfering with endothelial function, and increasing arterial wall inflammation via oxidized phospholipids. Meta-analyses of prospective studies show increased risk of coronary heart disease when Lp(a) concentrations are greater than 30 mg/dL (>1.07 μmol/L). The American College of Cardiology and Endocrine Society clinical practice guidelines note that a Lp(a) concentration greater than or equal to 50 mg/dL (≥1.79 μmol/L) is an ASCVD risk-enhancing factor. The 2020 Endocrine Society clinical practice guidelines suggest its use only in persons with a familial risk for ASCVD, which this patient does not have. Furthermore, assays for Lp(a) are not standardized and risk cutoff points have not been established. Thus, measurement of Lp(a) is not the best way to further stratify risk.

C-reactive protein is a serum biomarker for inflammation. Elevated high-sensitivity serum C-reactive protein greater than or equal to 2.0 mg/L (≥19.0 nmol/L) is an independent risk predictor for atherosclerosis in apparently healthy men and women. However, the incremental predictive value of C-reactive protein measurement (Answer B) for ASCVD is small and controversial, so its measurement is not the best step in this case.

In asymptomatic patients, cardiac stress testing (Answer D) is generally not indicated or appropriate.

Coronary artery calcium assessment with noncontrast CT (Answer E) has emerged as a useful predictor of coronary heart disease and ASCVD risk, including in persons with diabetes. This tool allows for evaluation of subclinical atherosclerosis. If no coronary calcium is detected, the patient is said to have a score of 0. Malik et al used a large multiethnic cohort without ASCVD at baseline and found that in patients with diabetes mellitus, a score of 0 was associated with annual coronary heart disease event rates of 0.4 for persons with diabetes mellitus over a 6.4-year follow-up period. By comparison, event rates were 2.3, 2.9, and 4.1 for scores of 1-99, 100-399, and ≥400, respectively. An important consideration in younger persons with type 2 diabetes mellitus is that they may have noncalcified plaques. Because of concern regarding this relatively short period of follow-up, subsequent studies from the MESA cohort have been performed and have documented an annual coronary heart disease event rate of 0.37. This rate did not differ significantly between participants who had diabetes for more or less than 10 years. Therefore, while the risk is not zero, such information is helpful for defining this patient's individual risk. South Asian patients were not included in the MESA cohort. Haque et al used the MASALA cohort, a community-based, observational, prospective study of individuals of south Asian ancestry to determine prevalence of coronary artery calcium in at-risk individuals. Investigators found that among patients at intermediate risk, 30% had a score of 0, and in those at low risk, 54% had a score of 0. Finally, of the advanced risk assessment strategies, coronary artery calcium assessment, high-sensitivity C-reactive protein measurement, and carotid ultrasonography are considered the most promising to detect subclinical atherosclerosis. Comparative-effective analysis suggests that the coronary artery calcium score is the single best tool to improve risk assessment. The 2020 Endocrine Society clinical practice guidelines recommend assessing the coronary artery calcium score in persons with borderline (5.0%-7.4%) or intermediate (7.5%-19.9%) ASCVD risk based on pooled cohort equations to help inform shared decision-making. Therefore, based on extensive evidence that a coronary artery calcium score of 0 has a strong negative predictive value for coronary heart disease events in persons with diabetes and studies suggest that such a finding is prevalent in individuals of south Asian descent, ordering coronary artery calcium scoring with noncontrast CT would be the most meaningful step to help inform appropriate management for this patient. Indeed, this patient had a score of 0 and chose to forgo statin treatment.

Educational Objective

Explain the role of coronary artery calcium scoring in stratifying heart disease risk and in clinical decision-making for persons with type 2 diabetes mellitus.

Reference(s)

American Diabetes Association Professional Practice Committee; Draznin B, Aroda VR, Bakris G, et al. 10. Cardiovascular disease and risk management: standards of medical care in diabetes-2022. *Diabetes Care.* 2022;45(Suppl 1):S144-S174. PMID: 34964815

Malik S, Zhao Y, Budoff M, Nasir K, et al. Coronary artery calcium score for long-term risk classification in individuals with type 2 diabetes and metabolic syndrome from the Multi-Ethnic Study of Atherosclerosis. *JAMA Cardiol.* 2017;2(12):1332-1340. PMID: 29117273

Haque W, Grandhi GR, Kanaya AM, et al. Implications of the 2019 American College of Cardiology/American Heart Association primary prevention guidelines and potential value of the coronary artery calcium score among South Asians in the US: the Mediators of Atherosclerosis in South Asians Living in America (MASALA) study. *Atherosclerosis.* 2021;334:48-56. PMID: 34481175

Grundy SM, Stone NJ, Bailey AL, et al. 2018 AHA/ACC/AACVPR/AAPA/ABC/ACPM/ADA/AGS/APhA/ASPC/NLA/PCNA guideline on the management of blood cholesterol: a report of the American College of Cardiology/American Heart Association Task Force on Clinical Practice Guidelines. *Circulation.* 2019;139:e1082-e1143. PMID: 30586774

Newman CB, Blaha MJ, Boord JB, et al. Lipid management in patients with endocrine disorders: an Endocrine Society clinical practice guideline. *J Clin Endocrinol Metab.* 2020;105(12):dgaa674. PMID: 32951056

73 ANSWER: D) Thyroxine-binding globulin measurement

The patient's serum TSH is normal, total T_3 is near the lower end of the reference range, and total T_4 is frankly low. These biochemical findings could be suggestive of central hypothyroidism in the right clinical context; however, her serum free T_4 level is normal and she has no symptoms suggestive of hypothyroidism (thyroid testing was ordered to evaluate for *hyper*thyroidism in the context of weight loss and increased anxiety). Given these findings and the patient's normal serum cortisol concentration, performing pituitary MRI with and without contrast (Answer B) would not be the most appropriate next step in her evaluation.

Her clinical presentation is consistent with euthyroid hypothyroxinemia, which is defined by normal free thyroid hormone concentrations in the setting of abnormal levels of total T_4 and T_3 resulting from perturbations in thyroid hormone–binding proteins. Most T_4 (99.96%) and T_3 (99.6%) is bound to proteins in serum with approximately 70% bound to thyroxine-binding globulin (TBG) and the remainder bound to albumin and transthyretin. Thyroid hormone–binding proteins have a role in both hormone storage and transport, creating a physiologic buffer to protect against day-to-day fluctuations in thyroid hormone levels.

Hereditary TBG deficiency is an X-linked recessive disorder that can result in complete or partial deficiency. Affected individuals have low total T_4 and T_3 levels and normal TSH and free thyroid hormone levels. Affected individuals are clinically euthyroid and do not require treatment. Heterozygous females tend to have less pronounced abnormalities than affected males because of random X chromosome inactivation. It is possible that the patient's maternal aunt was misdiagnosed with hypothyroidism in the context of low T_4 and/or T_3 values. Newborn screening includes measurement of serum TSH and T_4 to evaluate for congenital hypothyroidism. The patient described in this vignette had initially been found to have a low T_4 concentration on newborn screening, and further evaluation at the time confirmed TBG deficiency as the cause.

When TBG deficiency is suspected, as in this case, serum TBG (Answer D) should first be measured, followed by gene sequencing if an inherited disorder seems likely. Acquired TBG deficiency can be observed in the context of androgen excess (increased glycosylation and clearance), glucocorticoid therapy or endogenous Cushing syndrome, severe hepatic dysfunction, and nephrotic syndrome (due to urinary loss of TBG).

THRB gene sequencing (Answer C) is indicated in cases of suspected resistance to thyroid hormone. Resistance to thyroid hormone is characterized by elevated serum total and free T_4 and usually T_3 in the context of normal or slightly high serum TSH. Inherited defects in the *THRB* gene account for most cases of resistance to thyroid hormone β, the most common defect in thyroid hormone action. Although most patients with resistance to thyroid hormone β are clinically euthyroid, some have symptoms of hyperthyroidism or hypothyroidism. Central hyperthyroidism from a thyrotrope adenoma (TSHoma) should be considered as part of the differential diagnosis for any patient suspected to have resistance to thyroid hormone. In the described case, the biochemical findings are not consistent with resistance to thyroid hormone and thus testing for this disorder would not be indicated.

Heterophile antibody measurement (Answer A) would also be of low diagnostic utility. Heterophile antibodies are weak, polyspecific antibodies against animal antigens that are capable of causing positive or negative interference in common laboratory tests. Spurious TSH, thyroglobulin, hCG, and PTH values due to interference from heterophile antibodies have all been described. Although spurious free T_4 levels have also been reported in the literature, these appear to be extremely rare. Interference is most common with noncompetitive immunometric assays that use murine monoclonal antibodies. To rule out interference due to heterophile antibodies, the biochemical measurement in question should be repeated using a heterophile-blocking tube, rather than simply assessing for the presence of heterophile antibodies in serum, which lacks diagnostic specificity.

TPO antibody measurement (Answer E) is not needed in this patient with a normal serum TSH concentration.

Educational Objective

Identify thyroxine-binding globulin deficiency as a cause of abnormal thyroid function test results.

Reference(s)

Mimoto MS, Refetoff S. Clinical recognition and evaluation of patients with inherited serum thyroid hormone-binding protein mutations. *J Endocrinol Invest.* 2020;43(1):31-41. PMID: 31352644

74 ANSWER: C) Cystic prolactinoma

Hyperprolacinemia in the presence of a sellar lesion (and absence of pregnancy or prolactin-increasing drugs) can be due to the lesion secreting prolactin (prolactinoma) or to disruption of tuberoinfundibular dopamine release into the hypothalamic-pituitary portal vessels in the median eminence ("stalk effect"). Additionally, a mildly to moderately elevated prolactin (particularly if not associated with typical symptoms of hyperprolactinemia) can be caused by macroprolactinemia. Macroprolactinemia is characterized by a large molecular mass of prolactin (macroprolactin) as the main molecular form of prolactin in serum. Macroprolactin is largely a complex of prolactin and immunoglobulin G, especially prolactin autoantibodies. The prevalence of macroprolactinemia is 10% to 25% in patients with hyperprolactinemia and about 3.7% in the general population. This condition requires no further investigation or treatment.

Although a prolactin concentration greater than 100 ng/mL (>4.35 nmol/L) generally indicates the presence of a prolactin-secreting adenoma, pituitary stalk compression may occasionally cause higher serum prolactin, particularly if other factors are present such as renal insufficiency or macroprolactinemia. In this case, the patient has a sellar lesion with a maximal diameter of 1.1 cm. Additionally, deviation of the stalk toward the right is noticeable. If this were a solid macroprolactinoma, one would expect a prolactin concentration above 200 ng/mL (>8.70 nmol/L). However, this lesion is mostly cystic, so a lower prolactin level is expected than if the lesion were solid. In summary, before treatment, it is impossible to determine whether this is a cystic prolactinoma or a nonprolactin-secreting cystic lesion causing hyperprolactinemia by stalk compression. Starting cabergoline was therefore reasonable. Her periods resumed, showing prolactin responsiveness and normal anterior pituitary function. Six months later, while the lesion has not shrunk (a cystic prolactinoma is not expected to shrink rapidly), the fact that the prolactin concentration is not frankly low strongly suggests that this is indeed a cystic prolactinoma (Answer C). One year later (18 months after medical therapy was initiated), the patient's prolactin concentration remained normal and significant shrinkage of the lesion was observed. These findings are consisent with recent literature suggesting that cystic prolactinomas can shrink significantly with dopaminergic therapy (with median time to shrinkage of 24 months from initiation of dopaminergic agent therapy).

Rathke cleft cyst (Answer E), nonfunctioning pituitary adenoma with cystic degeneration (Answer D), arachnoid cyst (Answer A), or craniopharyngioma (Answer B) would be unlikely diagnoses, as they would have caused hyperprolactinemia by stalk compression, a scenario in which prolactin would drop much more dramatically, and would most likely be frankly low or even not measurable after 6 months of dopaminergic therapy. While mass shrinkage may be seen in cystic prolactinomas after dopaminergic therapy, it may also occur spontaneously in nonfunctioning adenomas that have bled. Therefore, the prolactin response to dopaminergic therapy is more informative than imaging (although growth despite prolactin normalization would strongly argue against the prolactinoma diagnosis).

Educational Objective

Distinguish between cystic prolactinoma and hyperprolactinemia due to stalk compression.

Reference(s)

Samperi I, Lithgow K, Karavitaki N. Hyperprolactinaemia. *J Clin Med.* 2019;8(12):2203. PMID: 31847209

Samson SL, Hamrahian AH, Ezzat S; AACE Neuroendocrine and Pituitary Scientific Committee; American College of Endocrinology (ACE). American Association of Clinical Endocrinologists, American College of Endocrinology disease state clinical review: clinical relevance of macroprolactin in the absence or presence of true hyperprolactinemia. *Endocr Pract.* 2015;21(12):1427-1435. PMID: 26642103

Faje A, Chunharojrith P, Nency J, Biller BMK, Swearingen B, Klibanski A. Dopamine agonists can reduce cystic prolactinomas. *J Clin Endocrinol Metab.* 2016;101(10):3709-3715. PMID: 27459530

Vilar CF, Lyra R, Freitas MDC. Pitfalls in the diagnostic evaluation of hyperprolactinemia. *Neuroendocrinology.* 2019;109(1):7-19. PMID: 30889571

75 ANSWER: E) Saxagliptin

Bullous pemphigoid is an autoimmune dermatologic disorder, and its idiopathic form often occurs in the sixth and seventh decade of life. Autoantibodies develop against 2 hemidesmosomal proteins. The process can be idiopathic or drug induced. Bullous pemphigoid starts as a pruritic rash that can develop into bullous lesions over time.

A recent systematic review lists at least 90 medications that have been implicated in the development of bullous pemphigoid. Although multiple antihypertensive agents are on the list, including ACE inhibitors, calcium channel blockers, and diuretics, the strongest association has been seen with (in order of strength of association) DPP-4 inhibitors, PD-1 and PD-L1 inhibitors, loop diuretics, penicillin, nonsteroidal antiinflammatory drugs, and thiazide diuretics.

This patient is on multiple agents on the list (amlodipine, lisinopril, and saxagliptin). Of these agents, saxagliptin (Answer E) is most strongly associated with bullous pemphigoid. These agents are associated with other skin conditions such as angioedema, exfoliative skin changes, and Stevens-Johnson syndrome. The precise mechanism by which DPP-4 inhibitors cause bullous pemphigoid has not been elucidated. On further questioning, the patient reported that saxagliptin was the most recent medication added to his regimen for glycemic control.

A number of cutaneous reactions can occur with ACE inhibitors, including pruritus, urticaria, photosensitivity, bullous eruptions, and life-threatening angioedema. Calcium channel blockers can be associated with eczema, and the reaction may be delayed. There are also reports of bullous lesion formation with use of calcium channel blockers. However, with both ACE inhibitors and calcium channel blockers, bullous skin changes are much less likely than with DPP-4 inhibitors. Therefore, neither the ACE inhibitor (Answer C) nor calcium channel blocker (Answer A) would be the first drug to discontinue.

Metformin (Answer D) can be associated with urticaria and lichenoid eruption, and SGLT-2 inhibitors (Answer B) can lead to generalized rash, urticaria, and eczema. Bullous pemphigoid is not listed as an associated disorder with either of these agents.

Educational Objective

Identify medications that are associated with the development of bullous pemphigoid.

Reference(s)

Verheyden MJ, Bilgic A, Murrell DF. A systematic review of drug-induced pemphigoid. *Acta Derm Venereol.* 2020;100(15):adv00224. PMID: 32176310

76 **ANSWER: A) Genetic testing for pathogenic variants in the androgen receptor gene**

This patient presents with lack of adequate virilization despite a serum testosterone concentration above the normal range. Despite the high serum testosterone, his LH is elevated. This presentation indicates resistance to testosterone's actions both at the somatic level (undervirilization), as well as at the hypothalamic-pituitary level (increased LH). Given that testosterone acts via the androgen receptor, the logical next step is to perform genetic testing for pathogenic variants in the androgen receptor gene (*AR*) (Answer A). Indeed, this patient had a pathogenic variant in the ligand-binding domain of the *AR* gene.

These findings are parallel to those in patients with resistance to thyroid hormone due to an inactivating pathogenic variant in the thyroid hormone receptor β gene, a clinical syndrome presenting with somatic features of hypothyroidism in tissues where the thyroid hormone β receptor is expressed in the context of elevated thyroid hormones and (inappropriately) normal or elevated TSH. Resistance to androgen action, usually referred to as androgen insensitivity syndrome, occurs with an estimated frequency of 1 in 20,000 to 1:100,000 male births. Since the *AR* gene is encoded by a single-copy gene on the X chromosome, *AR* pathogenic variants are inherited in an X-linked recessive fashion. Affected individuals have a 46,XY karyotype, with a hemizygous *AR* pathogenic variant. X-linked disorders are associated with a relatively high rate of de novo variants, and they account for about 30% of androgen insensitivity syndrome cases.

The clinical phenotype depends on the residual transcriptional activity of the *AR* gene. The phenotype of complete androgen insensitivity syndrome is that of a female with normal breast development (testosterone is aromatized to estradiol) despite the presence of a 46,XY karyotype, formation of normal testes, and male-range testosterone (ie, complete androgen resistance). Due to the absent uterus, individuals with complete androgen insensitivity syndrome present with primary amenorrhea and have a blind vaginal pouch on examination. Individuals with partial androgen insensitivity syndrome present, depending on the residual transcriptional activity of the *AR* gene, with a wide spectrum of (under)virilization of the external genitalia, which may involve perineoscrotal hypospadias, micropenis, and bifid scrotum. When androgen receptor function is only mildly impaired (mild androgen insensitivity syndrome), men such as the patient in this vignette have a male genital phenotype but have gynecomastia, infertility, and reduced beard and pubic hair. Because men with mild androgen insensitivity syndrome respond to estradiol, and given that estradiol is primarily responsible for closing epiphyses, body proportions are usually normal, in contrast to the eunuchoidal proportions seen in men with congenital hypogonadotropic hypogonadism (eg, Kallmann syndrome) who lack both testosterone and estradiol. For reasons not understood, there are no strong genotype-phenotype correlations, and there is considerable heterogeneity in the phenotypic expression of a given pathogenic variant, sometimes even within the same family.

Patients with mild androgen insensitivity syndrome typically present either with gynecomastia in adolescence or with infertility in adulthood. Because of elevations in serum estradiol's substrate (serum testosterone), serum estradiol is elevated, which leads to gynecomastia, as there is no resistance to the actions of estradiol. Thus, genetic testing for pathogenic variants in the estradiol α gene (Answer B) is incorrect. Given that testosterone reduces SHBG and estradiol increases SHBG, men with mild androgen insensitivity syndrome may have a relatively high serum SHBG concentration, as in this patient, although this is not universal. In mild androgen insensitivity syndrome, FSH concentrations are usually normal because FSH is mainly regulated by gonadal inhibin. Of note, men with a pathogenic variant in the estrogen receptor α gene (*ESR1*) (ie, estradiol resistance, an extremely rare condition) also present with elevations in LH, serum testosterone, and estradiol, because the central negative feedback that sex steroids in men have on LH is mediated by both testosterone and estradiol via the androgen receptor and estrogen receptor α. However, the clinical phenotype of men with *ESR1* pathogenic variants is different from that of mild androgen insensitivity syndrome and is characterized by tall stature, delayed bone age, osteoporosis, and central adiposity/insulin resistance.

Functioning pituitary gonadotroph adenomas (ie, adenomas that express and secrete gonadotropins) could present with a biochemical picture similar to that of partial androgen insensitivity syndrome. However, functioning pituitary gonadotroph adenomas are extremely rare in men, and, in the handful of cases reported, patients present with FSH elevations, whereas elevations in LH and testosterone are variable. Affected men do not present with clinical features of androgen deficiency (there is no resistance to androgen receptor actions), but they may have testicular enlargement due to trophic effects of FSH (and/or mass effects depending on adenoma size). The clinical presentation does not suggest a functioning pituitary gonadotroph adenoma, and pituitary imaging (Answer E) is not indicated.

DHEA-S (Answer C) is an adrenally produced testosterone precursor; there is no suspicion of endogenous adrenal androgen excess in this case and DHEA-S measurement is therefore not indicated.

Given the clinical picture of partial androgen insensitivity syndrome, there is no rationale to request a free testosterone measurement (Answer D).

Educational Objective

Recommend genetic testing to confirm a suspected diagnosis of partial androgen insensitivity due to pathogenic variants in the androgen receptor gene causing reduced androgen receptor activity.

Reference(s)

Migeon CJ, Brown TR, Lanes R, Palacios A, Amrhein JA, Schoen EJ. A clinical syndrome of mild androgen insensitivity. *J Clin Endocrinol Metab.* 1984;59(4):672-678. PMID: 6434576

Hughes IA, Deeb A. Androgen resistance. *Best Pract Res Clin Endocrinol Metab.* 2006;20(4):577-598. PMID: 17161333

Smith EP, Boyd J, Frank GR, Takahashi H, et al. Estrogen resistance caused by a mutation in the estrogen-receptor gene in a man. *N Engl J Med.* 1994;331(16):1056-1061. PMID: 8090165

Ntali G, Capatina C, Grossman A, Karavitaki N. Clinical review: functioning gonadotroph adenomas. *J Clin Endocrinol Metab.* 2014;99(12):4423-4433. PMID: 25166722

77

ANSWER: C) Measurement of serum copeptin

Polyuria is defined as the passage of more than 3 L of urine over 24 hours. Typically, this is associated with a similar volume of fluid intake. The workup of a patient with frequent urination must begin with measurement of the 24-hour urine volume to distinguish polyuria from pollakiuria (frequent urination without increased urine volume). Once polyuria is confirmed, common causes of osmotic diuresis such as hyperglycemia and hypercalcemia must be ruled out. This patient has polyuria and normal glucose and calcium concentrations. In a patient without diabetes or hypercalcemia, determining whether polyuria is causing polydipsia or vice versa (primary polydipsia) is sometimes difficult. Typically, but not always, patients with diabetes insipidus can point out quite accurately when the problems started. The second step is to determine whether the kidneys are appropriately concentrating the urine. This can be done with a formal water-deprivation test, usually performed during hospital admission with frequent measurements of weight and serum sodium, or in the outpatient setting by asking patients to note the longest period they can go without drinking.

In this case, after 12 hours of water deprivation, the patient's serum osmolality increased above 295 mOsm/kg. A simultaneus urine osmolality measurement of 380 mOsm/Kg was abnormal, showing a defect in urine concentration (urine osmolality should have reached a level about 2 times that of serum osmolality). While this is consistent with diabetes inspidus, it does not completely rule out primary polydipsia because chronic polyuria itself can affect the kidneys' urine concentrating capacity through washout of renal gradient and/or downregulation of aquaporin receptor expression in the kidneys. Additionally, patients with acquired nephrogenic diabetes insipidus are often only partially resistant to antidiuretic hormone, resulting in a clinical presentation that is similar to that of partial central diabetes inspidus.

While serum antidiuretic hormone measurement (Answer B) may assist in differentiating among central and renal causes of urine concentration defects, significant limitations of the antidiuretic hormone assay and instability of antidiuretic hormone in samples greatly reduce its utility.

Copeptin (Answer C), the C-terminal segment of antidiuretic hormone prohormone, is an easy-to-measure arginine vasopressin surrogate that is very stable, reflecting the circulating antidiuretic hormone concentration. A copeptin concentration greater than 21.4 pmol/L identifies nephrogenic diabetes inspidus even prior to water deprivation. More challenging is distinguishing between primary polydipsia and partial central diabetes inspidus. A study published in 2018 described 144 patients with hypotonic polyuria who underwent both water-deprivation testing and hypertonic saline infusion. An osmotically stimulated copeptin concentration lower than 4.9 pmol/L after infusion of 3% saline had an overall diagnostic accuracy of 96.5% (93.2% sensitivity and 100% specificity) in distinguishing central diabetes insipidus (copeptin <4.9 pmol/L) from primary polydipsia, while the accuracy was 76% for the water-deprivation test (using the same cutoff). The patient in this vignette had been on long-term lithium therapy, and therefore may have nephrogenic diabetes inspidus. Measurement of serum copeptin after water deprivation would distinguish nephrogenic diabetes inspidus from partial central diabetes inspidus, and most likely from primary polydipsia as well.

Performing pituitary MRI (Answer E) is premature, as this would not be indicated in nephrogenic diabetes inspidus.

Kidney anatomy is usually not abnormal in nephrogenic diabetes inspidus, and therefore kidney ultrasonography (Answer A) is incorrect.

Measurement of urinary sodium (Answer D) is sometimes helpful in diagnosing syndrome of inappropriate antidiuretic hormone secretion, but it is generally not helpful in the differential diagnosis of polyuria.

This patient's low prolactin level is most likely due to aripiprazole, an antipsychotic medication that acts as dopamine partial agonist. His borderline-low testosterone may be due to obesity, and it does not necessarily indicate a pituitary pathology.

Educational Objective

Explain the utility of copeptin measurement in distinguishing between central and nephrogenic diabetes insipidus.

Reference(s)

Christ-Crain M. Vasopressin and copeptin in health and disease. *Rev Endocr Metab Disord.* 2019;20(3):283-294. PMID: 31656992

Christ-Crain M, Bichet DG, Fenske WK, et al. Diabetes insipidus. *Nat Rev Dis Primers.* 2019;5(1):54. PMID: 31395885

Fenske W, Refardt J, Chifu I, et al. A copeptin-based approach in the diagnosis of diabetes insipidus. *N Engl J Med.* 2018;379(5):428-439. PMID: 30067922

78 ANSWER: B) Intravenous iron-induced hypophosphatemia

The patient described in this vignette has symptomatic hypophosphatemia following iron infusions for anemia. Some intravenous iron formulations, in particular ferric carboxymaltose, have been recognized to induce renal phosphate wasting. This has been shown to be mediated by FGF-23, a phosphatonin, which results in hypophosphatemia through renal phosphate wasting by reducing expression of the sodium phosphate cotransporters NaPi2a and NaPi2c, as well as decreasing serum calcitriol thought to be due to decreased expression of 1α-hydroxylase and increased catabolism of 1,25-dihydroxyvitamin D. The decrease in calcitriol leads to mild hypocalcemia, which subsequently causes secondary hyperparathyroidism that may in turn aggravate the hypophosphatemia. Clinical manifestations include generalized weakness, fatigue, and bone and muscle pain. Although the peak occurrence of hypophosphatemia is at 2 to 3 weeks after the dose, some studies show that a large percentage of patients continue to manifest severe hypophosphatemia weeks and even months after the last dose of the iron treatment. Patients with impaired kidney function have a significantly lower risk of developing hypophosphatemia because the reduced glomerular filtration rate limits the amount of phosphate that can be excreted in the urine.

Accordingly, the US FDA updated the "warning and precautions" section for ferric carboxymaltose to acknowledge that symptomatic hypophosphatemia requiring clinical intervention has been reported in patients at risk of low serum phosphate. The label also states that these cases have occurred mostly after repeated exposure in patients with no reported history of kidney impairment. In most patients, hypophosphatemia resolves within 3 months. The updated label also notes that serum phosphate levels should be monitored in patients at risk for hypophosphatemia who require a repeated course of iron treatment. Therefore, in this clinical scenario, the most likely diagnosis is intravenous iron-induced hypophosphatemia (Answer B).

X-linked hypophosphatemia (Answer E), or XLH, is an inherited condition with an X-linked dominant pattern of inheritance. The gene responsible for XLH, *PHEX* (phosphate-regulating endopeptidase on the X chromosome), is expressed predominantly in bone and teeth. Inactivating pathogenic variants in *PHEX* cause XLH by increasing the level of FGF-23 relative to the ambient phosphorus level. Clinical features of XLH in adults include fatigue, muscle weakness, stiffness, bone pain, and gait abnormalities. The major clinical findings are short stature, leg deformities, teeth defects, and osteomalacia. Accelerated osteoarthritis and enthesopathy are very common, usually beginning in the second or third decade of life.

Tumor-induced osteomalacia (Answer D), also known as oncogenic osteomalacia, is an acquired paraneoplastic syndrome in which mesenchymal tumors secrete FGF-23 and other phosphaturic proteins. Most affected patients have increased circulating FGF-23 levels, and the biochemical and bone mineralization abnormalities closely resemble those in genetic forms of hypophosphatemic rickets.

While XLH and tumor-induced osteomalacia may have similar laboratory findings to those of this patient, they are both rare conditions and neither is the most likely diagnosis given the clinical scenario.

Nutritional osteomalacia (Answer C) is typically characterized by a very low serum 25-hydroxyvitamin D level (<10 ng/mL [<25.0 mmol/L]), which this patient does not have. Other manifestations include low to low-normal serum calcium and phosphate levels, high PTH and alkaline phosphatase levels, and low urinary calcium excretion. The serum concentration of 1,25-dihydroxyvitamin D may be normal, low, or high, depending on the severity and duration of vitamin D deficiency.

Finally, hereditary resistance to vitamin D (Answer A) is caused by end-organ resistance to 1,25-dihydroxyvitamin D most often because of loss-of-function pathogenic variants in the gene encoding the vitamin D receptor (*VDR*). The typical laboratory abnormalities in this scenario include hypocalcemia, hypophosphatemia, high serum PTH levels, and high serum 1,25-dihyroxyvitamin D levels, which are not consistent with the findings in this case.

Educational Objective

Identify intravenous iron therapy as the cause of hypophosphatemia in a patient being treated for iron deficiency.

Reference(s)

Schaefer B, Tobiasch M, Wagner S, et al. Hypophosphatemia after intravenous iron therapy: comprehensive review of clinical findings and recommendations for management. *Bone.* 2022;154:116202. PMID: 34534708

Ifie E, Oyibo SO, Joshi H, Akintade O. Symptomatic hypophosphataemia after intravenous iron therapy: an underrated adverse reaction. *Endocrinol Diabetes Metab Case Rep.* 2019;2019(1):19-0065. PMID: 31385673

Wolf M, Chertow GM, Macdougall IC, Kaper R, Krop J, Strauss W. Randomized trial of intravenous iron-induced hypophosphatemia. *JCI Insight.* 2018;3(23):e124486. PMID: 30518682

Glaspy JA, Wolf M, Strauss WE. Intravenous iron-induced hypophosphatemia: an emerging syndrome. *Adv Ther.* 2021;38(7):3531-3549. PMID: 34053011

79 ANSWER: D) Reduce basal insulin by 20%, reduce prandial insulin by 20%, and start an SGLT-2 inhibitor

A previous consensus report established continuous glucose monitoring metrics and goals and generated a standard format (ambulatory glucose profile [*see figure*]) for reporting metrics for time-in-range, hypoglycemia, hyperglycemia, and glycemic variability.

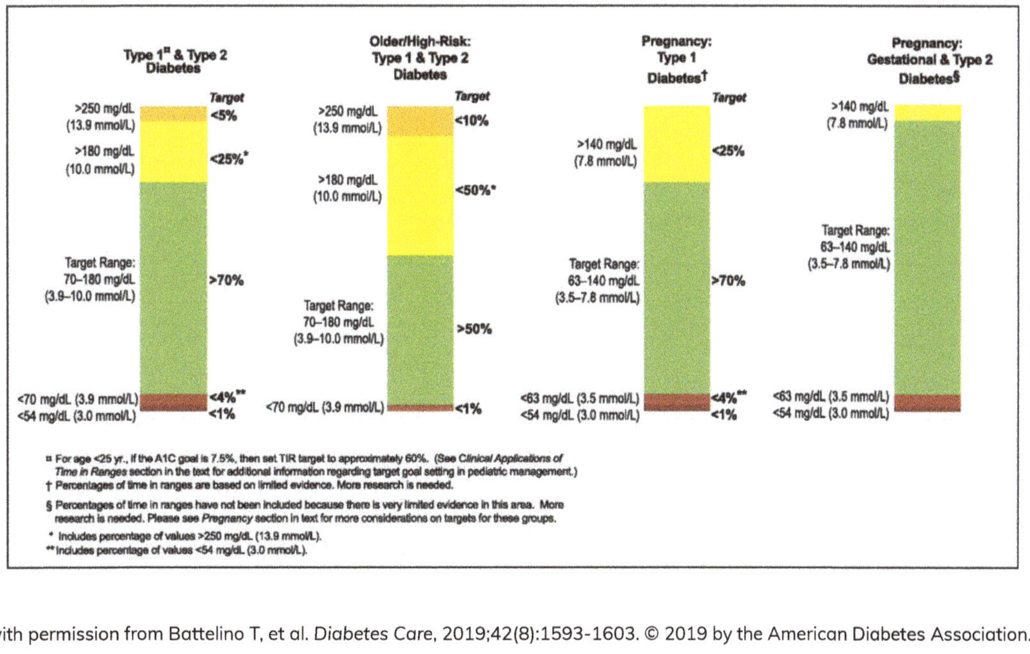

The standardized continuous glucose monitoring report in the stem shows that this patient has significant hyperglycemia, hypoglycemia, and glycemic variability. Given his age and comorbidities, as well as his absence of hypoglycemic symptoms despite evidence of hypoglycemia on the report, hypoglycemia is his main risk. The goal for this patient is to spend less than 1.0% of the time in hypoglycemia (<70 mg/dL [<3.9 mmol/L]) given his age and kidney disease, which contribute to his risk. Thus, the focus in this vignette is to recommend medication changes to reduce his risk of hypoglycemia, while also addressing his comorbidities.

The timing of hyperglycemia and hypoglycemia was not provided in this vignette (although this is one of the main advantages of a continuous glucose monitor, which provides data about glucose patterns 24 hours a day). While reducing his basal insulin dosage (Answer A) or reducing his basal insulin dosage and increasing his prandial insulin dosage (Answer B) may reduce hypoglycemia, these are not the best next steps, as neither option addresses his kidney disease. The American Diabetes Association guidelines stress the use of insulin-sparing agents such as SGLT-2 inhibitors for reasons in addition to glycemic control, especially in patients with kidney disease who have an estimated glomerular filtration rate greater than 25 mL/min per 1.73 m^2 and a urinary albumin-to-creatinine ratio greater than 30 mg/g creat (especially greater than 300 mg/g creat). The best strategy to decrease this patient's risk for hypoglycemia and preserve his kidney function is to reduce his insulin dosage and add an SGLT-2 inhibitor (Answer D).

There are promising data on GLP-1 receptor agonists and kidney disease, but no trials have yet been published with a primary endpoint of kidney events. However, several studies are ongoing (eg, FLOW [Effect of Semaglutide versus Placebo on the Progression of Renal Impairment in Subjects With Type 2 Diabetes and Chronic Kidney Disease]). The primary composite kidney outcome for this study a persistent ≥50% reduction in estimated glomerular filtration rate or a persistent rate less than 15 mL/min per 1.73 m^2 or the initiation of renal replacement therapy (dialysis or renal transplant) or death of renal or cardiovascular causes. Reducing basal and prandial insulin doses and adding a GLP-1 receptor agonist (Answer C) would be useful for weight loss if weight were the primary concern, but this patient's BMI is normal and he has chronic kidney disease. Given the more limited data on GLP-1 receptor agonists and chronic kidney disease, this is not the best choice.

Metformin has a low risk for causing hypoglycemia; his dosage takes into consideration his kidney disease, and his estimated glomerular filtration rate remains greater than 30 mL/min per 1.73 m^2. Thus, stopping metformin (Answer E) is not recommended.

Table. Metformin Prescribing in the Setting of Chronic Kidney Disease

Chronic kidney disease stage	Estimated glomerular filtration rate, mL/min per 1.73 m^2	Maximum total daily metformin dose, mg
1	≥90	2550
2	60-<90	2550
3A	45-<60	2000
3B	30-<45	1000
4	15-<30	Do not use
5	<15	Do not use

Adapted from Lazarus B, Wu A, Shin J-I, Sang Y, et al. Association of metformin use with risk of lactic acidosis across the range of kidney function: a community-based cohort study. *JAMA Intern Med.* 2018;178(7):903-910.

Educational Objective

Determine glycemic goals in older patients with type 2 diabetes mellitus.

Reference(s)

Beck RW, Bergenstal RM, Cheng P, et al. The relationships between time in range, hyperglycemia metrics, and HbA1c. *J Diabetes Sci Technol.* 2019;13(4):614-626. PMID: 30636519

Yoo JH, Choi MS, Ahn J, et al. Association between continuous glucose monitoring-derived time in range, other core metrics, and albuminuria in type 2 diabetes. *Diabetes Technol Ther.* 2020;22(10):768-776. PMID: 32167394

Battelino T, Danne T, Bergenstal RM, et al. Clinical targets for continuous glucose monitoring data interpretation: recommendations from the International Consensus on Time in Range. *Diabetes Care.* 2019;42(8):1593-1603. PMID: 31177185

Lazarus B, Wu A, Shin J-I, Sang Y, et al. Association of metformin use with risk of lactic acidosis across the range of kidney function: a community-based cohort study. *JAMA Intern Med.* 2018;178(7):903-910. PMID: 29868840

Piperidou A, Sarafidis P, Boutou A, et al. The effect of SGLT-2 inhibitors on albuminuria and proteinuria in diabetes mellitus: a systematic review and meta-analysis of randomized controlled trials. *J Hypertens.* 2019;37(7):1334-1343. PMID: 31145707

Górriz JL, Soler MJ, Navarro-González JF, et al. GLP-1 receptor agonists and diabetic kidney disease: a call of attention to nephrologists. *J Clin Med.* 2020;9(4):947. PMID: 32235471

80 ANSWER: C) Left adrenalectomy

Bilateral macronodular adrenal hyperplasia (BMAH) is a rare cause of ACTH-independent or primary hypercortisolism. As in this case, most patients with BMAH present in their 50s or 60s with mild hypercortisolism. BMAH can be sporadic or familial. Germline pathogenic variants in the tumor suppressor gene *ARMC5* are found in approximately 25% of patients with apparently sporadic BMAH.

Low morning ACTH and DHEA-S concentrations are suggestive of autonomous hypercortisolism. The patient's abnormal cortisol concentration after the 1-mg overnight dexamethasone-suppression test (despite an undetectable ACTH) and mildly elevated 24-hour urinary cortisol excretion further support the diagnosis. She also has several comorbidities that can be promoted or worsened by cortisol excess, including type 2 diabetes mellitus, hypertension, dyslipidemia, and osteopenia. Surgical treatment is typically offered to patients with BMAH. In patients with mild hypercortisolism, the adrenal gland with the largest nodule(s) (in this case the left [Answer C], not right [Answer D]) is removed first, and this intervention might be sufficient for many years. If overt hypercortisolism reoccurs, medical therapy or second adrenalectomy can be considered.

Because this patient has mild hypercortisolism, pursuing bilateral adrenalectomy (Answer B) is too aggressive and potential complications exceed the benefits.

Adrenal venous sampling (Answer A) is not necessary in cases of BMAH, and surgery should target the largest nodules.

In patients presenting with bilateral adrenal hyperplasia and adrenal insufficiency, serum 17-hydroxyprogesterone measurement (Answer E) is useful to screen for congenital adrenal hyperplasia. This patient, however, has cortisol excess.

Educational Objective

Guide the management of bilateral macronodular adrenal hyperplasia.

Reference(s)

Meloche-Dumas L, Mercier F, Lacroix A. Role of unilateral adrenalectomy in bilateral adrenal hyperplasias with Cushing's syndrome. *Best Pract Res Clin Endocrinol Metab.* 2021;35(2):101486. PMID: 33637447

Bourdeau I, El Ghorayeb N, Gagnon N, Lacroix A. Management of endocrine disease: differential diagnosis, investigation and therapy of bilateral adrenal incidentalomas. *Eur J Endocrinol.* 2018;179(2):R57-R67. PMID: 29748231

81 ANSWER: D) Start atenolol

The patient in this vignette has a history of hepatitis C, and interferon alfa treatment was started 4 months ago. Now, several months after initiating this medication, she has developed symptoms of thyrotoxicosis (weight loss, palpitations, fatigue, bilateral hand tremor, and tachycardia). The most common differential diagnoses are Graves disease, toxic adenoma, toxic multinodular goiter, and thyroiditis. Thyroid-stimulating immunoglobulin was not elevated, making Graves disease less likely. Toxic multinodular goiter and toxic adenoma are unlikely based on her age and physical findings. Thyroiditis is the most likely diagnosis, and interferon alfa could be the culprit. Several drugs in addition to interferon alfa have been reported to induce thyroiditis, including lithium, amiodarone, immune-checkpoint inhibitors, interleukin-2, and tyrosine kinase inhibitors. Thyroiditis associated with interferon alfa is usually painless.

Interferon alfa has immunomodulatory effects and can lead to the development of antithyroid antibodies without a clinical disorder in 5% to 40% of patients. Painless thyroiditis, Hashimoto thyroiditis, or Graves disease develops in approximately in 5% to 10% of patients taking interferon alfa. The changes in thyroid function often occur after 3 months of therapy but can happen as long as the patient is being treated with this medication. Cessation of interferon alfa resolves thyroiditis. The presence of antithyroid antibodies before starting interferon alfa is a significant risk factor for developing thyroid dysfunction in patients taking this medication. In a study of 422 patients with chronic viral hepatitis C, B, or D, antithyroid antibodies were higher in women than in men (8.7% vs 3.4%) and in patients with chronic hepatitis C (11.2% vs 3.6%). Interferon alfa therapy increased the prevalence of antithyroid antibodies and thyroid dysfunction.

In patients with hepatitis C, baseline serum TSH and TPO antibodies should be measured before the initiation of interferon alfa, and serum TSH should be monitored every several months while on treatment.

Patients with thyroiditis should be monitored for the development of hypothyroidism, which usually follows the hyperthyroid phase within a few weeks. Corticosteroids are generally contraindicated in patients with chronic hepatitis C infection. If the workup of hyperthyroidism reveals the diagnosis of Graves disease, treatment with radioactive iodine or thyroid surgery should be considered. Antithyroid drugs should be avoided because they can worsen the liver dysfunction. Interruption of interferon alfa is recommended if symptomatic thyrotoxicosis develops in patients on this medication.

As thyroiditis is a self-limited condition, the best treatment option is to initiate atenolol (Answer D) to control sympathetic override during the hyperthyroid phase.

Methimazole (Answer E) is not indicated for thyroiditis, as there is no overproduction of thyroid hormones.

Total thyroidectomy (Answer C) should not be offered because her thyroid gland is not enlarged and she has no compressive symptoms.

Performing thyroid ultrasonography (Answer B) is unnecessary due to the size of her thyroid gland on physical examination.

A radioiodine scan and uptake (Answer A) is not currently indicated, as thyroiditis is the most likely diagnosis and thyroid-stimulating immunoglobulin is not elevated. If she remains hyperthyroid with no improvement in thyroid blood test results over the next few months, a radioiodine scan and uptake might be necessary.

Educational Objective

Diagnose and manage thyroiditis in a patient with hepatitis C who is on interferon alfa therapy.

Reference(s)

Deutsch M, Dourakis S, Manesis EK, et al. Thyroid abnormalities in chronic viral hepatitis and their relationship to interferon alfa therapy. *Hepatology.* 1997;26(1):206-210. PMID: 9214471

Mandac JC, Chaudhry S, Sherman KE, Tomer Y. The clinical and physiological spectrum of interferon-alpha induced thyroiditis: toward a new classification. *Hepatology.* 2006;43(4):661-672. PMID: 16557537

Tomer Y, Menconi F. Interferon induced thyroiditis. *Best Pract Res Clin Endocrinol Metab.* 2009;23(6):703-712. PMID: 19942147

82 ANSWER: A) Check for blood ketones

This patient with preexisting diabetes is now in the third trimester of pregnancy and calls the clinic with a change in clinical status. In addition, her glycemic control is not optimized for pregnancy. The key point is that despite being relatively euglycemic, she remains at risk for diabetic ketoacidosis. Euglycemic diabetic ketoacidosis refers to metabolic acidosis that occurs when blood glucose levels are less than 200 mg/dL (<11.1 mmol/L) in the presence of ketonemia. Diabetic ketoacidosis has a higher incidence in pregnant vs nonpregnant individuals. Multiple mechanisms contribute to this higher risk. Increased insulin resistance occurs, particularly in the second and third trimesters due to increased placental lactogen and progesterone. As compared with the metabolic rate before pregnancy, the maternal metabolic rate is increased by as much as 30%, resulting in predisposition for ketosis with even short periods of starvation. For example, after a 12-hour fast, concentrations of free fatty acids and β-hydroxybutyrate are higher in pregnant women than in nonpregnant women. Finally, bicarbonate levels in pregnancy are lower, presumably to compensate for respiratory alkalosis of pregnancy. All of these factors may be worse in the third trimester of pregnancy, and most cases of diabetic ketoacidosis are reported at that time. Relevant to this case is that diabetic ketoacidosis occurs at lower blood glucose levels due to physiologic hemodilution of glucose, increased glomerular filtration rate contributing to osmotic diuresis, and placental sequestration of glucose due to increased expression of GLUT1, GLUT4, and GLUT9 transporters by the placenta. Multiple case reports suggest that pregnancy is a risk factor for euglycemic diabetic ketoacidosis.

Diabetic ketoacidosis is an obstetric and medical emergency and carries a risk of stillbirth. Immediate complications include high rates of fetal demise (27%-35%), fetal hypoxia, reduced uterine perfusion, and recurrent late decelerations. Acidosis is a major contributing factor, and anecdotally many maternal-fetal medicine physicians treat with bicarbonate when pH is less than or equal to 7, which is more aggressive than the typical approach in nonpregnant individuals. Resolution of acidosis reduces risk of fetal complications. Later complications include delayed mental development with studies showing inverse relationships between degree of ketone elevation and lower mental development scores at 2 years of age. Emergency caesarean delivery is only performed if the maternal condition becomes critical, and it is associated with high rates of maternal morbidity and mortality. For these reasons, assessing for blood ketones (Answer A) is urgently necessary, so that prompt treatment can be instituted to prevent maternal and fetal complications. Obviously, avoiding ketoacidosis is a high priority in pregnancy, and patients should be counseled ahead of time about the importance of checking for ketones during any illness and if glucose levels rise above baseline (even if the values are not elevated per se).

This patient's glucose levels are not optimally controlled. The postprandial glucose target is usually less than 140 mg/dL (<7.8 mmol/L) after 1 hour, so increasing the insulin-to-carbohydrate ratio is required, particularly at lunch and dinner (Answer C), but it is not the most urgent priority.

Reducing the basal rate overnight (Answer E) and increasing the correction factor (Answer B) would not be supported by the reported glucose levels, as her fasting glucose values are not routinely less than 70 mg/dL (<3.9 mmol/L), and there is not enough evidence to suggest that the correction factor is inadequate.

Measuring serum amylase (Answer D) is done to assess for acute pancreatitis. Its sensitivity for patients who present 24 hours after onset of pancreatitis is lower and nonspecific because of production of amylase in other conditions, including ketoacidosis. Therefore, measurement of amylase is not the best next test.

Educational Objective

Assess for euglycemic diabetic ketoacidosis in pregnancy.

Reference(s)

Jaber JF, Standley M, Reddy R. Euglycemic diabetic ketoacidosis in pregnancy: a case report and review of current literature. *Case Rep Crit Care.* 2019;2019:8769714. PMID: 31531246

American Diabetes Association Professional Practice Committee, Draznin B, Aroda VR, et al. 15. Management of diabetes in pregnancy: standards of medical care in diabetes-2022. *Diabetes Care.* 2022;45(Suppl 1):S232-S243. PMID: 34964864

83 **ANSWER: C) Referral for chest surgery**

Transgender and gender-diverse individuals are persons whose sex assigned at birth differs from their gender identity, including individuals who do not identify with a specific gender or whose gender might be considered more fluid along, within, or outside of a spectrum. Instead of identifying as male, female, man, or woman, an individual might describe their gender as nonbinary, gender fluid, genderqueer, agender, or bigender, among many possible terms. Nonbinary gender-diverse individuals should not be considered as undecided or uncertain in their gender identity. They should have the same considerations for their gender identity and affirming treatments as binary individuals. In this vignette, body dysphoria is triggered by their chest, and they have established that an androgynous appearance will be affirming as supported by a letter from their therapist. Gender-affirming surgery (Answer C) will help improve health outcomes for this individual just as in transgender individuals. The updated World Professional Association for Transgender Health (WPATH) Standard of Care (SOC) 8 guidelines emphasize the importance of understanding and recognizing gender-diverse individuals and affirming their gender identity.

In both binary and nonbinary gender-diverse individuals, gender-affirming hormone therapy (Answers B and E) is not required or recommended before consideration of chest surgery for chest dysphoria. Although 12 months of hormone therapy might be recommended before breast augmentation, as it could affect the result, hormone therapy is not necessary prior to mastectomy or masculinizing chest surgery. It is only for gender-affirming gonadectomy that guidelines recommend a year of gender-affirming hormone therapy, which is also beneficial to establish and avoid hypogonadism and effects on cardiovascular and bone health.

This patient has had a mental health evaluation and treatment with a gender therapist who has provided a letter of support consistent with WPATH guidelines recommendations before proceeding with gender-affirming masculinizing chest surgery (often required for insurance coverage). Therefore, this patient does not need a follow-up visit before referral for chest surgery (Answer A) or referral for a second letter of support or mental health assessment (Answer D). The WPATH SOC guidelines (Version 8) recommend a second mental health assessment or letter of support prior to gonadectomy because of the irreversible nature of this surgery.

Educational Objective

Apply the criteria for gender-affirming chest surgery for nonbinary/gender-fluid individuals.

Reference(s)

Deutsch MB, ed. *Guidelines for the Primary and Gender-Affirming Care of Transgender and Gender Nonbinary People.* 2nd ed. 2016. Available at: www.transhealth.ucsf.edu/guidelines. Accessed for verification January 2022.

Hembree WC, Cohen-Kettenis PT, Gooren L, et al. Endocrine treatment of gender-dysphoric/gender-incongruent persons: an Endocrine Society clinical practice guideline. *J Clin Endocrinol Metab.* 2017;102(11):3869-3903. PMID: 28945902

Coleman E, Radix AE, Bouman WP, et al. Standards of care for the health of transgender and gender diverse people, version 8. *Int J Transgend Health.* 2022;23(Suppl 1):S1-S259. PMID: 36238954

84

ANSWER: C) Start intravenous calcium therapy

Denosumab is a fully human monoclonal antibody to the receptor activator of nuclear factor kappaB ligand (RANKL). By blocking the binding of RANKL to RANK, denosumab reduces the formation, function, and survival of osteoclasts, which results in decreased bone resorption and increased bone density. Denosumab is administered by subcutaneous injection once every 6 months. It is not excreted by the kidneys; therefore, it can be used in patients with reduced kidney function without the need for a dosage change. Denosumab is eliminated through an immunoglobulin clearance pathway via the reticuloendothelial system and has a mean elimination half-life of 25 to 30 days. Denosumab may induce significant hypocalcemia in patients with kidney impairment and should not be given to patients with preexisting hypocalcemia until it is corrected. To avoid hypocalcemia with denosumab use, it is important to ensure that patients maintain an adequate amount of calcium and vitamin D supplementation, especially with conditions that predispose to hypocalcemia, such as chronic kidney disease or malabsorption syndromes. Patients with vitamin D deficiency should receive vitamin D replacement before denosumab is administered. Monitoring serum calcium is required in patients with risk factors for hypocalcemia. In such patients, serum calcium should be measured approximately 1 to 2 weeks after denosumab administration, as this is when the nadir in serum calcium typically occurs.

The patient described in this vignette has acute severe symptomatic hypocalcemia following denosumab injection. Her laboratory workup reveals secondary hyperparathyroidism in the setting of hypocalcemia, stage 3 chronic kidney disease, and a normal 25-hydroxyvitamin D level. She is currently treated with calcium and vitamin D supplementation, although she is not taking these consistently. She also has a prolonged QTc interval on electrocardiography.

While increasing her oral elemental calcium intake (Answer B) would be helpful in the long run, the most appropriate next step in the management of this patient who has acute severe symptomatic hypocalcemia with electrocardiographic changes is to start intravenous calcium therapy (Answer C). Intravenous calcium is started with an initial bolus administered over 10 to 20 minutes, followed by a calcium infusion that should be continued until she is taking an effective regimen of oral calcium and vitamin D. Patients typically require 0.5 to 1.5 mg/kg of elemental calcium per hour, and the infusion is usually prepared using calcium gluconate diluted in dextrose and water or saline.

Calcitriol (Answer D) is the preferred preparation of vitamin D for patients with severe acute hypocalcemia because of its rapid onset of action (hours). While intravenous calcium is the initial therapy of choice in this case, for the reasons listed above, oral calcitriol should be initiated as soon as possible to assist with the management of her hypocalcemia, at least in the short-term.

This patient's 25-hydroxyvitamin D level is suboptimal, most likely due to lack of adherence to her daily cholecalciferol supplement. She would benefit from taking her supplement consistently in the long-run, but increasing her oral cholecalciferol intake (Answer A) is not the most appropriate next step in the management of her hypocalcemia.

Finally, teriparatide or PTH (1-34) therapy (Answer E), an osteoanabolic agent used in the treatment of osteoporosis, has no role in the treatment of hypocalcemia.

It is important to remember that low magnesium levels may impair PTH release in response to hypocalcemia and may also cause hypocalcemia by impairing PTH action, leading to functional hypoparathyroidism. Risk factors for hypomagnesemia include diarrhea, malabsorption, proton-pump inhibitor therapy, diuretic use, alcoholism, malnutrition, and severe illness. Clinical manifestations of hypomagnesemia include refractory hypocalcemia or hypokalemia, neuromuscular disturbances, and cardiac arrhythmias. In patients with hypomagnesemia, hypocalcemia is difficult to correct without normalizing the serum magnesium concentration. Patients with severe hypomagnesemia should receive intravenous magnesium, while oral repletion may be given to patients with mild symptoms. In addition, the underlying cause of low magnesium should be corrected if possible.

Educational Objective

Recognize hypocalcemia due to denosumab and recommend the appropriate treatment.

Reference(s)

Cooper MS, Gittoes NJL. Diagnosis and management of hypocalcaemia. *BMJ.* 2008;336(7656):1298-1302. PMID: 18535072

Pepe J, Colangelo L, Biamonte F, et al. Diagnosis and management of hypocalcemia. *Endocrine.* 2020;69(3):485-495. PMID: 32367335

85 ANSWER: D) Initiation of doxazosin

Pheochromocytomas are catecholamine-producing tumors arising from the adrenal medulla. Typical clinical features of pheochromocytomas include hypertension, episodic headache, sweating, and tachycardia. Many patients with pheochromocytoma have anxiety. Due to overlapping clinical manifestations and high prevalence of anxiety within the general population, the diagnosis of pheochromocytoma can be overlooked, as it was in this patient. Her hypertension, episodes of palpitation, and substantially elevated plasma metanephrines support the diagnosis of pheochromocytoma. Worsening of symptoms in the supine position can occur in pregnancy due to compression of the tumor by the enlarged uterus, particularly late in pregnancy. This patient had prophylactic thyroidectomy in childhood because one of her biological parents was reported to have had medullary thyroid cancer. The patient was later adopted and was not aware of the association with pheochromocytoma as part of multiple endocrine neoplasia (MEN) type 2 syndrome. As in this case, pheochromocytomas associated with MEN type 2 lead to disproportionate elevation of serum metanephrine concentrations due to abundant expression of phenylethanolamine N-methyltransferase (PNMT, the enzyme that converts norepinephrine to epinephrine).

Medical treatment with an α-adrenergic blocking agent should be immediately initiated in this patient. Although data are limited, both nonselective α-adrenergic blockers (eg, phenoxybenzamine) or α_1-selective blockers (eg, doxazosin [Answer D]) have been associated with favorable maternal and fetal outcomes. Both nonselective and selective α-adrenergic blockers cross the placenta, and phenoxybenzamine has been reported to cause perinatal depression and transient hypotension. Labetalol (Answer E) is a β-adrenergic blocker with α_1-blocking activity; it is one of the preferred antihypertensive agents in pregnancy, regardless of etiology. Rarely, labetalol can cause maternal hepatotoxicity. Reports on safety of β-adrenergic blockers during pregnancy have been inconsistent, and in part confounded by the overlapping adverse effects of these agents with symptoms of untreated hypertension. In patients with pheochromocytoma, β-adrenergic blockade should be initiated a few days after α-blockade because blockade of vasodilatory peripheral β-adrenergic receptors can precipitate hypertension.

Abdominal MRI without gadolinium (Answer A) is the imaging test of choice in pregnant women with pheochromocytoma. Abdominal ultrasonography (Answer B), while noninvasive, has poor performance for detecting adrenal masses in any patient. The diagnosis of pheochromocytoma is well established clinically and hormonally in this patient, and the role of imaging at this point would be to assist with surgical intervention.

As this patient is in her third trimester, a reasonable approach would be to first attempt to medically control blood pressure and symptoms. In selected patients, surgery might be considered during the second trimester, but medical treatment should always precede surgery. For more advanced pregnancies, cesarean delivery followed by postpartum tumor removal is the preferred approach. Preoperative blood pressure and heart rate control are important to prevent a hypertensive crisis. An α-adrenergic blocker must be initiated at least 7 days before surgery; adequate α-adrenergic blockade is suggested by orthostasis, nasal congestion, and fatigue. Before treatment, patients with pheochromocytoma have a relative intravascular volume deficit, due to chronic vasoconstriction. The use of α-adrenergic blockers must be followed by aggressive hydration and dietary salt supplementation (>5000 mg sodium daily), which aids with intravascular volume reexpansion. β-Adrenergic blockade is typically added 3 to 4 days before surgery, and the dosage is titrated to achieve a resting heart rate less than 90 beats/min. Calcium channel blockers are an alternative preoperative treatment when α- and β-blockers are not covered by insurance or are not tolerated. Oral nicardipine can be used to control blood pressure preoperatively, and intravenous infusion might be used intraoperatively. Metyrosine (α-methyl-para-tyrosine) inhibits catecholamine synthesis, and it can be used when other agents are ineffective or when marked tumor manipulation or destruction is anticipated (eg, radiofrequency ablation of metastases). Data regarding pregnancy safety are not available for metyrosine, and its use is not recommended in pregnant women. Emergent cesarean delivery (Answer C) is not necessary in this case, as the patient and fetus are in no imminent danger.

Educational Objective

Diagnose pheochromocytoma and guide management during pregnancy.

Reference(s)

Bancos I, Atkinson E, Eng C, Young WF Jr, Neumann HPH, International Pheochromocytoma and Pregnancy Study Group. Maternal and fetal outcomes in phaeochromocytoma and pregnancy: a multicentre retrospective cohort study and systematic review of literature. *Lancet Diabetes Endocrinol.* 2021;9(1):13-21. PMID: 33248478

86 **ANSWER: A) CT imaging of the neck and chest**

This patient has a large right-sided thyroid nodule without suspicious findings on ultrasonography that has gradually increased in size over time. He has undergone FNA biopsy on 2 occasions with negative cytology results, making thyroid malignancy very unlikely. However, he is now reporting symptoms that could potentially be attributable to tracheal and/or esophageal compression from the large nodule. Dysphagia/globus sensation is the most common compressive symptom reported by patients with thyroid nodules, and it is associated with nodule size greater than 3 cm or location over the trachea. Because the patient is reporting globus sensation, a referral for upper endoscopy (Answer E) or a swallow study could be ordered to help determine the underlying cause and evaluate for extrinsic compression of the esophagus. However, the patient also has symptoms that raise concern for possible mass effect on the trachea (dyspnea and cough), and thus performing CT of the neck and chest (Answer A) would be a more appropriate next step to evaluate both concerns simultaneously. CT of the chest is indicated specifically because substernal extension is suspected based on physical examination findings. Both CT and MRI are superior to neck ultrasonography for defining anatomic relationships between the thyroid gland and adjacent structures and can help to inform surgical planning in the context of known or suspected mediastinal extension.

A flow-volume loop study (Answer B) is indicated in patients with symptoms of airway compression or when the tracheal lumen measures less than 1 cm in diameter on CT. Performing this study is not the best next step in this patient's evaluation given his concomitant dysphagia. Although referral for surgery or radiofrequency ablation would be considered in this patient's case, specifically if 1 or more of his symptoms is proven to be related to his large thyroid nodule, a right lobectomy would be the most appropriate surgical approach. There is no compelling indication for total thyroidectomy (Answer D) given the absence of contralateral nodules or suspicion for malignancy.

Although neck ultrasonography in 12 months (Answer C) could be used to assess for continued growth of the patient's right thyroid nodule, the nodule is almost certainly benign based on ultrasonography findings and history of 2 negative biopsies, and thus clinical follow-up (ongoing assessment of symptoms plus clinical neck examination) would probably be sufficient and a more cost-effective approach. Furthermore, recommending follow-up neck ultrasonography in 12 months would not answer the clinical question of whether his current symptoms could be attributed to the thyroid nodule.

This patient's CT imaging demonstrated leftward deviation of the subglottic trachea without airway narrowing, as well as narrowing of the esophagus at the thoracic inlet secondary to leftward mass effect from the thyroid nodule and posterior mass effect from an aberrant retroesophageal right subclavian artery. He underwent uneventful right lobectomy with benign histopathology results and symptom resolution.

Educational Objective

Recommend appropriate diagnostic testing to evaluate the etiology of compressive symptoms in the presence of goiter.

Reference(s)

Nam I-C, Choi H, Kim E-S, Mo E-Y, Park Y-H, Sun D-I. Characteristics of thyroid nodules causing globus symptoms. *Eur Arch Otorhinolaryngol.* 2015;272(5):1181-1188. PMID: 25636252

Wong R, Farrell SG, Grossmann M. Thyroid nodules: diagnosis and management. *Med J Aust.* 2018;209(2):92-98. PMID: 29996756

87 ANSWER: E) *USP8*

This patient has obvious evidence of ACTH-dependent Cushing syndrome. In a young woman with a visible pituitary adenoma, the most likely diagnosis is Cushing disease.

Somatic (not inherited) pathogenic variants in the deubiquitinase gene (*USP8*) (Answer E) are associated with ACTH-secreting adenomas. *USP8* pathogenic variants have been identified in about 50% of ACTH-secreting adenomas, with a higher prevalence in adults, as well as in females. In response to epidermal growth factor, the epidermal growth factor receptor is activated in corticotroph cells to trigger multiple downstream signaling pathways, including MAP kinase, and subsequently undergoes polyubiquitination for lysosomal degradation to switch down its signaling. The *USP8* pathogenic variants increase epidermal growth factor receptor deubiquitination, inhibiting epidermal growth factor–induced receptor downregulation, and leading to augmented and more sustained receptor signaling. Patients with Cushing disease who have adenomas carrying *USP8* pathogenic variants are diagnosed at an earlier age than those without these variants. Additionally, they have higher preoperative 24-hour urinary free cortisol levels and seem to have a higher recurrence risk after surgical remission.

While most cases of pituitary adenomas occur sporadically, a few familial forms due to germline (ie, inherited) pathogenic variants exist. Multiple endocrine neoplasia (MEN) type 1 syndrome (in which pituitary adenomas can be associated with primary hyperparathyrodism and neuroendocrine gastric or pancreatic tumors and skin abnormalities) is caused by pathogenic variants in the gene encoding menin (*MEN1*). Cyclin-dependent kinase inhibitor 1B (*CDKN1B*) pathogenic variants are a rare cause of MEN type 4 syndrome, in which pituitary adenomas can occur in conjunction with tumors of the parathyroid glands and tumors of the adrenal glands, kidneys, and reproductive organs. Germline pathogenic variants in the aryl hydrocarbon receptor-interacting protein gene (*AIP*) (Answer A) are found in familial isolated pituitary adenoma (FIPA) syndrome. In FIPA syndrome, adenomas often secrete GH and/or prolactin and the condition has an early onset and aggressive clinical course. Nonfunctioning adenomas are also seen in FIPA syndrome, which rarely includes Cushing disease. Somatic *AIP* pathogenic variants have not been described in ACTH-secreting adenomas. Xq26.3 duplications involving the gene *GPR101* are a cause of X-linked acrogigantism (X-LAG syndrome), with very early onset of aggressive G-secreting adenomas. Somatic (not inherited) pathogenic activating variants in the gene encoding the stimulatory α subunit of the guanine nucleotide-binding protein (*GNAS*) (Answer B) are identified in about 40% of sporadic GH-secreting adenomas but have not been reported as a cause of Cushing disease. Postzygotic pathogenic variants in this gene underlie the development of McCune-Albright syndrome, characterized by a triad of gonadotropin-independent precocious puberty, café-au-lait skin pigmentation, and fibrous dysplasia of bone. While acromegaly may be part of this syndrome, Cushing disease is not.

Inherited pathogenic variants in the *PRKAR1A* gene (Answer C), which encodes the regulatory subunit type 1α of protein kinase A, cause Carney complex, a rare autosomal dominant multiple endocrine neoplasia and lentiginosis syndrome. This syndrome includes skin abnormalities and a variety of endocrine and nonendocrine tumors. Endocrine manifestations include Cushing syndrome due to primary pigmented micronodular adrenocortical disease, acromegaly caused by either GH-secreting pituitary adenomas or pituitary somatotropic hyperplasia, and gonadal and thyroid tumors. Nonendocrine tumors include myxomas of the heart, schwannomas, breast ductal adenomas, osteochondromyxomas, and a predisposition to a number of malignancies. Cushing disease due to a pituitary adenoma is not part of Carney complex.

Germline *RET* pathogenic variants (Answer D) cause MEN type 2, a rare autosomal dominant syndrome associated with medullary thyroid carcinoma, pheochromocytoma, and primary hyperparathyroidism. Pituitary adenomas are not commonly present in individuals with MEN type 2.

Educational Objective

Determine which somatic pathogenic variant is the most likely culprit for the development of ACTH-secreting pituitary adenomas.

Reference(s)

Chang M, Yang C, Bao X, Wang R. Genetic and epigenetic causes of pituitary adenomas. *Front Endocrinol (Lausanne).* 2021;11:596554. PMID: 33574795

Vandeva S, Daly AF, Petrossians P, Zacharieva S, Beckers A. Somatic and germline mutations in the pathogenesis of pituitary adenomas. *Eur J Endocrinol.* 2019;181(6):R235-R254. PMID: 31658440

Kamilaris CDC, Faucz FR, Voutetakis A, Stratakis CA. Carney complex. *Exp Clin Endocrinol Diabetes.* 2019;127(2-03):156-164. PMID: 30428497

Albani A, Theodoropoulou, Reincke M. Genetics of Cushing's disease. *Clin Endocrinol (Oxf).* 2018;88(1):3-12. PMID: 28850717

88

ANSWER: C) Oral glucose tolerance test (75 g) now

Women with polycystic ovary syndrome are at increased risk for complications during pregnancy, and the presence of obesity further increases complication rates, which include gestational diabetes, preterm delivery, and preeclampsia. Preconception assessment and management is recommended in persons with polycystic ovary syndrome. The Endocrine Society guideline recommends assessment of BMI, blood pressure, and oral glucose tolerance. An international evidence-based guideline also recommends preconception assessment, including glycemic status. For initial evaluation, hemoglobin A_{1c} measurement, fasting glucose measurement, or oral glucose tolerance testing is acceptable. If other risk factors are present (eg, BMI >25 kg/m^2 [>23 mg/kg^2 in Asian patients], impaired fasting glucose, impaired glucose tolerance, history of gestational diabetes, family history of type 2 diabetes, or ethnicity at high risk), then oral glucose tolerance testing is recommended. This patient has a BMI higher than 30 kg/m^2 and has a family history of type 2 diabetes. A review of impaired glucose tolerance and diabetes in 122 women with polycystic ovary syndrome demonstrated good correlation between fasting glucose and 2-hour glucose in the whole group; however, there was poor correlation between these 2 measures in women with impaired glucose tolerance. Therefore, oral glucose tolerance testing (Answer C) is the test of choice in those at higher risk of impaired glucose tolerance and is preferred over measuring fasting glucose (Answer B) and hemoglobin A_{1c} (Answer A).

Screening for impaired glucose tolerance should be performed right away and not delayed until she is pregnant (Answers D and E).

Educational Objective

Evaluate glucose intolerance in patients with polycystic ovary syndrome.

Reference(s)

Teede HJ, Misso ML, Costello MF, et al; International PCOS Network. Recommendations from the international evidence-based guideline for the assessment and management of polycystic ovary syndrome. *Clin Endocrinol (Oxf).* 2018;89(3):251-268. PMID: 30024653

Legro RS, Arslanian SA, Ehrmann DA, et al; Endocrine Society. Diagnosis and treatment of polycystic ovary syndrome: an Endocrine Society clinical practice guideline. *J Clin Endocrinol Metab.* 2013;98(12):4565-4592. PMID: 24151290

Ehrmann DA, Barnes RB, Rosenfield RL, Cavaghan MK, Imperial J. Prevalence of impaired glucose tolerance and diabetes in women with polycystic ovary syndrome. *Diabetes Care.* 1999;22(1):141-146. PMID: 10333916

89

ANSWER: E) Testosterone treatment

This man presents with clinical features of androgen deficiency and a clear-cut biochemical picture of primary hypogonadism. While his serum testosterone concentration is only borderline-low, the reference range for total testosterone is wide. His elevated LH clearly indicates a pituitary response to Leydig-cell failure. As with any hormonal value, an individual's normal range is much narrower than the normal range in the population, and this man's premorbid serum testosterone concentration may well have been significantly higher than it is currently. Not only his sexual symptoms, but also his fatigue, low motivation, low mood (although depression is in the differential diagnosis), and weight gain, are quite possibly related to androgen deficiency. He has several plausible reasons for primary hypogonadism. First, some data suggest that testicular tumors may represent a feature of the so-called testicular dysgenesis syndrome. Accordingly, observational studies have reported that testicular cancer may be associated with poorer gonadal function in the remaining testis even before other treatments. Second, although Sertoli cells are generally more sensitive to chemoradiation than Leydig cells (note the relatively higher elevation of FSH than LH in this case), the evidence suggests that Leydig cells are also vulnerable to chemotherapy (especially platinum-based) and radiotherapy (especially more than 20-Gy dose of radiation at the testicular level). For example, in one prospective controlled study of 1235 testicular cancer survivors with 11-year follow-up, the age-adjusted odds ratio for primary hypogonadism (defined as serum testosterone concentration <231 ng/dL [<8.0 nmol/L] and LH concentration >12.0 mIU/mL [>12.0 IU/L]) was 3.8 (3.5 for surgery alone, 4.8 for surgery and radiotherapy, and 7.9 for surgery and high-dosage chemotherapy). In controlled studies, testicular cancer survivors had 2- to 4-fold increased risk of erectile dysfunction, with higher risks in those receiving radiotherapy and/or chemotherapy, and a 2.2-fold increased risk of developing metabolic syndrome (increasing to 4.1-fold in those with a serum testosterone concentration <432 ng/dL [<15.0 nmol/L]). While these observational studies, by design, cannot prove that sexual dysfunction and metabolic syndrome are causally related to hypogonadism, they are recognized manifestations of organic hypogonadism that have, in men with organic hypogonadism (not related to testicular cancer), been shown to respond to testosterone treatment. Therefore, this man was started on testosterone treatment (Answer E), which improved his sexual function and energy and enabled him to lose weight (11 lb [5.0 kg]) during the first 12 months of testosterone treatment.

While optimization of lifestyle measures to achieve a healthy body weight (Answer C) is an important component of cancer survivorship care, obesity is associated with secondary hypogonadism, and primary hypogonadism does not improve with weight loss.

Given his primary hypogonadism, the first-line treatment of his sexual dysfunction should be testosterone replacement, rather than increasing the phosphodiesterase 5 inhibitor dosage (Answer C). Indeed, following testosterone treatment, the phosphodiesterase 5 inhibitor was successfully discontinued.

While depression is always a consideration in cancer survivors, whether low testosterone is causally associated with depression is unknown, and men with depression typically present with nonelevated gonadotropins. Primary hypogonadism does not respond to antidepressive treatment (Answer D).

Selective estrogen receptor modulators such as clomiphene (Answer A) lead (via antagonizing estradiol-mediated negative hypothalamic-pituitary feedback) to an increase in LH and consequently serum testosterone in men with functional hypothalamic-pituitary axis suppression (eg, due to obesity, ill health). However, there is no rationale for using them in the setting of primary hypogonadism, where the LH concentration is already high. No studies report clinically meaningful health benefits of selective estrogen receptor modulators in men, and long-term risks are unknown.

Given the unequivocal clinical and biochemical picture of primary hypogonadism, requesting a free testosterone measurement (Answer B) will not add any useful information. In general, the Endocrine Society clinical practice guideline recommends requesting free testosterone measurement only in situations where the biochemical diagnosis of hypogonadism is not clear cut, especially if abnormalities in SHBG are suspected.

Educational Objective

Diagnose and manage primary hypogonadism in survivors of testicular cancer.

Reference(s)

Nord C, Bjøro T, Ellingsen D, et al. Gonadal hormones in long-term survivors 10 years after treatment for unilateral testicular cancer. *Eur Urol.* 2003;44(3):322-328. PMID: 12932930

La Vignera S, Cannarella R, Duca Y, et al. Hypogonadism and sexual dysfunction in testicular tumor survivors: a systematic review. *Front Endocrinol (Lausanne).* 2019;10:264. PMID: 31133982

Bhasin S, Brito JP, Cunningham GR, et al. Testosterone therapy in men with hypogonadism: an Endocrine Society clinical practice guideline. *J Clin Endocrinol Metab.* 2018;103(5):1715-1744. PMID: 29562364

90 ANSWER: B) Prescribe potassium citrate, 20 mEq twice daily

Kidney stones are common and affect nearly 10% of adults in the United States during their lifetime. Hypercalciuria is one of many factors that can contribute to the formation of calcium oxalate kidney stones. Diets high in sodium and animal protein increase urinary calcium excretion. This patient's urinary calcium is not elevated, so reducing sodium intake (Answer D) and reducing animal protein intake (Answer C) may have some benefit, but there are other interventions that may have a greater effect on reducing formation of kidney stones.

The calcium carbonate supplements that this patient takes are most likely reducing her risk of stone formation by sequestering dietary oxalate and thus reducing oxalate gut absorption. Thus, stopping calcium supplements (Answer E) is not the best next step. Changing her supplement from calcium carbonate to calcium citrate (Answer A) would be unlikely to significantly affect her risk.

This patient was found to have low urinary citrate excretion. Roux-en-Y gastric bypass has been linked to metabolic changes that can alter urine chemistry profiles, resulting in higher urinary oxalate, lower urinary citrate, and higher calcium oxalate supersaturation. Hypocitraturia can significantly increase the risk for stone formation. Urine citrate complexes with calcium in the renal tubules and thus reduces free calcium and binding to urine oxalate. Alkalinizing the urine with potassium citrate (Answer B) can increase urinary citrate excretion and thus reduce kidney stone formation.

Educational Objective

Manage hypocitraturia in a patient with kidney stones.

Reference(s)

Pearle MS, Goldfarb DS, Assimos DG, et al; American Urological Association. Medical management of kidney stones: AUA Guideline. *J Urol.* 2014;192(2):316-324. PMID: 24857648

Barcelo P, Wuhl O, Servitge E, Rousaud A, Pak CY. Randomized double-blind study of potassium citrate in idiopathic hypocitraturic calcium nephrolithiasis. *J Urol.* 1993;150(6):1761-1764. PMID: 8230497

91 ANSWER: B) Familial dysalbuminemic hyperthyroxinemia

The patient in this vignette has abnormal thyroid blood test results with elevated total T_4 and free T_4 concentrations but normal TSH, free T_3, and total T_3 concentrations. In addition, she has no symptoms of hyperthyroidism. This constellation of findings should prompt consideration of familial dysalbuminemic hyperthyroxinemia (Answer B). Familial dysalbuminemic hyperthyroxinemia is an inherited autosomal dominant disorder that most commonly occurs in Hispanic populations (0.2%). This disorder is characterized by abnormal albumin molecules with a high capacity for T_4 but not for T_3. Single point variants in exon 7 of the human serum albumin gene (*ALB*) can change arginine in position 218 or 222 in the mature protein to another amino acid. Usually, these genetic variants lead to an increased affinity for T_4. Therefore, affected individuals have a high serum total T_4 concentration but a normal serum TSH concentration and are clinically euthyroid. Serum free T_4 is usually normal, but it may be elevated due to the assay measuring free T_4, which in turn is likely to reflect different assay conditions (including buffer composition). Interestingly, individuals from the same kindred harboring the same pathogenic variant may have different results: for example, one individual with elevated free T_4 and another individual with normal free T_4. Familial dysalbuminemic hyperthyroxinemia has also been reported in Japanese, Korean, and Swedish populations.

A Thai individual with familial dysalbuminemic hypertriiodothyroninemia and an elevated total T_3 concentration has been described. This condition has also been reported in Japanese families. However, the prevalence of this disorder remains unknown. Familial dysalbuminemic hypertriiodothyroninemia is caused by a change from leucine to proline in position 66 of the ALB protein, which results in increased binding affinity for T_3 but not for T_4. Patients with this disorder are euthyroid; their total T_3 is elevated, but other thyroid laboratory values are within the reference range.

Familial dysalbuminemic hyperthyroxinemia is a common cause of euthyroid hyperthyroxinemia. Hyperthyroxinemia due to this syndrome may be confused with thyroid hormone resistance syndromes or a TSH-secreting pituitary tumor, leading to unnecessary workup and treatment. A resin (or charcoal) uptake test using radiolabeled T_4 rather than radiolabeled T_3 would detect excessive thyroxine binding to serum albumin and establish the diagnosis. Serum T_4 binding is increased in affected patients. Protein sequencing and/or sequencing of the albumin gene may be performed.

The thyroid function test results in this vignette are not consistent with biotin interference (Answer A). High-dosage biotin intake can cause artifactual thyroid function results. High circulating levels of biotin result in (1) falsely low ligand measurement in an immunometric sandwich assay (such as for TSH) and (2) falsely high ligand measurements in a competitive immunoassay (such as for free T_3, free T_4, and thyroid-stimulating immunoglobulin). Biotin must be withheld for at least 2 to 7 days to prevent its effect on various assays. Patients who are ingesting more than 5000 mcg of biotin daily may have spurious results in certain assays.

Thyroxine-binding globulin deficiency (Answer D) may be present in patients with chronic liver failure, as thyroxine-binding globulin is secreted by the liver. In the case of thyroxine-binding globulin deficiency, total T_4 and total T_3 are low. In this patient, total T_4 is elevated and total T_3 is normal. Therefore, thyroxine-binding globulin deficiency is incorrect.

A TSH-secreting pituitary tumor (Answer E) or resistance to thyroid hormone (caused by germline pathogenic variants in the thyroid hormone receptor ß gene [*THRB*]) (Answer C) is unlikely, as this patient is clinically euthyroid and both free thyroid hormones are not elevated. In the setting of both of these diagnoses, serum TSH is measurable, or even elevated, and free thyroid hormones are elevated. Patients with either of these entities have clinical symptoms of hyperthyroidism. To distinguish between the 2 conditions, serum α-subunit can be measured, which is elevated in patients with TSH-secreting pituitary tumors and normal in patients with resistance to thyroid hormone. However, a normal serum α-subunit value does not exclude a TSH-secreting pituitary tumor. An α-subunit-to-TSH molar ratio less than 1.0 favors resistance to thyroid hormone, and a ratio greater than 1.0 favors a TSH-producing pituitary tumor. Serum SHBG is usually elevated in patients with TSH-secreting pituitary tumors and normal in patients with resistance to thyroid hormone. Pituitary MRI typically shows a pituitary adenoma in a patient with a TSH-secreting pituitary tumor; most such tumors are macroadenomas, but microadenomas are possible as well.

Educational Objective

Diagnose familial dysalbuminemic hyperthyroxinemia.

Reference(s)

Pannain S, Feldman M, Eiholzer U, Weiss RE, Scherberg NH, Refetoff S. Familial dysalbuminemic hyperthyroxinemia in a Swiss family caused by a mutant albumin (R218P) shows an apparent discrepancy between serum concentration and affinity for thyroxine. *J Clin Endocrinol Metab.* 2000;85(8):2786-2792. PMID: 10946882

Khoo S, Lyons G, McGowan A, et al. Familial dysalbuminaemic hyperthyroxinaemia interferes with current free thyroid hormone immunoassay methods. *Eur J Endocrinol.* 2020;182(6):533-538. PMID: 32213658

Kragh-Hansen U, Galliano M, Minchiotti L. Clinical, genetic, and protein structural aspects of familial dysalbuminemic hyperthyroxinemia and hypertriiodothyroninemia. *Front Endocrinol (Lausanne).* 2017;8:297. PMID: 29163366

92 ANSWER: D) Pravastatin

New dyslipidemia after initiation of highly active antiretroviral therapy (HAART) commonly occurs. Protease inhibitor–containing regimens are associated with increases in total cholesterol, LDL cholesterol, and triglycerides and decreases in HDL cholesterol. The risk of hypercholesterolemia in patients treated with a protease inhibitor is 4 to 20 times higher than that of patients not taking a protease inhibitor (depending on the protease inhibitor used). Nonnucleoside reverse transcriptase inhibitors are also associated with increases in LDL cholesterol and triglycerides; however, increases in HDL cholesterol are also observed. Neither nucleoside reverse transcriptase inhibitors nor integrase inhibitors have an adverse effect on lipid profiles.

A lipid panel is recommended before HAART initiation and 3 to 6 months after starting or changing medications. When lipid levels are stable, annual follow-up testing is recommended. Patients with dyslipidemia should work on lifestyle changes, including dietary modification (lower fat intake for patients with hypercholesterolemia or lower carbohydrate intake for patients with hypertriglyceridemia), increased physical activity, and cessation of cigarette smoking.

Evaluation of cardiovascular risk in HIV-infected persons on HAART is similar to that for HIV-negative persons. The first step is to calculate the patient's 10-year risk of atherosclerotic cardiovascular disease. If the patient's risk is 5% or higher over 10 years, starting a moderate-intensity statin should be considered given that HIV infection is a risk enhancer for atherosclerotic cardiovascular disease. The patient in this vignette has a 10-year risk of 9.3% for atherosclerotic cardiovascular disease.

When selecting which statin to prescribe, one must remember which cytochrome P450 enzyme metabolizes each medication (*see table*). Atorvastatin (Answer A), simvastatin (Answer E), and lovastatin (Answer C) are metabolized by CYP3A4, and protease inhibitors are inhibitors of this enzyme. If these statins are used with a protease inhibitor, their concentration will increase. Pravastatin (Answer D) is metabolized by a sulfation reaction and by CYP3A4 to a minimal degree. Rosuvastatin and fluvastatin (not offered as an answer option) are metabolized by CYP2C9. Pravastatin, rosuvastatin and fluvastatin are considered safer for patients who are taking a protease inhibitor.

Table. Cytochrome P450 Metabolism of Statins

Statin	CYP enzyme
Atorvastatin	CYP3A4
Fluvastatin	CYP2C9
Lovastatin	CYP3A4
Pravastatin	CYP3A4 minor
Rosuvastatin	CYP2C9
Simvastatin	CYP3A4

Ezetimibe, a cholesterol absorption inhibitor, can be used in patients on a HAART regimen. Bile acid sequestrants are usually not recommended, as they may interfere with the absorption of antiretroviral agents.

Fibrates (Answer B) are indicated to lower triglycerides when the concentration is greater than 500 mg/dL (>5.65 mmol/L). Both gemfibrozil and fenofibrate have been used in combination with HAART. Nelfinavir and ritonavir, both protease inhibitors, can lower the concentration of gemfibrozil, so fenofibrate is the preferred agent when patients are on either of these protease inhibitors.

Educational Objective

Prescribe a statin while considering its interaction with highly active antiretroviral therapy.

Reference(s)

Grundy SM, Stone NJ, Bailey AL, et al. 2018 AHA/ACC/AACVPR/AAPA/ABC/ACPM/ADA/AGS/APhA/ASPC/NLA/PCNA Guideline on the management of blood cholesterol: a report of the American College of Cardiology/American Heart Association Task Force on Clinical Practice Guidelines. *Circulation.* 2019;139:e1082-e1143. PMID: 30586774

Manuel O, Thiébaut R, Darioli R, Tarr PE. Treatment of dyslipidaemia in HIV-infected persons. *Expert Opin Pharmacother.* 2005;6(10):1619-1645. PMID: 16086650

Ballocca F, D'Ascenzo F, Gili S, Grosso Marra W, Gaita F. Cardiovascular disease in patients with HIV. *Trends Cardiovasc Med.* 2017;27(8):558-563. PMID: 28779949

93 ANSWER: B) Mifepristone

Numerous therapies are now available for the medical management of Cushing syndrome. These therapies are particularly useful for patients who either decline surgery or are considered to be at too high risk to undergo a surgical procedure, as well as for patients in whom remission has not been achieved through surgical management.

The etiology of hypercortisolism (ACTH independent vs ACTH dependent) and the presence or absence of dysglycemia are important factors to consider when selecting medical therapy. Whereas medications such as mifepristone (Answer B), mitotane (Answer C), and ketoconazole (Answer A) can be used in patients with either ACTH-independent or ACTH-dependent hypercortisolism, some medications are only useful in patients with ACTH-dependent Cushing syndrome for lowering ACTH levels and therefore cortisol (ie, pasireotide [Answer E]). Such a medication would have little value in ACTH-independent Cushing syndrome where ACTH is already suppressed. Pasireotide has a higher affinity for somatostatin receptor type 5 and a slightly lower affinity for somatostatin receptor type 2 compared with octreotide and lanreotide. As a result, in patients with dysglycemia, initiation of pasireotide often worsens glycemic control by reducing insulin secretion through agonism of somatostatin type receptor 5 located on the β cells.

Osilodrostat (Answer D) is a cortisol synthesis inhibitor that inhibits 11β-hydroxylase, the enzyme responsible for the final step of cortisol biosynthesis: converting 11-deoxycortisol to cortisol. While this drug would certainly be expected to be effective in patients with either ACTH-independent or ACTH-dependent hypercortisolism, it is currently only approved for the treatment of adults with Cushing disease who either cannot undergo pituitary gland surgery or have undergone surgery but still have the disease. Off-label use in some patients may be warranted, but given its currently approved indication, it is not the best answer. If used, it would be expected to have a positive effect on glycemic control.

Given this patient's underlying liver disease, ketoconazole (Answer A) is contraindicated. Mitotane (Answer C) should be administered with care to patients with liver disease other than metastatic lesions from the adrenal cortex, since the metabolism of mitotane may be affected and the drug could accumulate. Considering his underlying liver disease, and given alternative options, mitotane is not the best choice.

Mifepristone (Answer B) is a cortisol receptor blocker indicated to control hyperglycemia secondary to hypercortisolism in adult patients with endogenous Cushing syndrome who have type 2 diabetes or glucose intolerance and have undergone unsuccessful surgery or are not surgical candidates (which includes patients who do not want to undergo surgery). In the SEISMIC study (Study of the Efficacy and Safety of Mifepristone in the Treatment of Endogenous Cushing Syndrome), mifepristone demonstrated a reduction in the area under the curve glucose by 25% or more in 60% of patients ($P < .0001$). The secondary endpoint was significant reduction in hemoglobin A_{1c} of 1.1% ($P < .001$). These improvements were also observed with simultaneous reductions in antidiabetes treatments. The insulin daily dose was reduced by greater than 50% in 5 of 12 patients, and antidiabetes treatments were reduced in 7 of 15 patients. The best next step in this patient's care is mifepristone therapy because he has hypercortisolism and uncontrolled type 2 diabetes and is not a good surgical candidate (and he also declined to pursue surgical intervention).

The blocking of cortisol action via mifepristone will also help to ameliorate additional adverse effects of hypercortisolism, but it is important to note that there are no laboratory markers to monitor to help gauge the patient's response. ACTH and cortisol actually increase while receiving mifepristone because of blockade of the glucocorticoid receptor. Thus, the response to mifepristone (and dosage escalation) is determined based on the patient's clinical response (improvement in glycemia, reduction in the dose or number of diabetes therapies, improvement in other comorbidities, etc). Important adverse events include abortion and/or endometrial hypertrophy because of the antiprogesterone effects of mifepristone. Thus, women of childbearing age must understand this risk and be using nonhormonal forms of contraception. Endometrial hypertrophy can lead to vaginal bleeding, which requires evaluation by an obstetrician/gynecologist if it occurs. Lastly, through blockade of the cortisol receptor, cortisol binding to the mineralocorticoid receptor is increased. Cortisol has a higher binding affinity for the mineralocorticoid receptor than for the glucocorticoid receptor. Thus, affected patients often develop hypokalemia and hypervolemia, and sometimes worsening hypertension. These effects must be considered and addressed at baseline and during therapy. Spironolactone or eplerenone is recommended for patients with potassium levels that are already at the lower end of the reference range, and the drug should be titrated judiciously to maintain adequate potassium levels. Potassium supplementation is sometimes required. Hypervolemia and worsening hypertension can be managed using diuretics and/or additional antihypertensive therapies, if required. Lastly, antidiabetes therapies should be preemptively adjusted before initiation of mifepristone or dosage increases to avoid hypoglycemia (in patients receiving insulin secretogogues or insulin therapy). Reduction or cessation of all antidiabetes may be considered, when appropriate, depending on the patient's response to mifepristone.

Mifepristone can be used in mild-to-moderate hepatic impairment, but it should not be used in severe hepatic impairment. This patient has nonalcoholic fatty liver disease with only a slight elevation of transaminase values, so the use of mifepristone would be appropriate.

Educational Objective

Recommend medical treatment options for Cushing syndrome, particularly in the setting of dysglycemia/suboptimally controlled type 2 diabetes mellitus, and describe the medications' indications and contraindications.

Reference(s)

Hinojosa-Amaya JM, Cuevas-Ramos D, Fleseriu M. Medical management of Cushing's syndrome: current and emerging treatments. *Drugs.* 2019;79(9):935-956. PMID: 31098899

Brown DR, East HE, Eilerman BS, et al. Clinical management of patients with Cushing syndrome treated with mifepristone: consensus recommendations. *Clin Diabetes Endocrinol.* 2020;6(1):18. PMID: 33292727

94 **ANSWER: C) Radioactive iodine therapy with 100 mCi ^{131}I and recombinant human TSH**

Differentiated thyroid cancer is the only malignancy for which staging is determined based on the patient's age at diagnosis. Using the 8th edition of the American Joint Committee on Cancer (AJCC)/tumor-node-metastasis (TNM) staging system, thyroid cancers in persons younger than 55 years are categorized as either stage I or II, depending on whether distant metastases are present or absent, while cancers in persons 55 years and older are classified as stages I through IV. The patient described in this vignette has AJCC/TNM stage I (T2N1bMx) papillary thyroid carcinoma.

While staging is a good predictor of disease-specific survival, it does not accurately predict recurrence-free survival. Risk of recurrence is thus separately determined using systems such as the American Thyroid Association (ATA) recurrence risk stratification system, which includes low-, intermediate-, and high-risk categories. The patient described in this vignette has clinical lymph node metastases, which confer a recurrence risk of approximately 20%. Thus, her thyroid cancer would be classified as intermediate risk, for which the estimated recurrence risk ranges from 5% to 20%.

Radioactive iodine therapy (^{131}I) is recommended for 1 or more of the following reasons: (1) ablation of the postoperative thyroid remnant, (2) adjuvant therapy (ie, treatment of suspected but unconfirmed residual, usually microscopic, cancer), and/or (3) treatment of known structural disease. It is important to weigh the risks and benefits of radioactive iodine for each individual patient. Risk stratification systems, such as that proposed by the ATA, should be used to inform treatment decisions. Adjuvant radioactive iodine should be considered in patients who are designated as having an intermediate risk of structural recurrence, such as in the described case, with the goal of decreasing recurrence risk.

TSH stimulation is required for ^{131}I uptake by tumor cells, which can be achieved either through temporary withdrawal of thyroid hormone or through the administration of human recombinant TSH (rhTSH). The ATA thyroid nodule and cancer guidelines recommend rhTSH as an acceptable alternative to temporary withdrawal of thyroid hormone when radioactive iodine is being used as adjuvant therapy, although insufficient data are available for high-risk disease. As compared with withdrawal of thyroid hormone, the use of rhTSH is associated with the prevention of hypothyroid symptoms, improved quality of life, lower rates of hyponatremia in the context of a low-iodine diet, and a shorter mean total-body effective half-life of ^{131}I (lower total-body radiation exposure). In this patient with intermediate recurrence risk and low suspicion for gross residual disease or distant metastasis (postoperative serum thyroglobulin <2 ng/mL), using rhTSH instead of withdrawal of thyroid hormone would be preferable given the better adverse event profile and similar efficacy. Therefore, any option that incorporates withdrawal of thyroid hormone as the method of TSH stimulation (Answers B and D) is incorrect.

When radioactive iodine is being administered as adjuvant therapy, the ATA guidelines recommend administered activities above those used for remnant ablation (ie, >30 mCi) up to a maximum of 150 mCi. Therefore, recommending ^{131}I activities of 30 mCi (Answer A) or 200 mCi (Answer E) would not be the most appropriate treatment approach. A retrospective study of 204 patients at intermediate risk (97% papillary thyroid cancer) demonstrated that patients who received 30 mCi ^{131}I had a higher rate of biochemical or structural incomplete response to therapy after 10 years, as compared with patients who received 100 or 150 mCi (25% vs 10%), respectively. However, other studies have found that adjuvant radioactive iodine doses greater than 100 mCi do not appear to improve the response to therapy for patients with N1b disease, especially for younger patients. Thus, the most appropriate treatment option for this patient is radioactive iodine with 100 mCi ^{131}I and rhTSH (Answer C). Administering 30 mCi ^{131}I would be appropriate if radioactive iodine were being given solely for the purpose of thyroid remnant ablation. An activity of 200 mCi could be recommended for the treatment of known distant metastatic disease. However, whole-body dosimetry should be used if the administered ^{131}I activity exceeds 200 mCi or 150 mCi in adults older than 70 years. Dosimetry estimates an effective dose that maximizes uptake by tumor cells but limits potential toxicity to other tissues (eg, bone marrow).

Educational Objective

Recommend radioactive iodine therapy and determine the most appropriate administered activity in a patient with intermediate-risk differentiated thyroid cancer.

Reference(s)

Haugen BR, Alexander EK, Bible KC, et al. 2015 American Thyroid Association management guidelines for adult patients with thyroid nodules and differentiated thyroid cancer: the American Thyroid Association Guidelines Task Force on Thyroid Nodules and Differentiated Thyroid Cancer. *Thyroid.* 2016;26(1):1-133. PMID: 26462967

Iizuka Y, Katagiri T, Ogura K, Inoue M, Nakamura K, Mizowaki T. Comparison of thyroid hormone withdrawal and recombinant human thyroid-stimulating hormone administration for adjuvant therapy in patients with intermediate- to high-risk differentiated thyroid cancer. *Ann Nucl Med.* 2020;34(10):736-741. PMID: 32643022

Mayson SE, Chan CM, Haugen BR. Tailoring the approach to radioactive iodine treatment in thyroid cancer. *Endocr Relat Cancer.* 2021;28(10):T125-T140. PMID: 34254949

95 ANSWER: B) Administer zoledronic acid infusion

The patient in this vignette is an elderly African American postmenopausal woman hospitalized after sustaining a left hip fragility fracture, consistent with a clinical diagnosis of osteoporosis. This patient has never had a DXA scan, but a clinical diagnosis of osteoporosis may be made in the presence of a fragility fracture, particularly at the spine or hip, without measurement of bone mineral density. Risk factors for osteoporosis include her age, surgical menopause, and family history. She also has inadequate calcium and vitamin D intake, with evidence of vitamin D insufficiency on her laboratory evaluation. Nutritional osteomalacia would be highly unlikely in this case since this would typically present with very low serum 25-hydroxyvitamin D levels (<10 ng/mL [<25.0 nmol/L]), which this patient does not have.

She is at high risk for future fracture and should be counseled on fall prevention, started on adequate calcium and vitamin D intake, and treated with pharmacologic therapy for osteoporosis. It is critical to consider her barriers to health care when choosing the best therapeutic intervention. In addition, it is important to realize that African American women with postmenopausal osteoporosis are less likely than White women to receive osteoporosis-related health care. Compared with White women, African American women with postmenopausal osteoporosis also seem to have significantly higher rates of mortality, debility, and destitution after fracture.

An intravenous bisphosphonate such as zoledronic acid (Answer B) would be the ideal option given her difficulty in accessing health care, provided she is agreeable. Zoledronic acid is administered as an annual infusion and would be recommended as long as her estimated glomerular filtration rate remains above 35 mL/min per 1.73 m^2. In addition to decreasing her fracture risk, an annual infusion of zoledronic acid within 90 days after repair of a low-trauma hip fracture is associated with a reduction in all-cause mortality, with no clinically evident effect on fracture healing, even when the drug is infused in the immediate postoperative period. Since vitamin D deficiency is associated with increased risk of hypocalcemia when bisphosphonates are administered, this should ideally be corrected prior to treatment. The most common adverse effect of zoledronic acid treatment is an acute-phase reaction that is transient and usually mild. 25-Hydroxyvitamin D concentrations lower than 30 ng/mL (<74.9 nmol/L) seem to correlate with a higher risk of developing this flulike reaction. Furthermore, infusing zoledronic acid over a longer duration (45 to 60 minutes instead of 15 to 30 minutes) can minimize the risk of both kidney toxicity and this acute-phase reaction.

Raloxifene (Answer D) is a selective estrogen receptor modulator approved for the treatment of postmenopausal osteoporosis; however, it is considered a second-line agent because it only decreases the risk of vertebral fractures and has no effect on hip or other nonvertebral fracture risk. This option would not be the best choice in this patient who has just sustained a hip fracture. Safety concerns with raloxifene include an increased risk of venous thromboembolism.

While alendronate (Answer C) is an FDA-approved treatment option, it would require adherence to a weekly dosing regimen. Poor adherence appears to be a major limiting factor in clinical practice, with advancing age predicting a greater risk of nonadherence, in addition to adverse effects, patient health beliefs, and inadequate patient education. Furthermore, there are no data showing that alendronate would offer the same mortality benefit as zoledronic acid following a hip fracture.

Teriparatide (PTH 1-34) (Answer E), an anabolic agent used in the treatment of osteoporosis, is administered as a daily subcutaneous injection. Contraindications to its use include history of skeletal irradiation, Paget disease of bone, or unexplained elevation in alkaline phosphatase due to potential risk of osteosarcoma. This would not be recommended in this case given the patient's history of radiation exposure.

Denosumab (Answer A) is a fully human monoclonal antibody to the receptor activator of nuclear factor kappaB ligand (RANKL). It reduces the formation, function, and survival of osteoclasts, which results in decreased bone resorption and increased bone density. Denosumab is administered by subcutaneous injection once every 6 months. It is not excreted by the kidneys; therefore, it can be used in patients with reduced kidney function without the need for dosage adjustment. Because of emerging concerns about an increased risk of vertebral fracture after delaying or discontinuing denosumab, this would not be the best option for a patient who does not follow-up consistently with her physician due to transportation difficulties. Similar to bisphosphonate use, it is important to ensure that patients maintain adequate calcium and vitamin D supplementation to avoid hypocalcemia with denosumab use.

Educational Objective

Consider social determinants of health care and racial disparities in osteoporosis management and recommend the most appropriate intervention after hip fracture.

Reference(s)

Colón-Emeric C, Nordsletten L, Olson S, et al; HORIZON Recurrent Fracture Trial. Association between timing of zoledronic acid infusion and hip fracture healing. *Osteoporos Int.* 2011;22(8):2329-2336. PMID: 21153021

Wright NC, Chen L, Saag KG, Brown CJ, Shikany JM, Curtis JR. Racial disparities exist in outcomes after major fragility fractures. *J Am Geriatr Soc.* 2020;68(8):1803-1810. PMID: 32337717

Noel SE, Santos MP, Wright NC. Racial and ethnic disparities in bone health and outcomes in the United States. *J Bone Miner Res.* 2021;36(10):1881-1905. PMID: 34338355

Mikuls TR, Saag KG, George V, Mudano AS, Banerjee S. Racial disparities in the receipt of osteoporosis related healthcare among community-dwelling older women with arthritis and previous fracture. *J Rheumatol.* 2005;32(5):870-875. PMID: 15868624

Eriksen EF, Lyles KW, Colón-Emeric CS, et al. Antifracture efficacy and reduction of mortality in relation to timing of the first dose of zoledronic acid after hip fracture. *J Bone Miner Res.* 2009;24(7):1308-1313. PMID: 19257818

Lyles KW, Colón-Emeric CS, Magaziner JS, et al; HORIZON Recurrent Fracture Trial. Zoledronic acid and clinical fractures and mortality after hip fracture. *N Engl J Med.* 2007;357(18):1799-1809. PMID: 17878149

Crotti C, Watts NB, De Santis M, et al. Acute phase reactions after zoledronic acid infusion: protective role of 25-hydroxyvitamin D and previous oral bisphosphonate therapy. *Endocr Pract.* 2018;24(5):405-410. PMID: 29498910

96 **ANSWER: E) Reduce the insulin glargine dosage by 20%**

Based on this patient's hemoglobin A_{1c} level, his glycemic control appears to be excellent. However, given his age, such strict control is unlikely to provide significant benefit in terms of preventing microvascular complications. Indeed, he is at risk for hypoglycemia because of his age, kidney status, and recent weight loss; safety should be prioritized in this patient. The laboratory finding of anemia and notation of iron sulfate in his medication list suggests that he is being treated for iron deficiency anemia. Iron deficiency anemia may be associated with prolongation of red cell turnover, and in this setting hemoglobin A_{1c} levels may therefore overestimate the degree of glycemia. He may be experiencing asymptomatic nocturnal hypoglycemia. While there are no well-established glycemic targets in persons with chronic kidney disease and diabetes mellitus, one study has suggested that hemoglobin A_{1c} levels greater than 9.0% (>75 mmol/mol) and less than 6.5% (<48 mmol/mol) are associated with increased mortality in persons with non–dialysis-dependent chronic kidney disease that is stage 3 or more advanced. Reducing his risk of severe hypoglycemia by decreasing the insulin glargine dosage by 20% (Answer E) would be the highest priority. He does not report postprandial hypoglycemia, so reducing the insulin aspart dosage (Answer D) is not highest priority right now.

Prescribing continuous glucose monitoring (Answer C) to evaluate whether he is experiencing nocturnal hypoglycemia is reasonable, but it may take time to get acquire this device. The most important immediate step is to reduce the risk of hypoglycemia.

Increased physical activity (Answer B) is certainly a good goal, but it may increase his risk for hypoglycemia without preemptively reducing the insulin dosage and would not be the most important next step.

An SGLT-2 inhibitor (Answer A) may be indicated to reduce this patient's risk of hospital readmission considering his history of heart failure, but it is not likely to help improve his blood glucose levels substantially given his reduced estimated glomerular filtration rate. Furthermore, in trials of SGLT-2 inhibitors aimed at reducing heart failure risk, the mean age of enrollment is 61 to 66 years and such data should be applied with caution in an 80-year-old patient, as in this vignette. For these reasons and because reducing the risk of nocturnal hypoglycemia is a more urgent priority, initiation of SGLT-2 inhibitors is not the best next choice.

Educational Objective

Prioritize reducing the risk for hypoglycemia in a patient with type 2 diabetes mellitus treated with insulin.

Reference(s)

Shurraw S, Hemmelgarn B, Lin M, et al. Association between glycemic control and adverse outcomes in people with diabetes mellitus and chronic kidney disease: a population-based cohort study. *Arch Intern Med.* 2011;171(21):1920-1927. PMID: 22123800

Hahr AJ, Molitch ME. Management of diabetes mellitus in patients with chronic kidney disease. *Clin Diabetes Endocrinol.* 2015;1:2. PMID: 28702221

97 **ANSWER: A) Discontinue the oral contraceptive and initiate spironolactone, 100 mg daily**

In this case, the change in therapy from an oral contraceptive to a progestin-eluting intrauterine device for contraception worsened hirsutism because ovarian androgen production was no longer suppressed by the oral contraceptive. A progestin-eluting intrauterine device exerts its contraceptive effect locally on the endometrium and does not achieve systemic concentrations or suppress ovarian hormone production. Usually, menstrual bleeding stops or decreases in quantity or frequency, so a progestin-eluting intrauterine device might also be recommended for women with heavy bleeding. Removing the intrauterine device alone (Answer C) would not affect hyperandrogenism and could worsen irregular bleeding while she is on the combined oral contraceptive, which is the most likely cause of her new irregular bleeding.

Spironolactone (Answer A) is an aldosterone antagonist that also acts as a competitive inhibitor of the androgen receptor. It is considered second-line therapy for the treatment of hirsutism or first-line therapy in a patient who cannot be prescribed combined oral contraceptives. Spironolactone is also an appropriate addition to a combined oral contraceptive when symptoms are not controlled by the oral contraceptive alone. However, spironolactone alone would be more likely to cause irregular or more frequent vaginal bleeding. It is recommended to use spironolactone in combination with a combined oral contraceptive or a progestin-eluting intrauterine device to prevent conception and irregular uterine spotting or bleeding that might occur with spironolactone alone. Because she already has a progestin-eluting intrauterine device, she is an ideal candidate to discontinue the oral contraceptive and initiate spironolactone.

Repeated hormone testing (Answer D) is not indicated and would not change management because her androgen excess symptoms have not changed or progressed. FSH and estradiol are undetectable because the synthetic estrogen in combined oral contraceptives is not detectable as estradiol and is meant to suppress the endogenous hypothalamic-pituitary-gonadal axis.

Changing the progestin (Answer E) is considered more often for patients who are experiencing adverse effects such as bloating or acne after starting the oral contraceptive and who might benefit from a different, less androgenic progestin. With ongoing symptoms of androgen excess while on oral contraceptives and persistently elevated DHEA-S, increased suppression might be helpful with either an increased estrogen dosage or continuous hormone suppression by eliminating the placebo week. However, both of these changes are less likely to eliminate the irregular bleeding. In this case, she has both irregular bleeding after starting the oral contraceptive and persistent hirsutism and acne. Stopping the oral contraceptive and starting spironolactone would be indicated to stop the irregular bleeding and treat the androgen excess symptoms not responding to the oral contraceptive.

Pelvic ultrasonography (Answer B) is helpful to exclude an anatomical cause of amenorrhea, to determine adequate estrogen in the setting of amenorrhea, and to detect polycystic ovarian morphology. It would be indicated in a woman presenting with abnormal uterine bleeding spontaneously or after menopause. This patient is experiencing irregular bleeding with oral contraceptives, so imaging is less important than changing the therapeutic intervention, both because of the probable association with the bleeding and the ongoing symptoms of androgen excess.

Educational Objective

Manage hirsutism.

Reference(s)

Martin KA, Anderson RR, Chang RJ, et al. Evaluation and treatment of hirsutism in premenopausal women: an Endocrine Society practice guideline. *J Clin Endocrinol Metab.* 2018;103(4):1233-1257. PMID: 29522147

Gallo MF, Nanda K, Grimes DA, Schulz KF. 20 mcg versus >20 mcg estrogen combined oral contraceptives for contraception. *Cochrane Database Syst Rev.* 2005;(2):CD003989. PMID: 15846690

Kaunitz AM, Burkman RT, Fisher AC, LaGuardia KD. Cycle control with a 21-day compared with a 24-day oral contraceptive pill: a randomized controlled trial. *Obstet Gynecol.* 2009;114(6):1205-1212. PMID: 19935020

98 ANSWER: B) basal setting: 12 AM to 3 AM = 0.6 units/h, 3 AM to 9 AM = 0.8 units/h, and 8 AM to 12 AM = 0.7 units/h; insulin-to-carbohydrate ratio = 1:12; correction factor = 1:50

Traditional teaching for calculating basal insulin pump settings is to take the total daily dose of insulin from the patient's multiple-dose insulin (prandial and basal) regimens and use 75% to 80% of the total daily needs for the insulin pump calculations. Fifty percent of this reduced dose will be the initial basal hourly rate of insulin. In this vignette, the patient's total daily dose using injections is 45 units. With the initiation of pump therapy, a reduction to 75% of total daily dose indicates a need for about 34 units daily. Fifty percent of this dose would become the basal rate. In this patient, the total basal dose would be 17 units. Seventeen divided by 24 gives an initial hourly rate of insulin = 0.7 units/h.

Typically, one would not alter this patient's insulin-to-carbohydrate ratio upon pump initiation unless there were a clear clinical indication (thus, Answers D and E are incorrect). However, she is currently not using correctional insulin dosing appropriately. The formula of 1500 to 1800 mg/dL divided by total daily dose (using her new total daily dose of approximately 35 units daily) provides an estimate of 42 to 51. Thus, Answers C and E are incorrect, as these correction doses are too high and could lead to hypoglycemia.

When initiating pump therapy, a single basal rate is often used that comprises approximately 50% of the new calculated total daily dose; an hourly rate is calculated by dividing this by 24 hours. If this is selected, then a basal dose of 17 units is estimated, and a single rate would be 0.7 units/h. However, given the information provided in this case, a single basal rate may not be appropriate. This patient reports both frequent nocturnal hypoglycemia at 2 AM and fasting hyperglycemia. The nocturnal hypoglycemia is likely due to lower insulin needs overnight. Her fasting hyperglycemia may be due to the dawn phenomenon. Some studies demonstrate a 15 to 25 mg/dL blood glucose elevation from nocturnal nadir until breakfast. The most likely mechanism of the dawn phenomenon in type 1 diabetes is spikes in GH secretion. Observational studies also highlight that insulin sensitivity is higher after midnight until 3 AM as compared with the period from 4 AM to 8 AM. Patients with diabetes lack the natural rise in insulin in the morning that is seen in patients without diabetes.

Thus, a single hourly insulin rate may not be the best starting point for this patient's insulin pump. In Answer A, the hourly rate does not account for her predicted lower total daily dose and could be expected to cause hypoglycemia. In Answer D, the basal rate is appropriately reduced; however, the single basal rate does not address her reported swings in glucose overnight. Additionally, the insulin-to-carbohydrate ratio is inappropriately increased in this answer option, which may lead to higher glucose values. This case is an example of individualizing treatment plan/pump settings based on the patient's current glycemic indices. Given that she reports hypoglycemia overnight but rising early-morning blood glucose, the best choice would be to decrease the hourly insulin rate after midnight and then increase her hourly rate in the early morning (Answer B).

Educational Objective

Calculate initial insulin pump settings for a patient with type 1 diabetes mellitus when transitioning from multiple daily insulin injections.

Reference(s)

Porcellati F, Lucidi P, Bolli GB, Fanelli CG. Thirty years of research on the dawn phenomenon: lessons to optimize blood glucose control in diabetes. *Diabetes Care.* 2013;36(12):3860-3862. PMID: 24265365

Chow N, Shearer D, Tildesley HG, Aydin Plaa J, et al. Determining starting basal rates of insulin infusion for insulin pump users: a comparison between methods. *BMJ Open Diabetes Res Care.* 2016;4(1):e000145. PMID: 26977305

99 **ANSWER: C) Adrenal myelolipoma**

Adrenal incidentalomas are commonly encountered during cross-sectional imaging studies of the abdomen (found in 4% to 7% of all patients older than 40 years). Adopting a systematic approach to assessment is important, and the clinician must answer 2 important questions:

1. Could this be a primary (eg, adrenocortical carcinoma) or secondary (eg, metastasis) malignant tumor?
2. Is the lesion functioning?

With modern imaging techniques (unenhanced ± triple-phase CT; chemical shift MRI), most adrenal incidentalomas are readily classified as benign in nature. Both unenhanced CT and chemical shift MRI provide an assessment of lipid content within the adrenal mass. In a homogeneous lesion, a Hounsfield unit (HU) value less than 10 on noncontrast CT identifies a lipid-rich lesion and confidently excludes malignancy, even in larger adrenal masses.

In this patient, the lesion is larger than 4 cm in diameter, which, based on size criteria alone might raise concerns. However, it is well circumscribed, with no evidence of local invasion, and has a distinctive pathognomonic appearance, being composed mostly of low-density tissue, which is typical of a macroscopic fat-containing adrenal myelolipoma (Answer C). Higher attenuating myeloid elements within the lesion may have a cloudy appearance (as in this case, *see image, arrowheads*) as solid strands or forming a discrete solid nodule within the fat. The remaining normal adrenal gland may be visible, albeit displaced (*see image, dashed arrow*).

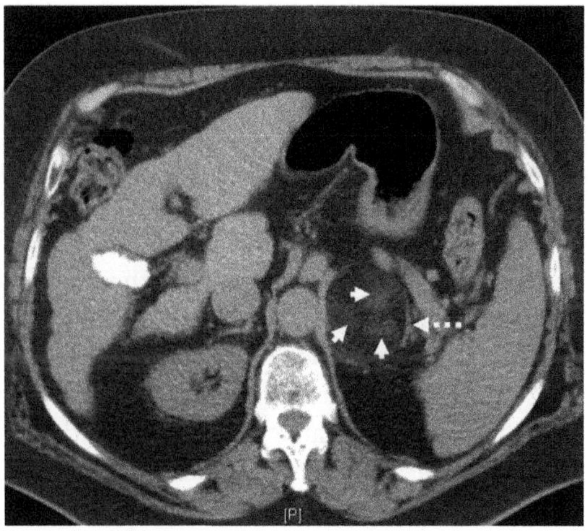

The amount of fat can vary, ranging from only a few small regions in an otherwise largely soft-tissue density mass (~10%), to lesions containing roughly equal proportions of fat and soft tissue (~50%), to those that are almost completely composed of fatty tissue (~40%). In the latter, CT attenuation, measured in HU, is very low (even reaching −100 HU). With increasing myeloid components, density progressively increases (eg, −50 to 0 HU). However, in predominantly solid lesions with minimal macroscopic fat, attenuation values may not exclude other diagnoses. Myeloid elements typically demonstrate contrast enhancement. Occasionally, small areas of calcification are seen.

Large adrenal myelolipomas (>10 cm) can cause local symptoms due to mass effect and are occasionally complicated by acute hemorrhage. However, this patient's lesion is 6 cm in diameter, with no evidence of intralesional hemorrhage, and his symptoms are on the contralateral side to the radiologic abnormality. A concomitant adrenal adenoma is estimated to occur in approximately 5% of cases and may be associated with adrenal hormone (eg, cortisol) excess. In this vignette, the postdexamethasone cortisol value is marginally above the traditional threshold for excluding autonomous hypercortisolism (<1.8 μg/dL [<50 nmol/L]) and merits further investigation.

While some clinicians recommend measurement of plasma free metanephrines or 24-hour urinary fractionated metanephrines in all adrenal incidentalomas to exclude pheochromocytoma (Answer E), recent data suggest that if the imaging findings effectively exclude pheochromocytoma (eg, homogeneous mass with unenhanced CT density <10 HU, or typical appearance of myelolipoma), then this assessment is not necessary unless other clinical concerns dictate. Indeed, in this case, measurement of plasma metanephrines only served to cause confusion, as the mildly elevated normetanephrine level was subsequently shown to be secondary to amitriptyline treatment.

Although cortisol (± androgen) secretion may be a feature of adrenocortical carcinoma (Answer D), the radiologic appearance in this case is not consistent with this diagnosis.

Adrenal metastasis (Answer B) has been estimated to account for 8% to 9% of all adrenal incidentalomas; however, the radiologic appearance is not consistent with a malignant lesion.

Adrenal hemorrhage (hematoma) (Answer A) may result from a variety of traumatic and nontraumatic causes. Risk factors for adrenal hemorrhage include anticoagulation, disseminated intravascular coagulation, sepsis (including meningococcemia—Waterhouse-Friderichsen syndrome), primary antiphospholipid syndrome, or an underlying adrenal tumor. On CT, adrenal hematomas characteristically appear round or oval and are often accompanied by stranding of periadrenal fat. The attenuation value of an adrenal hematoma depends on its age, with high attenuation (eg, >50 HU) in the acute/subacute phase but reduced attenuation (and size) over time. Some resolve completely, while others remain visible as a nonenhancing mass with a hypoattenuating center, with or without calcification(s). The radiologic findings in this case are not suggestive of adrenal hemorrhage.

Educational Objective

Identify the typical radiologic appearance of an adrenal myelolipoma and describe causes of mild abnormalities in biochemical screening tests for adrenal incidentalomas.

Reference(s)

Fassnacht M, Arlt W, Bancos I, et al. Management of adrenal incidentalomas: European Society of Endocrinology clinical practice guideline in collaboration with the European Network for the Study of Adrenal Tumors. *Eur J Endocrinol.* 2016;175(2):G1-G34. PMID: 27390021

Hamidi O, Raman R, Lazik N, et al. Clinical course of adrenal myelolipoma: a long-term longitudinal follow-up study. *Clin Endocrinol (Oxf).* 2020;93(1):11-18. PMID: 32275787

Calissendorff J, Juhlin CC, Sundin A, Bancos I, Falhammar H. Adrenal myelolipomas. *Lancet Diabetes Endocrinol.* 2021;9(11):767-775. PMID: 34450092

100 **ANSWER: E) Recommend external-beam radiation to the neck**

This patient has had incomplete resection of his thyroid cancer based on surgeon report. Furthermore, his pathology report revealed a more aggressive thyroid cancer (tall-cell features) than classic papillary thyroid cancer, with vascular invasion, extrathyroidal extension, and cervical node metastases. In addition, his posttherapy radioiodine scan did not show any iodine uptake in his neck or anywhere else. Therefore, he has non–iodine-avid disease confirmed by a negative posttherapy scan. According to the 2015 American Thyroid Association thyroid cancer guidelines, external-beam radiation (Answer E) should be recommended to treat this patient's nonresected persistent thyroid cancer in his neck and to reduce his recurrence risk.

According to the aforementioned guidelines for thyroid cancer, routine adjuvant external-beam radiation therapy is not recommended for patients with differentiated thyroid cancer following initial complete surgical resection. External-beam radiation therapy may be considered in patients undergoing multiple and frequent neck reoperations for palliation of locoregional recurrent disease. Persistent nonresectable/or gross residual disease in the neck that is iodine refractory is an indication for external-beam radiation therapy. Per the National Comprehensive Cancer Network, external-beam radiation therapy is recommended for patients with gross or recurrent locoregional or distant metastatic disease unamenable to radioiodine treatment. Adverse effects seen after external-beam radiation therapy include skin erythema; mucositis of the esophagus, trachea, and larynx; and dysphagia. Further surgeries can be challenging after receiving external-beam radiation therapy to the neck.

This patient's serum TSH concentration of 1.8 mIU/L is not within target range considering his high recurrence risk. Therefore, his levothyroxine dosage should be increased to achieve a target TSH concentration below 0.1 mIU/L. There is no indication to prescribe liothyronine (Answer A) in addition to levothyroxine, as his target TSH level can be achieved by further adjustment of his levothyroxine dosage.

As this patient's posttherapy scan did not show iodine-avid uptake in his neck or elsewhere, there is no indication for him to receive additional radioiodine treatment (Answer D).

Ordering PET/CT scan (Answer C) or performing neck ultrasonography (Answer B) is not yet indicated, but these imaging modalities will be required in this patient's follow-up (eg, at 6 months follow-up) given his iodine-refractory thyroid cancer.

Educational Objective

List the indications for external-beam radiation in patients with differentiated thyroid cancer.

Reference(s)

Haugen BR, Alexander EK, Bible KC, et al. 2015 American Thyroid Association management guidelines for adult patients with thyroid nodules and differentiated thyroid cancer: the American Thyroid Association Guidelines Task Force on Thyroid Nodules and Differentiated Thyroid Cancer. *Thyroid.* 2016;26(1):1-133. PMID: 26462967

Kiess AP, Agrawal N, Brierley JD, et al. External-beam radiotherapy for differentiated thyroid cancer locoregional control: a statement of the American Head and Neck Society. *Head Neck.* 2016;38(4):493-498. PMID: 26716601

101 **ANSWER: C) Initiate a 10-day course of progesterone to induce a withdrawal bleed**
Primary ovarian insufficiency (POI) refers specifically to hypergonadotropic hypogonadism that develops before age 40 years. POI can result from oophorectomy, chemotherapy, or radiotherapy or can occur spontaneously. POI was previously referred to as premature ovarian failure with insufficiency a more appropriate description due to fluctuating ovarian function, estrogen status, menses, and fertility that can be observed over a prolonged period as illustrated in this case. FSH and estrogen status can normalize spontaneously, as indicated by this patient's normal FSH and sufficient endometrial lining. Women with POI might conceive during fertile/ ovulatory cycles, so contraception is still indicated if pregnancy is not desired. POI can develop spontaneously secondary to autoimmune oophoritis associated with other autoimmune endocrinopathies such as autoimmune thyroid disease and primary autoimmune adrenal insufficiency (Addison disease). Screening for autoimmune thyroid disease with TSH and TPO antibodies (elevated in this case) and autoimmune adrenal insufficiency with cortisol +/- ACTH and 21-hydroxylase antibodies is recommended. As opposed to screening for hypothyroidism, evaluation for adrenal insufficiency (Answer A) would not be considered when looking for a cause of secondary amenorrhea unless there was significant weight loss or other suggestive symptoms. Additional testing in the evaluation of hypergonadotrophic hypogonadism would include karyotype analysis, although Turner syndrome would be unlikely in a patient who experienced normal puberty. When POI is diagnosed, testing for a premutation in the *FMR1* gene is also recommended because of the association of POI with fragile X syndrome. Fragile X syndrome is an X-linked disorder that is the most common cause of genetic intellectual impairment.

In this patient, the primary clinical question is whether amenorrhea is due to hyperprolactinemia or POI. An additional important clinical consideration is whether she has enough estrogen present or requires estrogen replacement regardless of the diagnosis. This patient's prolactin concentration is minimally elevated, her FSH concentration is now normal, and her endometrial lining is sufficient (>4 mm), which is consistent with normal estrogen concentrations. This means that the elevated prolactin is not causing hypogonadotropic hypogonadism, and increasing the cabergoline dosage (Answer B) is unlikely to restore menses. If she were trying to conceive and had elevated prolactin concentrations, increasing the cabergoline dosage might be recommended to further improve chances of ovulation, fertilization, and implantation by normalizing prolactin. During the progesterone withdrawal test, the equivalent of luteal-phase progesterone is administered to determine whether there is enough endogenous estrogen present to develop an endometrial lining and result in a menstrual period within 10 days of completing the 10-day progesterone. With prolonged absent menses and estrogen present, this patient is also at risk for endometrial hyperplasia with a thickened endometrial lining. Progesterone withdrawal can also be a treatment for women with anovulatory amenorrhea with estrogen present, and it is recommended to induce a withdrawal bleed every 3 months if there are no spontaneous menses. Therefore, the best next step would be to initiate a 10-day course of progesterone to induce a withdrawal bleed (Answer C), which would confirm adequate estrogen status and prevent endometrial hyperplasia.

In the management of POI, hormone replacement regimens that might be considered include more physiologic estradiol replacement regimens using transdermal estradiol (Answer E) or vaginal routes with possible lower risk compared with risk associated with oral estrogen based on data in postmenopausal women. However, in a woman with an intact uterus, progesterone should be added for endometrial protection, to prevent hyperplasia and the potential for cancer. Therefore, transdermal estradiol would not be recommended alone and would be combined with progesterone cyclically or daily.

Because this patient is not interested in conceiving and could conceive even with POI (as she has shown evidence of FSH normalization on recent laboratory results), a combined oral contraceptive (Answer D) would be a better choice than transdermal estradiol and progesterone hormone replacement. However, because she has not had a withdrawal bleed for 9 months and her endometrial lining is thickened on ultrasonography, she is more likely to have irregular bleeding when starting combined oral contraceptives now. Before considering a combined oral contraceptive, the best next step would be to initiate a 10-day course of progesterone to induce a withdrawal bleed.

Educational Objective

Evaluate and treat primary ovarian insufficiency in the setting of hyperprolactinemia.

Reference(s)

Giri R, Vincent AJ. Prevalence and risk factors of premature ovarian insufficiency/early menopause. *Semin Reprod Med*. 2020;38(4-05):237-246. PMID: 33434933

Melmed S, Casanueva FF, Hoffman AR, et al; Endocrine Society. Diagnosis and treatment of hyperprolactinemia: an Endocrine Society clinical practice guideline. *J Clin Endocrinol Metab*. 2011;96(2):273-288. PMID: 21296991

102 ANSWER: B) Continue metformin; decrease insulin glargine dosage to 40 units; titrate dulaglutide to maximum dosage tolerated

Hypoglycemia is associated with significant morbidity, mortality, and cost, and more hospital admissions are due to hypoglycemia than hyperglycemia. Hypoglycemia is more likely in patients with chronic kidney disease, so use of insulin-sparing agents and minimizing the insulin dosage is ideal. Previous recommendations included stopping metformin with an absolute creatinine concentration of 1.4 mg/dL (123.8 µmol/L) in women and 1.5 mg/dL (132.6 µmol/L) in men given the concern for increased risk of lactic acidosis. However, newer data have shown that lactic acidosis is rare, and current recommendations are to continue metformin at a reduced dosage unless the estimated glomerular filtration rate is less than 30 mL/min per 1.73 m^2. Additionally, metformin can be initiated if the estimated glomerular filtration rate is 45 mL/min per 1.73 m^2 or greater. Continuing metformin is appropriate for this patient, especially because it may promote modest weight loss and has a low risk for hypoglycemia (thus, Answers C, D, and E are incorrect).

Increasing the insulin dosage (Answer D) in a patient about to start an exercise program would not be the best choice, especially because her recent laboratory test results reveal a fasting glucose concentration of 80 mg/dL (4.4 mmol/L) and hint at the potential for hypoglycemia.

The American Diabetes Association guidelines now recommend GLP-1 receptor agonists as the first injectable medication for patients with type 2 diabetes unless the patient has symptoms of uncontrolled diabetes. This recommendation is based on this medication class's strong glycemic effect, lower risk of hypoglycemia, cardiovascular benefit, and potential for weight loss. Higher dosages of GLP-1 receptor agonists have now become available with more potential for lowering hemoglobin A_{1c} and inducing greater weight loss, although dosage escalation may be limited by the adverse effect profile, which includes nausea and other gastrointestinal issues. In this patient who has committed to small lifestyle changes and a personal weight-loss goal, escalating the dulaglutide dosage would support this goal and minimize risk for hypoglycemia. Thus, the best option for her is to continue metformin, decrease the insulin glargine dosage to 40 units, and titrate dulaglutide to the maximum dosage tolerated (Answer B). Not reducing her insulin dose while titrating dulaglutide (Answer A) would increase her risk for hypoglycemia. The *table* summarizes the weight-loss data for the higher dosage of dulaglutide and the head-to-head weight loss for typical dosages of the 2 newer GLP-1 receptor agonists, dulaglutide and semaglutide. Higher-dosage semaglutide will soon be available.

Table. Weight Loss in SUSTAIN-7 and AWARD-11 Trials

SUSTAIN-7	**Dulaglutide 1.5 mg**	**Semaglutide 1.0 mg**
Change in body weight 40 weeks	6.6 lb (3.0 kg)	14.3 lb (6.5 kg)
AWARD-11	**Dulaglutide 1.5 mg**	**Dulaglutide 4.5 mg**
Change in body weight 36 weeks	6.6 lb (3.0 kg)	10.1 lb (4.6 kg)

Educational Objective

Maximize GLP-1 receptor agonist therapy and minimize insulin use to reduce the risk for hypoglycemia in patients with type 2 diabetes mellitus.

Reference(s)

Lipska KJ, Ross JS, Wang Y, et al. National trends in US hospital admissions for hyperglycemia and hypoglycemia among Medicare beneficiaries, 1999 to 2011. *JAMA Intern Med.* 2014;174(7):1116-1124. PMID: 24838229

Inzucchi SE, Lipska KJ, Mayo H, Bailey CJ, McGuire DK. Metformin in patients with type 2 diabetes and kidney disease: a systematic review. *JAMA.* 2014;312(24):2668-2675. PMID: 25536258

Frias JP, Bonora E, Nevarez Ruiz L, et al. Efficacy and safety of dulaglutide 3.0 mg and 4.5 mg versus dulaglutide 1.5 mg in Metformin-Treated Patients With Type 2 Diabetes in a Randomized Controlled Trial (AWARD-11). *Diabetes Care.* 2021;44(3):765-773. PMID: 33397768

Pratley RE, Aroda VR, Lingvay I, et al; SUSTAIN 7 investigators. Semaglutide versus dulaglutide once weekly in patients with type 2 diabetes (SUSTAIN 7): a randomised, open-label, phase 3b trial. *Lancet Diabetes Endocrinol.* 2018;6(4):275-286. PMID: 29397376

103 ANSWER: B) Potassium iodide supplementation

This patient's serum TSH concentration is below the nonpregnant reference range, although only just below the lower limit of normal in the first trimester of pregnancy (which is 0.4 mIU/L lower than that of nonpregnant adults). Reduced serum TSH values in early pregnancy are common and inversely proportionate to the serum hCG concentration. In a small proportion of patients, serum TSH can be less than 0.01 mIU/L and still represent normal pregnancy. Subclinical hyperthyroidism has not been associated with adverse pregnancy outcomes. Neither methimazole (Answer A) nor propylthiouracil (Answer C) is indicated for this patient. The mild reduction in serum TSH is most likely related to normal pregnancy. Initiating treatment with antithyroid medication in the first trimester of pregnancy is associated with teratogenicity, and more serious birth defects have been observed in association with methimazole than with propylthiouracil.

The most appropriate treatment to recommend for this patient is potassium iodide supplementation (Answer B). She has been unable to tolerate taking a prenatal vitamin in the context of pregnancy-related nausea and vomiting and is instead taking a standalone folic acid supplement. Moreover, approximately one-quarter of commercially available prenatal vitamins do not contain supplemental iodine. Iodine is an essential dietary micronutrient that is required for thyroid hormone production. Severe iodine deficiency can lead to congenital hypothyroidism and impaired fetal/neonatal neurodevelopment; however, even mild maternal iodine deficiency has been associated with neurocognitive deficits. Iodine requirements are higher in pregnant and lactating women because of increased thyroid hormone production during gestation and the secretion of iodine into breast milk. Although the general US population is iodine sufficient, some populations, including pregnant and lactating women, are at risk for mild iodine deficiency. The most significant dietary sources of iodine are dairy products, eggs, seafood, and grains. Iodized salt is not used universally in the United States. A recent study demonstrated that nearly one-quarter of pregnant women were estimated to be at risk for iodine deficiency. The American Thyroid Association, Endocrine Society, and American Academy of Pediatrics recommend that women in the United States who are planning pregnancy, are pregnant, or are lactating should take supplemental iodine in the form of potassium iodide at a dosage of 150 mcg daily. In contrast, selenium supplementation (Answer D) is not recommended during pregnancy regardless of TPO-antibody status. There are conflicting data on the effect of selenium supplementation on TPO-antibody status and TPO-antibody titers in pregnancy. In addition, treatment with selenium may be associated with a higher risk of type 2 diabetes.

No additional treatment (Answer E) is incorrect, as iodine supplementation should be recommended for this patient.

Educational Objective

Provide counseling about increased iodine needs during pregnancy.

Reference(s)

Alexander EK, Pearce EN, Brent GA, et al. 2017 guidelines of the American Thyroid Association for the diagnosis and management of thyroid disease during pregnancy and the postpartum. *Thyroid.* 2017;27(3):315-389. PMID: 28056690

Kerver JM, Pearce EN, Ma T, et al. Prevalence of inadequate and excessive iodine intake in a US pregnancy cohort. *Am J Obstet Gynecol.* 2021;224(1):82.e1-82.e8. PMID: 32653458

Patel A, Lee SY, Stagnaro-Green A, MacKay D, Wong AW, Pearce EN. Iodine content of the best-selling United States adult and prenatal multivitamin preparations. *Thyroid.* 2019;29(1):124-127. PMID: 30266075

Snart CJP, Threapleton DE, Keeble C, et al. Maternal iodine status, intrauterine growth, birth outcomes and congenital anomalies in a UK birth cohort. *BMC Med.* 2020;18(1):132. PMID: 32522280

104 ANSWER: D) Screen for excess alcohol use

Post–gastric bypass hypoglycemia is estimated to occur in about 10% of patients who undergo gastric bypass surgery; about 1% of patients experience severe hypoglycemia as defined by a blood glucose concentration less than 40 mg/dL (<2.2 mmol/L), requiring an emergency department visit or hospitalization for hypoglycemia. Symptoms are always postprandial and typically occur 1 to 3 hours after eating. Symptoms are most often triggered by specific dietary choices and behaviors. The patient in this vignette has insulin-mediated hypoglycemia as evidenced by a low postprandial plasma glucose concentration in the setting of inappropriately normal insulin and C-peptide concentrations. As there is no indication that he has fasting hypoglycemia, there is no need to proceed with a 72-hour fast (Answer B).

Management of post–gastric bypass hypoglycemia starts with a careful dietary history performed by a bariatric dietitian. This is valuable to identify specific areas for change, for example, carbohydrate choice, speed of eating, or liquid consumption with meals, which can reduce the severity and/or frequency of these episodes. In general, high–glycemic index carbohydrates should be eliminated and the consumption of fat and protein with complex carbohydrates should be emphasized. Pharmacologic treatment with GLP-1 agonists and somatostatin analogues may be considered as adjunctive treatments. However, given the patient's known history of symptomatic gallstones, a somatostatin analogue (Answer A) would be relatively contraindicated.

The vignette gives no indication that the patient has bacterial overgrowth, so empiric treatment for this condition (Answer E) is not indicated. Patients with small intestinal bacterial overgrowth commonly have bloating, gas, diarrhea, and fat-soluble vitamin deficiencies.

Before considering gastric bypass reversal (Answer C), all modifiable risk factors should be addressed. Similar to what is observed in patients who have not undergone gastric bypass surgery, alcohol consumption in those who have undergone gastric bypass increases the risk of postprandial hypoglycemia by impairing hepatic glucose release. In this patient, alcohol consumption could be suspected based on the high-normal mean corpuscular volume (despite adequate vitamin B_{12} concentration) and elevated values on liver function tests. Hence, screening for excess alcohol use (Answer D) is appropriate. In this particular patient, excess alcohol use accounted for many of his severe symptoms. Alcohol use disorder is an increasingly recognized complication of gastric bypass surgery, and all patients should be screened for problematic alcohol consumption postoperatively.

Ultimately, a proportion of patients who experience post–gastric bypass hypoglycemia require reversal of gastric bypass when other treatment modalities are ineffective. However, in this particular patient, reestablishing the connection between his stomach and esophagus runs the risk of worsening Barrett esophagus, so this should only be considered once his alcohol use disorder is fully addressed.

Educational Objective

Diagnose alcohol use disorder after gastric bypass surgery and describe its effect on post–gastric-bypass hypoglycemia.

Reference(s)

Marsk R, Jonas E, Rasmussen F, Naslund E. Nationwide cohort study of post-gastric bypass hypoglycaemia including 5,040 patients undergoing surgery for obesity in 1986-2006 in Sweden. *Diabetologia.* 2010;53(11):2307-2311. PMID: 20495972

King WC, Chen J-Y, Courcoulas AP, et al. Alcohol and other substance use after bariatric surgery: prospective evidence from a U.S. multicenter cohort study. *Surg Obes Relat Dis.* 2017;13(8):1392-1402. PMID: 28528115

Davis DB, Khoraki J, Ziemelis M, et al. Roux en Y gastric bypass hypoglycemia resolves with gastric feeding or reversal: confirming a non-pancreatic etiology. *Mol Metab.* 2018;9:15-27. PMID: 29449181

105 ANSWER: C) Order 2-hour fasting urine for phosphate and creatinine measurements

Laboratory evaluation has documented that this patient has hypophosphatemia. Chronically low serum phosphate can lead to muscle weakness and osteomalacia due to defective bone mineralization. Elevated alkaline phosphatase may suggest osteomalacia, especially in the setting of hypophosphatemia, so a bisphosphonate (Answer D) would not be beneficial and may be harmful because of potential worsening of osteomalacia due to further inhibition of skeletal mineralization. Treatment of hypophosphatemia with phosphate supplements (Answer E) and calcitriol may be required, but the first step is to determine the etiology of the low serum phosphate. Causes of hypophosphatemia include decreased renal reabsorption, decreased intestinal absorption, and increased mobilization of phosphate into tissues.

This patient's history does not suggest refeeding syndrome or a reason for hungry bone syndrome, so increased mobilization of phosphate into tissues is unlikely. Measuring urine phosphate (Answer C) would be very helpful because increased urine phosphate would suggest renal phosphate wasting, and decreased urine phosphate would suggest a defect in intestinal absorption. Urine phosphate wasting is determined by first calculating the percentage of tubular reabsorption of phosphate (TRP): 100 × (1 –[urine phosphate/urine creatinine]) × (serum creatinine/ serum phosphate). Normal TRP is 85% to 95% when the serum phosphate concentration is normal. When serum phosphate is low, it would be expected that renal phosphate reabsorption and TRP would increase. TRP should be adjusted based on kidney function. The ratio of the tubular maximum reabsorption of phosphate (TmP) to glomerular filtration rate (GFR) is then calculated as TRP × serum phosphate when the TRP is less than or equal to 86%. When TRP is greater than 86%, the following calculation is used: TmP/GFR = 0.3 × TRP / (1 – 0.8 × TRP) × serum phosphate. Sex- and age-specific TmP/GFR normal values have been reported. Generally, a normal range for TmP/GFR for adults is 3.0 to 4.2 mg/dL. A detailed table for normal TmP/GFR values can be found in Chong et al.

If the patient indeed has renal phosphate wasting, then measuring serum FGF-23 (Answer B) may be important in the differential diagnosis, which would include tumor-induced osteomalacia and forms of Fanconi syndrome, but this measurement would be premature without knowing the renal response to hypophosphatemia. Furthermore, there are FGF-23–independent causes of hypophosphatemia (hereditary hypophosphatemic rickets with hypercalciuria) that require a different treatment approach (phosphorus supplements alone) from that used to address FGF-23–dependent disorders such as tumor-induced hypophosphatemia.

Measuring 1,25-dihydroxyvitamin D (Answer A) may assist in determining the cause, especially with FGF-23–mediated disease, which leads to inappropriately low 1,25-dihydroxyvitamin D, but its measurement is premature before determining whether renal phosphate wasting is present.

Educational Objective

Evaluate for renal phosphate wasting in a patient with hypophosphatemia.

Reference(s)

Gaasbeek A, Meinders AE. Hypophosphatemia: an update on its etiology and treatment. *Am J Med.* 2005;118(10):1094-1101. PMID: 16194637

Chong WH, Molinolo AA, Chen CC, Collins MT. Tumor-induced osteomalacia. *Endocr Relat Cancer.* 2001;18(3):R53-R77. PMID: 21490240

Weber TJ, Quarles LD. Molecular control of phosphorus homeostasis and precision treatment of hypophosphatemic disorders. *Curr Mol Biol Rep.* 2019;5(2):75-85. PMID: 31871877

106 ANSWER: D) Repeat serum testosterone measurement after recovery from acute illness

Major stress from any acute or chronic illness can suppress the hypothalamic-pituitary-gonadal (HPG) axis. The degree of HPG-axis suppression is usually proportional to the severity and duration of the offending illness. This man's serum testosterone is at a concentration that would be expected considering his illness severity, age, and comorbidities. Glucocorticoid treatment can further suppress the HPG axis. His previous testosterone treatment possibly contributed to HPG-axis suppression. Of note, his preillness serum testosterone concentration was modestly reduced, which was consistent with his age and comorbidities—especially obesity and diabetes. In cross-sectional studies of unselected older men with obesity and diabetes, whether from the United States, United Kingdom, or Australia, the median serum testosterone concentration was around 290 ng/dL (10.0 nmol/L), similar to this patient's preillness concentration. In this vignette, it is unclear whether the preillness sample was drawn in the morning in the fasting state (afternoon draw and food intake can reduce serum testosterone by up to 30%) and whether a repeated testosterone measurement was done. The Endocrine Society recommends that, in general, a clinical diagnosis of androgen deficiency be confirmed by at least 2 serum testosterone concentrations. If the serum testosterone is confirmed to be low, a further tailored workup including gonadotropins is needed, so that a clear diagnosis (eg, primary or secondary hypogonadism, the latter needing additional hormone testing and pituitary imaging in some cases) can be made before testosterone treatment is considered. Unfortunately, inappropriate testosterone prescribing is common, with one US study reporting that only 3.1% of men who received testosterone in the Veterans Health Administration underwent a guideline-conforming evaluation before starting testosterone therapy. Thus, the appropriateness of testosterone treatment in this man is doubtful.

Whether HPG-axis suppression in severe acute disease is adaptive (ie, beneficial), maladaptive (harmful), or neutral is not known. Androgens increase muscle mass, induce erythrocytosis, and improve bone density, and the catabolic state that occurs following sepsis presents a significant challenge. However, there have been no randomized controlled trials suggesting that in patients with sepsis (COVID-19–associated or otherwise) testosterone treatment has clinically meaningful outcomes. Therefore, testosterone treatment (either topical or intramuscular) (Answers B and E) is not indicated.

Measurement of free testosterone, SHBG, and gonadotropins (Answer C), which would be low in an acutely ill patient, would not add clinically useful information. Likewise, a full panel to assess pituitary function (Answer A) is not indicated. For example, cortisol and ACTH would be low due to glucocorticoid treatment. Evaluation of the thyroid axis would most likely show changes consistent with euthyroid sick syndrome (whether this is adaptive, maladaptive, or neutral is not known), and clinical trials of thyroid hormone treatment in acute illness have not shown benefits. The best course of action is to refrain from further investigations and treatment now and to repeat serum testosterone measurement after recovery from acute illness (Answer D).

Men are more susceptible than women to severe COVID-19 infection. While many factors have a role, some authorities have speculated whether testosterone is involved in COVID-19 pathogenesis. Data to date have been mixed. Androgens may facilitate viral entry into host cells by promoting the expression of a key serine protease (cell surface transmembrane protease serine 2, TMPRSS2), and clinical trials testing the hypothesis that androgen inhibition (using either GnRH or androgen receptor antagonists) improves clinical outcomes in men infected with COVID-19 are currently ongoing. However, it has also been speculated that androgens may confer protection against COVID-19 by attenuating inflammatory immune responses. This is based on evidence from several observational studies in men hospitalized with COVID-19 reporting that a low serum testosterone concentration is associated with poor clinical outcomes (including increased risk of intensive care unit admission and death). However, these studies have lacked a disease severity–matched control group of men with non–COVID-19 infections. Therefore, whether low serum testosterone in men with severe COVID-19 simply represents a marker of disease severity (rather than a causal mediator of poor outcomes) remains unknown.

Educational Objective

Guide the management of a patient with severe, acute illness that is suppressing the hypothalamic-pituitary-gonadal axis.

Reference(s)

Grossmann M. Low testosterone in men with type 2 diabetes: significance and treatment. *J Clin Endocrinol Metab.* 2011;96(8):2341-2453. PMID: 21646372

Jasuja GK, Bhasin S, Reisman JI, Berlowitz DR, Rose AJ. Ascertainment of testosterone prescribing practices in the VA. *Med Care.* 2015;53(9):746-752. PMID: 26196850

Bhasin S, Brito JP, Cunningham GR, et al. Testosterone therapy in men with hypogonadism: an Endocrine Society clinical practice guideline. *J Clin Endocrinol Metab.* 2018;103(5):1715-1744. PMID: 29562364

Mauvais-Jarvis F. Do anti-androgens have potential as therapeutics for COVID-19? *Endocrinology.* 2021;162(8):bqab114. PMID: 34089595

107 ANSWER: B) Hemoglobin A_{1c} measurement

This asymptomatic man presents for routine follow-up of hypothyroidism. His TSH concentration is in the normal range; there is no reason to think he has central hypothyroidism, so free T_4 measurement (Answer A) is not required.

Diabetes screening guidelines authored by the American Diabetes Association and US Preventive Services Task Force were revised in 2022 and 2021, respectively. The American Diabetes Association recommends universal screening, regardless of risk factor status, in all persons aged 35 years or older and in asymptomatic adults of any age who are overweight or obese who have 1 more risk factor: first-degree relative with diabetes, high-risk race or ethnicity, history of cardiovascular disease, blood pressure ≥140/90 mm Hg or therapy for hypertension, HDL-cholesterol concentration <35 mg/dL (<0.90 mmol/L) and/or triglyceride concentration >250 mg/dL (>2.82 mmol/L), history of polycystic ovary syndrome, physical inactivity, or other clinical findings associated with insulin resistance (severe obesity or acanthosis nigricans). Previously, the American Diabetes Association recommended screening persons without risk factors if they were 45 years or older and screening persons younger than 45 years only if they were overweight or obese with at least 1 additional risk factor.

In contrast, the US Preventive Services Task Force recommends screening adults 35 years or older who are overweight or obese, having previously recommended screening only in overweight and obese persons 40 years or older. Based on current American Diabetes Association guidelines, measurement of hemoglobin A_{1c} (Answer B) would be reasonable. Also, since a BMI value of 23 kg/m^2 or greater in Asian American individuals is considered overweight, one might argue that this patient's BMI of 22.9 kg/m^2 is a risk factor. Therefore, per US Preventive Services Task Force guidelines, screening for diabetes is reasonable. What were the drivers for changing the screening recommendations?

Chung et al designed a study to detect whether opportunistic universal screening of all adults older than 18 years would identify significantly more persons with diabetes or prediabetes than the previous American Diabetes Association and US Preventive Services Task Force guidelines, using NHANES data. The authors found that a sharp decrease in number needed to screen occurred between ages 30 and 34 years (number needed to screen = 80) vs ages 35 to 39 years (number needed to screen = 31). Per their estimates, if previous American Diabetes Association guidelines were strictly enforced, 206,455 cases of diabetes/prediabetes would have been missed (14.6% of positive tests) in persons 35 years and older. If previous US Preventive Services Task Force guidelines would have been strictly enforced, 5,508,164 cases (60.7% of positive tests) would have been missed in individuals 35 years and older. Based on estimated costs, it was proposed that adjustments to screening age be considered.

There are no agreed upon guidelines for measurement of lipoprotein(a) (Answer D) for the purposes of screening for cardiovascular disease. The American Heart Association does not explicitly recommend measurement of lipoprotein (a) but suggests that a concentration greater than 50 mg/dL (>125 nmol/L) is a risk-enhancing factor in persons aged 40 to 75 years without diabetes Endocrine Society lipid management guidelines suggest measurement of lipoprotein(a) only in persons with a familial risk for atherosclerotic cardiovascular disease, which this patient does not have. Therefore, there is no indication to measure lipoprotein (a).

High-sensitivity C-reactive protein (Answer C) is a serum biomarker for inflammation. An elevated concentration greater than or equal to 2.0 mg/L (≥19.0 nmol/L) is an independent risk predictor for atherosclerosis in apparently healthy men and women. However, the incremental predictive value of C-reactive protein measurement for atherosclerotic cardiovascular disease is small and controversial, so its measurement is not the best step in this case.

Given this patient's age, lack of other risk factors, and cholesterol panel that places him at a low 10-year risk for atherosclerotic cardiovascular disease, a repeated lipid panel (Answer E) is suggested every 4 to 6 years and is not necessary now.

Educational Objective

Review current recommendations for diabetes mellitus screening from major medical societies.

Reference(s)

American Diabetes Association Professional Practice Committee. 2. Classification and diagnosis of diabetes: standards of medical care in diabetes-2022. *Diabetes Care.* 2022;45(Suppl 1):S17-S38. PMID: 34964875

Chung S, Azar KMJ, Baek M, Lauderdale DS, Palaniappan LP. Reconsidering the age thresholds for type II diabetes screening in the U.S. *Am J Prev Med.* 2014;47(4):375-381. PMID: 25131213

US Preventive Services Task Force, Davidson KW, Barry MJ, et al. Screening for prediabetes and type 2 diabetes: US Preventive Services Task Force recommendation statement. *JAMA.* 2021;326(8):736-743. PMID: 34427594

Grundy SM, Stone NJ, Bailey AL, et al. 2018 AHA/ACC/AACVPR/AAPA/ABC/ACPM/ADA/AGS/APhA/ASPC/NLA/PCNA guideline on the management of blood cholesterol: a report of the American College of Cardiology/American Heart Association Task Force on Clinical Practice Guidelines. *Circulation.* 2019;139(25):e1082-e1143. PMID: 30586774

108 ANSWER: B) *CYP24A1*

The man described in this vignette has hypercalcemia associated with a PTH concentration less than 20 pg/mL (<20 ng/L), consistent with a PTH-independent etiology. He also has an inappropriately elevated 1,25-dihydroxyvitamin D level and hypercalciuria in the setting of kidney stones. Given his age and the family history of osteoporosis and nephrolithiasis, one must consider an inherited disorder of vitamin D metabolism. This patient most likely has loss-of-function pathogenic variants in the *CYP24A1* gene (Answer B), impairing the 24-hydroxylase enzyme. The 24-hydroxylase enzyme catabolizes calcitriol to the inert compound 24,25-dihydroxyvitamin D, and variants affecting its function lead to hypercalcemia, hypercalciuria, elevated 1,25-dihydroxyvitamin D, low-normal PTH, and nephrolithiasis. The recommended screening for this condition is determination of the ratio of serum 25-hydroxyvitamin D to 24,25-dihydroxyvitamin D, whereby a ratio of 99 or greater identifies patients who are candidates for genetic testing of the *CYP24A1* gene. A diet low in calcium and vitamin D is the cornerstone of therapy. Although treatment with antifungal agents such as ketoconazole and fluconazole, which inhibit 1α-hydroxylase, has proven beneficial, toxicity from these drugs limits their long-term use in many patients. Other causes of elevated calcitriol levels in PTH-independent hypercalcemia include extrarenal production of 1,25-dihydroxyvitamin D such as in granulomatous diseases or lymphoma.

Inactivating pathogenic variants in the *MEN1* gene (Answer C), which is a tumor suppressor gene, lead to multiple endocrine neoplasia (MEN) type 1, an autosomal dominant syndrome that predisposes to tumors of the parathyroid glands, anterior pituitary, and enteropancreatic endocrine cells. Activating pathogenic variants in the *RET* protooncogene (Answer D) lead to MEN type 2A, which is also inherited in an autosomal dominant pattern. MEN type 2A is characterized by medullary thyroid cancer, pheochromocytoma, and primary parathyroid hyperplasia. Both MEN type 1 and type 2A are associated with primary hyperparathyroidism, not PTH-independent hypercalcemia.

The *CASR* gene (Answer A) encodes the calcium-sensing receptor, which is expressed in multiple tissues, including the parathyroid glands and kidneys. Loss-of-function variants in this gene have been shown to cause a rare disorder called familial hypocalciuric hypercalcemia, which in most cases is a benign cause of mild hypercalcemia that is inherited in an autosomal dominant fashion. In patients with familial hypocalciuric hypercalcemia, serum PTH concentrations are typically inappropriately normal or high in the presence of mild hypercalcemia, and urinary calcium excretion is low with the calcium-to-creatinine clearance ratio typically less than 0.01, which is not consistent with the findings in this case.

Finally, the *VDR* gene (Answer E) encodes the vitamin D receptor. Inactivating pathogenic variants in this gene lead to vitamin D resistance, which results in markedly elevated calcitriol levels in the setting of hypocalcemia, not hypercalcemia.

Educational Objective

Suspect *CYP24A1* pathogenic variants as a cause of PTH-independent hypercalcemia.

Reference(s)

Roizen JD, Li D, O'Lear L, et al. CYP3A4 mutation causes vitamin D-dependent rickets type 3. *J Clin Invest.* 2018;128(5):1913-1918. PMID: 29461981

Bilezikian JP, Cusano NE, Khan AA, Liu J-M, Marcocci C, Bandeira F. Primary hyperparathyroidism. *Nat Rev Dis Primers.* 2016;2:16033. PMID: 27194212

Eastell R, Brandi ML, Costa AG, D'Amour P, Shoback DM, Thakker RV. Diagnosis of asymptomatic primary hyperparathyroidism: proceedings of the Fourth International Workshop. *J Clin Endocrinol Metab.* 2014;99(10):3570-3579. PMID: 25162666

Samander EH, Arnold A. Mutational analysis of the vitamin D receptor does not support its candidacy as a tumor suppressor gene in parathyroid adenomas. *J Clin Endocrinol Metab.* 2006;91(12):5019-5021. PMID: 17003089

Ketha H, Kumar R, Singh RJ. LC-MS/MS for identifying patients with CYP24A1 mutations. *Clin Chem.* 2016;62(1):236-242. PMID: 26585929

Tebben PJ, Singh RJ, Kumar R. Vitamin D-mediated hypercalcemia: mechanisms, diagnosis, and treatment. *Endocr Rev.* 2016;37(5):521-547. PMID: 27588937

109 **ANSWER: C) Day 21 progesterone measurement**

This patient's menses became more regular with metformin use, which is consistent with the diagnosis of polycystic ovary syndrome. She is wondering how to confirm whether ovulation is occurring. Corpus luteum secretion of progesterone rises after ovulation. Elevated progesterone increases the body temperature due to its effects on the hypothalamus. Daily temperature monitoring for a 0.5°F rise during the luteal phase is a method for detecting the increase in progesterone production. Measurement of basal body temperature requires the use of a special basal body temperature thermometer, which can discriminate one-tenth of a degree, usually not possible with standard electronic thermometers. The temperature rise begins 1 or 2 days after the LH surge and is observed for about 10 days. Therefore, this pattern can retrospectively confirm ovulation. Because of the difficulties involved in measurement and potential thermometer inaccuracy, basal body temperature (Answer A) is not considered the best indicator of ovulation. Since the probability of conception is greatest with intercourse 1 to 2 days prior to ovulation or the LH surge, basal body temperature is not as helpful as other methods for predicting timing of intercourse when trying to conceive.

In this case, the patient is more interested in confirming that ovulation is occurring than predicting ovulation for timing intercourse. Ovulation prediction for the timing of intercourse might be particularly important when cycle lengths are irregular (intervals <25 days or >35 days). Commercial home ovulation predictor kits (Answer D) identify an increase in LH that is detectable in the urine 12 hours after it can be seen in serum measurements. The serum LH rise occurs about 36 hours before the release of the oocyte from the follicle and persists for about 10 days. Therefore, these kits can be helpful for timing intercourse. However, polycystic ovary syndrome, primary ovarian insufficiency, and menopause can be associated with persistent LH elevations, resulting in false-positive results when ovulation is not occurring. For women with polycystic ovary syndrome, demonstrating a pattern of negative results before and after positive results increases the likelihood of true positive results. Therefore, the use of home ovulation predictor kits is less reliable than other measures for confirming ovulation, especially in women with polycystic ovary syndrome.

Serum progesterone concentrations rise in the midluteal phase, 18 to 24 days after the first day of menses in a 28-day cycle or 7 days before expected menses in a more prolonged or shortened cycle. Progesterone concentrations consistent with ovulation are 6 to 10 ng/mL (19.1 to 31.8 nmol/L) or at least greater than 3 ng/mL (>9.5 nmol/L). Because of the pulsatility of LH after ovulation, a single low value is not diagnostic and repeated measurements to confirm low levels are indicated. Alternatively, a single value above 3 ng/mL (>9.5 nmol/L) and, in particular, above 10 ng/mL (>31.8 nmol/L), is reassuring that ovulation is occurring. In this woman who now has 28-day regular menstrual cycles, day 21 progesterone measurement (Answer C) would be the best way to confirm occurrence of ovulation.

Day-3 FSH and estradiol measurements (Answer B) can assess ovarian reserve. An FSH concentration less than 10.0 mIU/mL (<10.0 IU/L) is consistent with sufficient ovarian reserve, and concentrations between 10.0 and 15.0 mIU/mL (10.0 and 15.0 IU/L) suggest declining ovarian reserve and declining fertility. The use of the estradiol measurement for this purpose is more controversial, although a day-3 estradiol concentration less than 80 pg/mL (<294 pmol/L) is consistent with sufficient ovarian reserve. Women undergoing in vitro fertilization have been noted to experience higher cycle cancellation rates and lower pregnancy rates when the day-3 estradiol concentration is greater than 80 pg/mL (>294 pmol/L) (although this could be due to multiple suboptimal parameters).

Mittelschmerz (Answer E) is a term used for pain that can occur with ovulation. Mittelschmerz in German translates to "middle pain" and describes pain that occurs unilaterally in the lower abdomen about 14 days before the first day of a period. It is a nonspecific symptom of ovulation, and other diagnoses of lower abdominal pain should be excluded first. Minor pain can be treated with nonsteroidal antiinflammatory agents, or an oral contraceptive might be used to prevent ovulation and Mittelschmerz. Although Mittelschmerz is considered to be consistent with pain with ovulation, it is not a reliable predictor for ovulation in most women compared with the other methods discussed.

Educational Objective

Evaluate for ovulation in a woman trying to conceive.

Reference(s)

Infertility workup for the women's health specialist: ACOG Committee Opinion, Number 781. *Obstet Gynecol.* 2019;133(6):e377-e384. PMID: 31135764

Practice Committee of the American Society for Reproductive Medicine in collaboration with the Society for Reproductive Endocrinology and Infertility. *Fertil Steril.* 2017;107(1):52-58. PMID: 28228319

Smotrich DB, Widra EA, Gindoff PR, Levy MJ, Hall JL, Stillman RJ. Prognostic value of day 3 estradiol on in vitro fertilization outcome. *Fertil Steril.* 1995;64(6):1136-1140. PMID: 7589666

110 ANSWER: C) 24-Hour urinary metanephrine measurement

Pheochromocytomas and paragangliomas are chromaffin-cell tumors arising from the adrenal medulla and the sympathetic ganglia, respectively. Pheochromocytomas and sympathetic paragangliomas typically produce catecholamines, while parasympathetic paragangliomas are usually nonsecretory. Pheochromocytomas can secrete all catecholamines. Paragangliomas lack phenylethanolamine-N-methyltransferase and do not produce epinephrine. Catecholamines are stress hormones, and they can be dramatically elevated (>3-fold) during acute illnesses. Thus, evaluation for pheochromocytoma should ideally be done in the outpatient setting.

Catecholamines are metabolized to metanephrine and normetanephrine within the tumor. Plasma fractionated metanephrines and 24-hour urinary metanephrines are both highly sensitive for the detection of secretory pheochromocytomas and paragangliomas, but plasma metanephrines have a lower specificity. Common causes of false-positive results include use of tricyclic antidepressants, decongestants, and amphetamines *(see table)*. Clonidine is a short-acting α_2-adrenergic agonist, and when taken orally, rebound of catecholamines might occur between doses. Medication-induced elevations of metanephrines are typically modest, while secretory pheochromocytomas and paragangliomas are often associated with metanephrine elevations at least 2-fold higher than the upper normal range. This patient had trivial elevations of metanephrines, which could have been a physiological response to her acute event, and/or a result of clonidine withdrawal. Measuring 24-hour urinary metanephrines (Answer C) has higher specificity than plasma metanephrines (Answer E), and it is the preferred test in this patient who takes oral clonidine.

Chromogranin A (Answer A) is a nonspecific biomarker of neuroendocrine tumors; however, it has numerous sources of false-positive results. In this patient with gastroesophageal reflux disease, one must consider that antacids, particularly proton-pump inhibitors, can cause substantial elevations of chromogranin A.

Imaging, either cross-sectional (Answer B) or functional (Answer D) should not be pursued unless the diagnosis of pheochromocytoma/paraganglioma is established clinically and hormonally.

Educational Objective

Identify causes of false-positive test results for pheochromocytoma.

Reference(s)

Lenders JWM, Duh QY, Eisenhofer G, et al; Endocrine Society. Pheochromocytoma and paraganglioma: an Endocrine Society clinical practice guideline. *J Clin Endocrinol Metab.* 2014;99(6):1915-1942. PMID: 24893135

Eisenhofer G, Goldstein DS, Walther MM, et al. Biochemical diagnosis of pheochromocytoma: how to distinguish true- from false-positive test results. *J Clin Endocrinol Metab.* 2003;88(6):2656-2666. PMID: 12788870

Table. Medications That Can Falsely Elevate Test Results for Plasma and Urinary Metanephrine Measurement

	Plasma		Urine	
	NMN	MN	NMN	MN
Acetaminophen[a]	++	–	++	–
Labetalol[a]	–	–	++	++
Sotalol[a]	–	–	++	++
α-Methyldopa[a]	++	–	++	–
Tricyclic antidepressants[b]	++	–	++	–
Buspirone[a]	–	++	–	++
Phenoxybenzamine[b]	++	–	++	–
MAO-inhibitors[b]	++	++	++	++
Sympathomimetics[b]	+	+	+	+
Cocaine[b]	++	+	++	+
Sulphasalazine[a]	++	–	++	–
Levodopa[c]	+	+	++	+

Abbreviations: MAO, monoamine oxidase; MN, metanephrine; NMN, normetanephrine; ++, clear increase; +, mild increase; –, no increase.

[a] Analytical interference for some but not all methods employing LC-ECD.

[b] Pharmacodynamic interference leading to increased levels affecting all analytical methods.

Reprinted from Lenders JWM et al. *J Clin Endocrinol Metab*, 2014;99(6):1915-1942. © Endocrine Society.

111 **ANSWER: B) Discontinue omeprazole**

Acquired hypocalcemia is unusual in patients without a history of neck surgery. In this patient, one would assume that this is indeed acquired given her older age and the recent development of hypocalcemic symptoms. While it remains important to inquire about a family history of disease (Answer A), it would be unusual for this 79-year-old woman to suddenly manifest a genetic cause of hypocalcemia. Causes of hypocalcemia include autoimmune polyglandular syndrome type 1 due to pathogenic variants in the *AIRE* gene, neck irradiation, and infiltrative disorders (eg, sarcoidosis, Wilson disease, and hemochromatosis).

Another cause of acquired hypocalcemia is hypomagnesemia. Magnesium is a critical mineral to ensure proper PTH release. Like calcium, magnesium also binds to the calcium-sensing receptor located on the parathyroid chief cells. While the molecular mechanisms remain unclear, hypomagnesemia reduces the effects of a low serum calcium level on the calcium-sensing receptor to increase PTH secretion and thus leads to hypoparathyroidism and hypocalcemia. In states of low serum magnesium, hypoparathyroidism and PTH resistance in target tissues can cause severe hypocalcemia.

The etiologies of hypomagnesemia are numerous, but the most obvious contributor in this patient is the combination of omeprazole and hydrochlorothiazide. Proton-pump inhibitors reduce intestinal magnesium absorption by altering the affinity of intestinal magnesium ion channels. However, hypomagnesemia only seems to result when combined with loop and thiazide diuretics that decrease renal magnesium reabsorption. Therefore, the combination of decreased intestinal absorption with an increase in renal excretion seems to be necessary to cause severe hypomagnesemia. Discontinuation of either omeprazole or hydrochlorothiazide are options, but since she is not having symptoms of gastroesophageal reflux disease, the correct intervention is to discontinue omeprazole (Answer B).

Treating hypocalcemia with calcitriol (Answer E) and evaluating with urine testing (Answer D) are certainly options, but these strategies would not address the underlying mechanism.

In the absence of focal and specific neurologic signs, brain MRI (Answer C) is unnecessary.

Educational Objective

Manage hypoparathyroidism in a patient with hypomagnesemia who is taking a proton-pump inhibitor and a diuretic.

Reference(s)

Danziger J, William JH, Scott DJ, et al. Proton-pump inhibitor use is associated with low serum magnesium concentrations. *Kidney Int.* 2013;83(4):692-699. PMID: 23325090

Perazella MA. Proton pump inhibitors and hypomagnesemia: a rare but serious complication. *Kidney Int.* 2013;83(4):553-556. PMID: 23538697

Zhang C, Zhang T, Zou J, et al. Structural basis for regulation of human calcium-sensing receptor by magnesium ions and an unexpected tryptophan derivative co-agonist. *Sci Adv.* 2016;2(5):e1600241. PMID: 27386547

Bai JPF, Hausman E, Lionberger R, Zhang X. Modeling and simulation of the effect of proton pump inhibitors on magnesium homeostasis. 1. Oral absorption of magnesium. *Mol Pharm.* 2012;9(12):3495-3505. PMID: 23051182

112 ANSWER: A) Add cabergoline

In general, surgery should be first-line therapy for acromegaly, particularly if the adenoma is small (microadenoma) or if it is an intrasellar macroadenoma. In expert surgical hands, surgical cure is achieved in about 80% of patients with microadenomas, in 70% of patients with intrasellar macroadenomas, and in only 30% of patients with invasive macroadenomas. However, surgery may have beneficial effects even when full surgical cure is not achievable, as lowering GH levels may increase the chance of successful control by medical therapy. Importantly, it may take up to 6 months for IGF-1 to reach its nadir after surgery, although in most cases it occurs within 3 months.

This patient underwent debulking surgery but could not be fully cured due to residual adenoma in the cavernous sinus, as shown by MRI findings and a persistently elevated serum IGF-1 level 6 months after surgery. However, surgery was successful in reducing GH and IGF-1 levels, increasing the likelihood of control by medical therapy. The somatostatin receptor ligand (lanreotide) dosage was increased to the maximum. While on lanreotide, his IGF-1 and GH levels have improved but have not reached target values (represented by normal age-adjusted serum IGF-1 and a fasting GH concentration <2.0 ng/mL). Therefore, some changes or additions should be made in his management.

Cabergoline (Answer A) is an orally active dopaminergic agent that may be effective (used off label) in treating acromegaly. It has been reported that the addition of cabergoline normalizes serum IGF-1 in about 40% of patients who have had a partial response to a somatostatin receptor agonist, and whose serum IGF-1 is elevated but less than 2 times normal (as is in this patient). Interestingly, and contrary to what one could expect, prolactin cosecretion by the adenoma is not a predictor of IGF-1 response to cabergoline.

Pasireotide (Answer E) is a newly approved somatostatin receptor agonist with high affinity for 4 of the 5 somatostatin receptor subtypes, including type 2 and 5 (while lanreotide and octreotide act principally on type 2). A pivotal study published in 2014 showed that pasireotide LAR was more effective than octreotide LAR in treatment-naïve patients with acromegaly (38.6% vs 23.6% achieved normal IGF-1, respectively). However, a significant percentage of patients (57%) treated with pasireotide LAR showed worsening glucose control. Hyperglycemia is indeed a common adverse effect of pasireotide, most likely due to inhibition of insulin secretion and incretin hormone response. This patient already has diabetes and would be at risk of developing worsening hyperglycemia with pasireotide treatment. However, pasireotide would be a logical second choice if the addition of cabergoline failed to achieve control.

Octreotide (Answer D) and lanreotide have very similar efficacy profiles and switching between these 2 drugs rarely changes the outcome.

Radiotherapy (Answer C) is a possible treatment for acromegaly. However, it typically takes several years to normalize GH secretion and is likely to cause hypopituitarism. Therefore, it would not be the best choice at this point, but it could be considered at a later stage if medical therapy fails.

The addition of the GH receptor pegvisomant (Answer B) would be another appropriate strategy in this case, and its use would most likely lead to acromegaly control. However, this would add another injectable drug to the patient's regimen and would significantly increase the economic burden of treatment. Therefore, adding pegvisomant, while not incorrect, is not the best next step.

Educational Objective

Select appropriate therapy for a patient with acromegaly who has had a partial response to somatostatin analogue therapy.

Reference(s)

Giustina A, Barkhoudarian G, Beckers A, et al. Multidisciplinary management of acromegaly: a consensus. *Rev Endocr Metab Disord.* 2020;21(4):667-678. PMID: 32914330

Starnoni D, Daniel RT, Marino L, Pitteloud N, Levivier M, Messerer M. Surgical treatment of acromegaly according to the 2010 remission criteria: systematic review and meta-analysis. *Acta Neurochir (Wien).* 2016;158(11):2109-2121. PMID: 27586125

Colao A, Bronstein MD, Freda P, et al; Pasireotide C2305 Study Group. Pasireotide versus octreotide in acromegaly: a head-to-head superiority study. *J Clin Endocrinol Metab.* 2014;99(3):791-799. PMID: 24423324

Jallad RS, Bronstein MD. Optimizing medical therapy of acromegaly: beneficial effects of cabergoline in patients uncontrolled with long-acting release octreotide. *Neuroendocrinology.* 2009;90(1):82-92. PMID: 19439914

Kuhn E, Chanson P. Cabergoline in acromegaly. *Pituitary.* 2017;20(1):121-128. PMID: 28025719

113 **ANSWER: E) Set up frequent visits with the local health coach**

Obesity disproportionately affects certain racial, ethnic, and socio-economic groups. Between 2017 and 2018 in the United States, the highest age-adjusted prevalence of obesity was in non-Hispanic Black adults (49.6%), followed by Hispanic adults (44.8%), non-Hispanic White adults (42.2%), and non-Hispanic Asian adults (17.4%). Within these racial and ethnic differences, the prevalence of obesity is further influenced by education attainment and income. A disproportionate number of Black communities live in "food deserts," ie, geographic areas where residents have few to no convenient options for securing healthy and affordable foods. Patients with obesity from within these groups often have a higher incidence of weight-related comorbidities such as hypertension, type 2 diabetes, and cardiovascular disease.

The gold-standard treatment of obesity incorporates an intensive lifestyle intervention program that focuses on calorie restriction, increased physical activity, and support for behavioral modification. However, this construct is often not readily available or acceptable to patients in socioeconomically disadvantaged groups, which further perpetuates health inequity. Furthermore, patients from minority ethnic groups and lower socioeconomic classes are not adequately represented in most large weight-loss trials.

Pragmatic weight-loss trials in real-world settings can help address this gap in patient care. The Be Fit, Be Well trial was conducted in a primary care setting and enrolled an ethnically diverse population with obesity (BMI = 30-50 kg/m^2) and hypertension. Approximately 40% of participants reported food insecurity. A total of 365 participants were randomly assigned to either usual care or to a behavioral intervention that promoted weight loss and hypertension self-management using eHealth components. The intervention arm received a prescription for 3 tailored goals to modify obesogenic lifestyle behaviors; self-monitoring and skills training; 18 telephone counseling calls; primary care provider endorsement; 12 optional group support sessions; and links to community resources. The completion rate at 24 months was 86%. At 24 months, there was a small but significant decrease in weight (1.03 kg) in the intervention arm, accompanied by improvement in self-management of hypertension. At a minimum, this trial showed that prevention of weight gain can be achieved with interventions that might be sustainable in resource-deprived practice settings.

More recently, the PROPEL trial reported on the effectiveness of a high-intensity, lifestyle-based obesity treatment program in low income, ethnically diverse patients with obesity (BMI = 30-50 kg/m^2) within primary care clinics. Patients were randomly assigned to either intensive lifestyle intervention (reduced caloric intake and increased physical activity) or usual care. Patients in the intervention group participated in a high-intensity program delivered by health coaches embedded in the clinics who met with participants weekly for the first 6 months, followed by monthly sessions for the remaining 18 months. A total of 803 adults with obesity were enrolled: 452 were assigned to the intensive-lifestyle group and 351 were assigned to the usual-care group. The completion rate at 24 months was 83.4%. The intensive-lifestyle group achieved a 5% decrease in body weight (vs 0.5% in the usual-care group). Weight loss of 5% is clinically significant and can lead to meaningful improvements in health.

As long as local health coaches (Answer E) are available and accessible (regarding timing, cost, and cultural sensitivity), pragmatic weight-loss strategies in low-income populations can be effective, as described in the trials discussed above. Local community centers and health clinics can often help identify these types of resources.

Increasing the levothyroxine dosage (Answer A) is highly unlikely to affect this patient's weight.

GLP-1 receptor agonists (Answer B), while effective, are expensive and are unfortunately not accessible to many patients. Generic weight-loss medications such as topiramate or phentermine (not offered here as options) may be considered in the appropriate clinical scenario.

Physical activity guidelines promote 150 minutes of moderate-intensity physical activity a week (Answer C). However, this patient with mechanical joint pain and trouble with activities of daily living cannot start at that goal. A graduated physical activity prescription, for example, using seated exercises, may be more acceptable to the patient.

Meal replacement programs (Answer D) can lead to weight loss, but they are also costly and difficult to sustain in the long-term.

Educational Objective

Summarize evidence-based weight-loss options for low-income patients.

Reference(s)

Bennett GG, Warner ET, Glasgow RE, et al; Be Fit, Be Well Study Investigators. Obesity treatment for socioeconomically disadvantaged patients in primary care practice. *Arch Intern Med.* 2012;172(7):565-574. PMID: 22412073

Katzmarzyk PT, Martin CK, Newton RL Jr, et al. Weight loss in underserved patients - a cluster-randomized trial. *N Engl J Med.* 2020;383(10):909-918. PMID: 32877581

114 ANSWER: E) Continue metformin; stop glimepiride; start empagliflozin; start basal insulin, 14 units daily

This patient's kidney disease has progressed to stage 3b (estimated glomerular filtration rate 30-44 mL/min per 1.73 m^2), and his hemoglobin A_{1c} level is currently 8.5% (69 mmol/mol). Caution is advised when using glimepiride in the setting of a glomerular filtration rate less than 60 mL/min per 1.73 m^2, and it is typically not recommended when the glomerular filtration rate is less than 30 mL/min per 1.73 m^2. This patient's kidney function is declining, and he has had a recent hypoglycemic episode while on glimepiride, 2 mg daily. Thus, continuing or increasing the current glimepiride dosage (Answers A, B, and D) is incorrect.

His metformin is appropriately renally dosed and this medication has a low risk for hypoglycemia, so it does not need to be stopped (Answers A and B) unless the patient's glomerular filtration rate decreases below 30 mL/min per 1.73 m^2.

His glycemic control is suboptimal, and additional agents are needed to address his hyperglycemia. SGLT-2 inhibitors have been shown to decrease cardiovascular events and improve kidney outcomes, especially in patients with macroalbuminuria (>300 mg/dL) and even in patients with a glomerular filtration rate in the range of 25 to 45 mL/min per 1.73 m^2. Thus, starting an SGLT-2 inhibitor (Answer E) is appropriate. SGLT-2 inhibitors inhibit the coupled reabsorption of sodium and glucose from the proximal tubules, promoting renal glucose and sodium excretion. Additional effects include inhibition of the sodium:proton exchanger, increased delivery of sodium to the loop of Henle, and correction of glomerular hyperfiltration. Although SGLT-2 inhibitors are appealing from a cardiac and kidney standpoint given their mechanism of action, there is unfortunately minimal glucose-lowering potential when a patient's glomerular filtration rate is less than 45 mL/min per 1.73 m^2, thus adding to the complexity of this question. Given this patient's individual characteristics, the best choice for medical management considering the answers provided would be to stop glimepiride and start empagliflozin. An additional agent is necessary, especially if glimepiride is stopped. A GLP-1 receptor agonist would be a good choice but was not offered as an option. Initiating weight-based insulin at a dosage of 0.15 units/kg daily (14 units) would be appropriate.

Educational Objective

Explain the renal benefit of SGLT-2 inhibitors and their minimal effect on glycemic control when the estimated glomerular filtration rate is less than 45 mL/min per m^2.

Reference(s)

Perkovic V, Jardine MJ, Neal B, et al; CREDENCE Trial Investigators. Canagliflozin and renal outcomes in type 2 diabetes and nephropathy. *N Engl J Med.* 2019;380(24):2295-2306. PMID: 30990260

Wilcox CS. Antihypertensive and renal mechanisms of SGLT2 (sodium-glucose linked transporter 2) inhibitors. *Hypertension.* 2020;75(4):894-901. PMID: 32114848

115 **ANSWER: B) Repeat DXA scan in 2 years**

Osteogenesis imperfecta (OI) describes a group of disorders whose main features are fragile bones with recurrent fractures. There are many different subtypes of OI based on genetic and clinical characteristics, and the most common and mildest form, type I OI, is typically caused by pathogenic variants in genes encoding the $\alpha 1$ and $\alpha 2$ chains of type I collagen. Clinical manifestations of OI can include blue-gray discoloration of the sclerae, short stature, scoliosis, bone deformities, hearing loss, and easy bruising. Individuals with type I OI usually do not begin to have fractures until they start walking. The frequency of fractures declines after puberty, but women may have premature or accelerated osteoporosis following menopause.

Patients with OI require regular surveillance for potential complications, including hearing loss and worsening of osteoporosis. Treatment requires a coordinated multidisciplinary team approach and consists of physical therapy, surgical interventions, and medications. Although not approved for this indication, bisphosphonates are the mainstay of pharmacologic therapy for fracture prevention for most forms of OI. Randomized controlled trials of bisphosphonates in OI have consistently shown that bone mineral density is increased and biochemical markers of bone turnover are decreased as compared with levels in patients who have received no treatment or placebo, but there have not been clear benefits in quality of life and functional status. The data on fracture are also conflicting, although studies performed so far have generally not been powered to detect a reduction in fracture incidence. There are limited data on the use of denosumab and teriparatide in OI. There have been some reports of denosumab use in OI but no randomized controlled trials. There has been 1 double-blind, randomized controlled trial of teriparatide in OI in which patients with type I OI exhibited robust bone mineral density increases with teriparatide compared with placebo; however, there was no difference in self-reported fractures between the 2 groups.

Decisions to start pharmacologic treatment in clinical practice mainly depend on disease progression as assessed by measured bone mineral density and fracture frequency. This premenopausal woman with type I OI has not had fragility fractures since puberty, and although her bone mineral density is abnormally low for her age, sex, and race, it has been stable for the past 2 years. Therefore, the best recommendation at this time is to repeat her DXA scan in 2 years (Answer B). There is no indication to initiate antifracture therapy now (Answers C, D, and E).

Waiting until age 65 years to repeat DXA (Answer A) would not be appropriate given her current Z-score and potential for premature or accelerated osteoporosis following menopause.

Educational Objective

Recommend the most appropriate intervention for a premenopausal woman with type I osteogenesis imperfecta and low bone mineral density.

Reference(s)

Scheres LJJ, van Dijk FS, Harsevoort AJ, et al. Adults with osteogenesis imperfecta: clinical characteristics of 151 patients with a focus on bisphosphonate use and bone density measurements [published correction appears in *Bone Rep.* 2021;14:101084]. *Bone Rep.* 2018;8:168-172. PMID: 29955635

Ralston SH, Gaston MS. Management of osteogenesis imperfecta. *Front Endocrinol (Lausanne).* 2020;10:924. PMID: 32117044

Forlino A, Marini JC. Osteogenesis imperfecta. *Lancet.* 2016;387(10028):1657-1671. PMID: 26542481

Orwoll ES, Shapiro J, Veith S, et al. Evaluation of teriparatide treatment in adults with osteogenesis imperfecta. *J Clin Invest.* 2014;124(2):491-498. PMID: 24463451

116 **ANSWER: A) β-adrenergic blocker**

This patient has muscle weakness, hypokalemia, and thyrotoxicosis. In addition, he is of Asian descent. This constellation of findings suggests the diagnosis of thyrotoxic periodic paralysis (TPP). Hyperthyroidism of any etiology can lead to TPP. TPP is a rare condition, and it predominantly occurs in men in the second to fourth decades of life and in Asian and Hispanic populations. TPP is an X-linked recessive condition, which explains its male preponderance. TPP is usually characterized by symmetric proximal muscle weakness and thyrotoxicosis. This patient presents with proximal muscle weakness in his lower extremities, sudden onset of hypokalemia, and thyrotoxicosis. The diagnosis of thyrotoxicosis differentiates TPP from hypokalemic periodic paralysis or familial periodic paralysis, an autosomal dominant disorder caused by pathogenic variants in the gene encoding Kir channels (L-type calcium channel 1-subunit [*CACNA1S*]). These conditions are caused by intermittent intracellular shift of potassium resulting in ineffective sacrolemmal activity within muscle fibrils. Potassium levels can return to normal between attacks. In TPP, thyroid hormone and adrenergic stimulation are known to stimulate the Na-K-ATPase pump, contributing to intermittent hypokalemia. Hypomagnesemia and hypophosphatemia are also present in some affected patients, which are features that distinguish TPP features from other forms of familial periodic paralysis. In addition, normal blood acid–base balance is usually seen in TPP as opposed to metabolic alkalosis often seen in individuals with hypokalemia. Early diagnosis is important, as β-adrenergic blockers can reverse the hypokalemia and treatment of hyperthyroidism can prevent further episodes. Other muscular disorders such as myasthenia gravis, Guillain-Barre syndrome, and transverse myelitis may be considered in patients presenting with acute muscle weakness.

During an episode of TPP with hypokalemia, potassium supplementation is required to help recover muscle function. The dosage of potassium supplementation should not exceed 50 mEq daily to prevent rebound hyperkalemia. Even lower doses of potassium supplementation may be beneficial to reduce the patient's risk of rebound hyperkalemia. β-Adrenergic blockers (Answer A) inhibit adrenergic simulation of the Na-K-ATPase pump, reverse hypokalemia, and prevent recurrent periodic paralysis.

Steroid treatment (Answer D) does not improve TPP but may be helpful in treating thyroiditis as a cause of hyperthyroidism. Steroids can be used in the management of myasthenia gravis. The most common cause of hyperthyroidism in patients with TPP is Graves disease, but other causes are also possible.

Methimazole (Answer C) or radioiodine treatment (Answer E) may be necessary once the etiology of hyperthyroidism is identified and the patient's preference is considered. In some cases, antithyroid drugs with a β-adrenergic blocker may need to be started if Graves disease seems to be the most likely diagnosis, but this option was not provided.

Definitive therapy for TPP includes treatment of hyperthyroidism depending on its cause. Prophylactic potassium supplementation between attacks has not been shown to be beneficial in TPP.

Immunoglobulin therapy (Answer B) is used to treat Guillain-Barre syndrome. As this patient has biochemical thyrotoxicosis, myasthenia gravis or Guillain-Barre syndrome is less likely to be the etiology of his muscle weakness in this context.

Educational Objective

Diagnose thyrotoxic periodic paralysis in a patient with hypokalemia and muscle weakness.

Reference(s)

Lin S-H. Thyrotoxic periodic paralysis. *Mayo Clin Proc.* 2005;80(1):99-105. PMID: 15667036

Lu K-C, Hsu Y-J, Chiu J-S, Hsu Y-D, Lin S-H. Effects of potassium supplementation on the recovery of thyrotoxic periodic paralysis. *Am J Emerg Med.* 2004;22(7):544-547. PMID: 15666258

117 ANSWER: C) Prescribe hybrid closed-loop therapy

This patient has had type 1 diabetes for more than 10 years and is at high risk for microvascular complications. She did have good glucose control for the first 6 years after her diagnosis. Persons in the age range of 18 to 26 or 30 years are termed *emerging adults.* This term is used to signify that in contemporary culture, individuals in that age group do not always take on typical adult roles such as work, marriage, or having children, in contrast to previous generations. Several lines of evidence show that emerging adults with diabetes may experience deterioration of glycemic control and increased risk for acute complications such as diabetic ketoacidosis.

In this patient, the main issue is to determine the best strategy to improve glycemic control. A regimen of premixed insulin (Answer A) is useful for persons with very fixed eating schedules who can commit to giving 2 injections daily and who would have difficulty with active management of a multiple daily injection regimen. In this patient, who describes an erratic lifestyle currently but who has previously managed a multiple daily injection regimen well, this option is not expected to be useful. Similarly, evidence from head-to-head trials suggests that insulin degludec (Answer B) is associated with lower rates of symptomatic or nocturnal hypoglycemia but not better hemoglobin A_{1c} levels. In this case, there might be a rationale to use degludec to offset the missed glargine doses, but better alternatives exist.

Many randomized controlled trials of hybrid closed-loop insulin delivery systems (Answer C) have been conducted. Two separate systematic reviews of randomized controlled trials comparing closed-loop systems with conventional insulin pump or sensor-augmented insulin pump therapy demonstrate that closed-loop systems result in 9% to 12% improvement in time spent in range, modest reductions in hemoglobin A_{1c} of approximately 0.3% without increased time spent in hypoglycemia. In other words, participants assigned to hybrid close-loop insulin delivery were in the target glycemic range approximately 2.5 hours longer per day than control participants. Importantly, one major study noted that the glycemic control benefits afforded by the hybrid closed-loop systems occurred irrespective of age, race, sex, and education level. Major society guidelines advise that insulin pumps be offered to persons with type 1 diabetes. Based on this, prescription of a hybrid closed-loop system is the best step to improve this patient's glycemic control. It is worthwhile to ponder why she may not have been offered insulin pump therapy in the past. Certainly, patient preference has a role. However, disparities in the care and outcomes of persons with diabetes have been well documented. Studies show that non-Hispanic Black and Hispanic young adults have substantially lower rates of use of diabetes technology. This inequity persists for Black young adults even after controlling for factors such as socioeconomic status and other health care factors. The reasons for this racial inequity are not known but may include implicit provider bias, patient preference, systemic racism, and mistrust of the medical community.

This patient has most likely previously met with a diabetes educator (Answer D). The fact that she previously had good blood glucose control suggests additional diabetes-specific education may not be required. Therefore, meeting with a diabetes educator, while possibly beneficial, is not the best next step. Similarly, while meeting with a psychologist (Answer E) may be an important part of this patient's care given the higher levels of diabetes distress reported by Black young adults, the evidence base does not suggest that it would be the best next step in improving her glycemic control.

This patient initiated a conventional insulin pump and continued to use continuous glucose monitoring. Approximately 5 months after this change, her hemoglobin A_{1c} level had decreased 2 percentage points.

Educational Objective

Identify reasons for disparity in use of diabetes technology.

Reference(s)

Agarwal S, Schechter C, Gonzalez J, Long JA. Racial-ethnic disparities in diabetes technology use among young adults with type 1 diabetes. *Diabetes Technol Ther.* 2021;23(4):306-313. PMID: 33155826

Karges B, Schwandt A, Heidtmann B, et al. Association of insulin pump therapy vs insulin injection therapy with severe hypoglycemia, ketoacidosis, and glycemic control among children, adolescents, and young adults with type 1 diabetes. *JAMA.* 2017;318(14):1358-1366. PMID: 29049584

Weisman A, Bai JW, Cardinez M, Kramer CK, Perkins BA. Effect of artificial pancreas systems on glycaemic control in patients with type 1 diabetes: a systematic review and meta-analysis of outpatient randomised controlled trials. *Lancet Diabetes Endocrinol.* 2017;5(7):501-512. PMID: 28533136

Bekiari E, Kitsios K, Thabit H, et al. Artificial pancreas treatment for outpatients with type 1 diabetes: systematic review and meta-analysis. *BMJ.* 2018;361:k1310. PMID: 29669716

Lane W, Bailey TS, Gerety G, et al; SWITCH 1. Effect of insulin degludec vs insulin glargine U100 on hypoglycemia in patients with type 1 diabetes: The SWITCH 1 Randomized Clinical Trial. *JAMA.* 2017;318(1):33-44. PMID: 28672316

118 ANSWER: D) Ionized calcium

Hypercalcemia is a common laboratory finding that is most often due to primary hyperparathyroidism in the outpatient setting. Other causes include hypercalcemia of malignancy, granulomatous disease due to increased 1,25-dihydroxyvitamin D, excessive dietary calcium, hyperthyroidism, and adrenal insufficiency. While hypercalcemia due to excessive bone resorption is in the differential diagnosis for this patient, the elevated total protein and the negative anion gap indicate the presence of substantial monoclonal paraproteinemia and another possible etiology.

Pseudohypercalcemia is an unusual but important peculiarity in some patients with multiple myeloma. Similar to albumin, calcium is bound to circulating substances including phosphate and sulfate. Changes in these binding factors affect total serum calcium, but the free ionized fraction remains unchanged assuming that no other diseases that affect calcium homeostasis are present. Monoclonal myeloma antibodies, when present in sufficient amounts, can also bind to circulating calcium with high affinity. Although ionized calcium initially decreases, homeostatic mechanisms, including PTH, normalize the ionized calcium level. Measuring ionized calcium (Answer D), especially in this patient with myeloma and in patients in whom the affinity of calcium to albumin is lower (eg, acidemia) or higher (eg, alkalemia), is important to avoid unnecessary evaluation. This patient may indeed have markedly increased bone resorption of multiple myeloma requiring additional testing for abnormalities in intact PTH (Answer C), phosphate (Answer E), urinary calcium (Answer B), and 1,25-dihydroxyvitamin vitamin D (Answer A). However, measuring ionized calcium is the best laboratory test to order now.

Educational Objective

Evaluate hypercalcemia in a patient with multiple myeloma.

Reference(s)

Ashrafi F, Iraj B, Nematollahi P, Darakhshandeh A. Pseudohypercalcemia in multiple myeloma: a case report. *Int J Hematol Oncol Stem Cell Res.* 2017;11(3):246-249. PMID: 28989592

Schwab JD, Strack MA, Hughes LD, Shaker JL. Pseudohypercalcemia in an elderly patient with multiple myeloma: report of a case and review of literature. *Endocr Pract.* 1995;1(6):390-392. PMID: 15251564

119 ANSWER: B) 24-Hour urinary cortisol and creatinine measurements

Hypercortisolism must be considered in this young woman with irregular menses, acne, central obesity, and abdominal and axillary pink striae. An early-morning ACTH concentration less than 10 pg/mL (<2.2 pmol/L), along with a serum cortisol value that is mildly elevated, is suggestive of ACTH-independent hypercortisolism. An overnight 1-mg dexamethasone-suppression test (Answer C) is sensitive for mild autonomous hypercortisolism. In this patient, however, the estrogen component of the oral contraceptive pill is expected to cause a false-positive result by increasing the cortisol-binding globulin. Assays for serum cortisol quantify total cortisol (protein-bound and free). Salivary and urinary cortisol assays measure free cortisol and would not be affected by oral estrogens. Thus, for this patient, measuring 24-hour urinary cortisol (Answer B) and creatinine excretion would be an excellent way to assess for clinically overt hypercortisolism.

Serum DHEA-S measurement (Answer E) can be a helpful adjunctive test in the evaluation of patients with signs and symptoms of hypercortisolism and androgen excess. A low serum DHEA-S concentration would further support the diagnosis of ACTH-independent hypercortisolism. Conversely, a very high serum DHEA-S concentration and ACTH-independent Cushing syndrome would suggest adrenal cortical carcinoma. Secretory adrenal cortical carcinomas typically lead to severe Cushing syndrome. The perioral and lip lentiginous lesions observed in this patient are suggestive of Carney complex, a disease that includes ACTH-independent hypercortisolism due to primary pigmented nodular adrenocortical disease. Carney complex is a rare autosomal dominant syndrome, most often caused by pathogenic variants in the *PRKAR1A* gene (encoding protein kinase cAMP-dependent type I regulatory subunit α). Affected patients might also develop GH excess, large-cell calcifying Sertoli-cell tumors, ovarian cysts, teratomas, endometrioid carcinomas, cardiac myxomas, and thyroid nodules.

Imaging should always be pursued after the diagnosis of hypercortisolism is firmly established. Abdominal CT (Answer A) is appropriate for patients with hormonal evidence of ACTH-independent hypercortisolism. Pituitary-directed MRI (Answer D) is indicated in patients with ACTH-dependent Cushing syndrome.

Educational Objective

Guide testing for clinically suspected hypercortisolism and recognize limitations of the dexamethasone-suppression test.

Reference(s)

Nieman LK, Biller BMK, Findling JW, et al. The diagnosis of Cushing's syndrome: an Endocrine Society clinical practice guideline. *J Clin Endocrinol Metab.* 2008;93(5):1526-1540. PMID: 18334580

Fassnacht M, Arlt W, Bancos I, et al. Management of adrenal incidentalomas: European Society of Endocrinology Clinical Practice Guideline in collaboration with the European Network for the Study of Adrenal Tumors. *Eur J Endocrinol.* 2016;175(2):G1-G34. PMID: 27390021

120 ANSWER: C) Continue current therapy but change lisinopril dosing to bedtime

All hypertensive patients with diabetes mellitus are advised to monitor their blood pressure at home. For patients with diabetes and hypertension who are at higher risk of atherosclerotic cardiovascular disease (ASCVD), including those with known cerebrovascular disease or patients whose 10-year risk for ASCVD is greater than 15%, a blood pressure target less than 130/80 mm Hg (or even 120/80 mm Hg based on different diabetes and kidney guidelines) may be appropriate if it can be safely attained. Currently, this patient appears to be achieving her blood pressure goals without reported orthostatic hypotension symptoms or falls, so reducing the dosage of her blood pressure medication (Answer E) is incorrect. However, adding amlodipine (Answer A), a third blood pressure medication, would be incorrect given her current tightly controlled blood pressure.

This patient has already had a cerebrovascular event. Semaglutide was a good choice for her management, not only to treat her diabetes, but also because GLP-1 receptor agonists have been shown to reduce cardiovascular events and nonfatal stroke in randomized controlled trials. A recent meta-analysis of 8 studies documented an overall 16% lower risk of all strokes (odds ratio 0.84; 95% CI, 0.75-0.93; $P = .001$; $I^2 = 0\%$) and reduced the risk of major adverse cardiac events (MACE) (odds ratio, 0.86; 95% CI, 0.80-0.92; $P < .0001$; $I^2 = 0\%$) among patients with a history of myocardial infarction or nonfatal stroke.

The physiological decrease in nocturnal blood pressure by 10% to 20% compared with daytime blood pressure is referred to as "nocturnal blood pressure dipping." There is evidence of an association between the absence of nocturnal blood pressure dipping and an increased incidence of ASCVD. A meta-analysis of randomized controlled trials found a small benefit of evening vs morning dosing of antihypertensive medications to ensure nocturnal dipping, but only 1 randomized controlled trial has shown that changing the administration time of antihypertensive medication to bedtime (Answer C) significantly reduced cardiovascular events. These results were limited by the small number of events. However, given this patient's cerebrovascular history, the best answer would be to move the timing of when she takes lisinopril to bedtime to optimize nocturnal blood pressure control. Moving the timing of when she takes her diuretic blood pressure medication to bedtime (Answer D) may improve nocturnal blood pressure, but it would most likely disturb sleep.

Finally, SGLT-2 inhibitors have been shown to confer cardiovascular event benefit, reduce all-cause mortality, and decrease hospitalization for congestive heart failure. Dapagliflozin (Answer B) may be a good addition to her medication regimen, but given her age, history of yeast infections, tight blood pressure control, and current diuretic use, adding an SGLT-2 inhibitor is incorrect. Also, when starting an SGLT-2 inhibitor, there is the potential need (as in this patient's case given currently tightly controlled blood pressure) to decease blood pressure medications, particularly the diuretic dosage, to reduce the risk for dehydration and orthostatic hypotension.

Educational Objective

Mitigate the risk for cerebrovascular accident associated with suboptimal nocturnal blood pressure control.

Reference(s)

Zhao P, Xu P, Wan C, Wang Z. Evening versus morning dosing regimen drug therapy for hypertension. *Cochrane Database Syst Rev.* 2011;(10):CD004184. PMID: 21975743

Hermida RC, Ayala DE, Mojón A, Fernández JR. Influence of time of day of blood pressure-lowering treatment on cardiovascular risk in hypertensive patients with type 2 diabetes. *Diabetes Care.* 2011;34(6):1270-1276. PMID: 21617110

Yano Y, Kario K. Nocturnal blood pressure and cardiovascular disease: a review of recent advances. *Hypertens Res.* 2012;35(7):695-701. PMID: 22378470

McGuire DK, Shih WJ, Cosentino F, et al. Association of SGLT2 inhibitors with cardiovascular and kidney outcomes in patients with type 2 diabetes: a meta-analysis. *JAMA Cardiol.* 2021;6(2):148-158. PMID: 33031522

Tomson CRV, Cheung AK, Mann JFE, et al. Management of blood pressure in patients with chronic kidney disease not receiving dialysis: synopsis of the 2021 KDIGO clinical practice guideline. *Ann Intern Med.* 2021;174(9):1270-1281. PMID: 34152826

Question-Mapping Index

ENDOCRINE SELF-ASSESSMENT PROGRAM 2023

Part III

This question-mapping index groups question topics according to the 8 umbrella sections of ESAP (Adrenal, Bone-Calcium, Diabetes, Lipids-Obesity, Pituitary, Reproduction [Female], Reproduction [Male], and Thyroid). Relevant **question numbers** *follow each topic.*

ADRENAL

CALCIUM-BONE

DIABETES

LIPIDS-OBESITY

PITUITARY

REPRODUCTION, FEMALE

REPRODUCTION, MALE

THYROID

www.ingramcontent.com/pod-product-compliance
Ingram Content Group UK Ltd.
Pitfield, Milton Keynes, MK11 3LW, UK
UKHW051040091026
15624UKWH00011B/614